Introduction to Exercise Science

Introduction to Exercise Science introduces undergraduate students to the foundational disciplines (e.g., anatomy, physiology) and subdisciplines (e.g., exercise physiology, biomechanics, motor behavior, nutrition, exercise psychology) of exercise science and is designed to provide an overview of individual areas of study versus an in-depth, exhaustive review. Exercise science continues to be among the most popular majors for post-secondary students interested in fitness, wellness, and strength and conditioning, as well as students interested in careers in medicine and the allied health professions.

In this fully updated and revised sixth edition, chapters are structured to include historical perspectives, key concepts, clinical and sports related applications, technology and equipment, educational preparation, and career pathways. Chapter features include learning objectives, keywords and definitions, journal abstracts, study questions, learning activities, suggested readings, and online resources. Chapters 1 through 3 provide introductory and foundational information about the field of exercise science and the remaining chapters focus on core areas of study in exercise science. Ancillary materials to support teaching include PowerPoint slides, hands-on learning/laboratory activities, and a test bank of questions for quizzes and examinations for each chapter.

Introduction to Exercise Science is a complete resource for a hands-on introduction to the core tenets of exercise science. It is an engaging and invaluable textbook for students beginning undergraduate degrees in Kinesiology, Exercise Science, Sports Coaching, Strength and Conditioning, Athletic Training, Sports Medicine, Sports Therapy, and Health and Fitness.

Dona J. McCanlies, PhD, FACSM, is a Professor in the Department of Oral Biology, College of Dentistry at the University of Nebraska Medical Center, USA. She teaches Human Physiology and Histology to dental hygiene, dental, doctoral, and postdoctoral students. Dr. McCanlies' research interests include muscle function, neuromuscular fatigue, and hypertrophic responses to various resistance training modalities.

Joan M. Eckerson, PhD, CSCS, FACSM, FNSCA, is Professor and Chair in the Department of Exercise Science and Pre-Health Professions at Creighton University in Omaha, NE, USA and currently serves on the editorial board for the *Journal of Strength and Conditioning Research* and the *Journal of the International Society of Sports Nutrition*.

Terry J. Housh, PhD, FACSM, FNSCA, is a Professor in the Department of Nutrition and Health Sciences, Director of the Exercise Physiology Laboratory, and Co-director of the Center for Youth Fitness and Sports Research at the University of Nebraska–Lincoln, USA.

Glen O. Johnson, PhD, FACSM, is a Professor Emeritus in the Department of Nutrition and Health Sciences at the University of Nebraska–Lincoln, USA and continues to advise Exercise Physiology doctoral students.

Introduction to Exercise Science

Scientific Foundations, Methodologies, and Career Opportunities

Sixth Edition

Edited by
Dona J. McCanlies, Joan M. Eckerson, Terry J. Housh, and Glen O. Johnson

Routledge
Taylor & Francis Group
NEW YORK AND LONDON

Designed cover image: Getty Images

Sixth edition published 2026
by Routledge
605 Third Avenue, New York, NY 10158

and by Routledge
4 Park Square, Milton Park, Abingdon, Oxon, OX14 4RN

Routledge is an imprint of the Taylor & Francis Group, an informa business

First edition published by Allyn & Bacon 2000
Fifth edition published by Routledge 2017

ISBN: 978-1-032-69719-2 (hbk)
ISBN: 978-1-032-69717-8 (pbk)
ISBN: 978-1-032-69718-5 (ebk)

DOI: 10.4324/9781032697185

Typeset in Sabon
by codeMantra

Access the Instructor and Student Resources: www.routledge.com/cw/McCanlies

Contents

List of Exhibits

About the Editors

Dona J. McCanlies and Joan M. Eckerson attended graduate school together at the University of Nebraska-Lincoln, USA. Although Dona is a professor at the University of Nebraska Medical Center and Joan is a professor at Creighton University, they have continued their friendship over the years and were happy to collaborate on the sixth edition of this textbook. Terry J. Housh is a professor and Director of the Human Performance and Body Composition Laboratory at the University of Nebraska-Lincoln. Glen O. Johnson is a Professor Emeritus at the University of Nebraska-Lincoln and was the doctoral advisor for Dona, Joan, and Terry.

Dona J. McCanlies, PhD, FACSM, is a Professor in the Department of Oral Biology, College of Dentistry at the University of Nebraska Medical Center (UNMC), USA. She teaches Human Physiology and General Histology to students across multiple levels, including dental hygiene, dental, doctoral, and postdoctoral programs. In recognition of her excellence in education, Dr. McCanlies has received numerous Outstanding Teaching Awards for her instruction of professional students at UNMC. Dr. McCanlies' research focuses on muscle function, neuromuscular fatigue, and hypertrophic adaptations to various resistance training modalities. Her work has been widely published in leading peer-reviewed physiology journals and her research presentations have been well received at the annual meetings of both the American College of Sports Medicine (ACSM) and the National Strength and Conditioning Association (NSCA). She has been a Fellow of the ACSM since 1997 and was recognized by the *Women in Sport and Physical Activity Journal* as one of the "most prolific scholars in Exercise Science." She has contributed to the field through her service on the National Strength and Conditioning Task Force on Women, has served on the editorial board of the *Journal of Strength and Conditioning Research*, the flagship journal of the NSCA, and currently serves as a reviewer for several journals in the fields of physiology and exercise science. *Introduction to Exercise Science (Sixth Ed.)* is her tenth college textbook.

Joan M. Eckerson, PhD, CSCS, FACSM, FNSCA, is a Professor and Chair in the Department of Exercise Science and Pre-Health Professions at Creighton University in Omaha, NE. She has over 150 publications and national presentations, primarily in the area of body composition assessment and the effect of sports supplements on athletic performance, and has received a number of awards acknowledging her accomplishments in teaching and research including the NSCA William J. Kraemer Outstanding Sport Scientist Award and the NSCA Nutritional Research Achievement Award. She is a Fellow of the NSCA and the ACSM and is a certified Strength and Conditioning Specialist (ACSM-CSCS) and certified Exercise Physiologist (ACSM-EP). She has served on several committees within the NSCA over her career, was Secretary/Treasurer and President of the NSCA Foundation, and currently serves on the editorial board for the *Journal of Strength and Conditioning Research* and the *Journal of the International Society of Sports Nutrition.*

Terry J. Housh, PhD, FACSM, FNSCA, is a Professor in the Department of Nutrition and Health Sciences and Director of the Exercise Physiology Laboratory at the University of Nebraska–Lincoln (UNL), USA. He has co-authored more than 400 peer-reviewed research articles and 12 college textbooks. He was the 1998 recipient of the NSCA Outstanding Sport Scientist Award, 2002 Doane College Honor D Award, 2006 NSCA Educator of the Year Award, 2008 NSCA President's Award, and 2008 Journal of Strength and Conditioning Research Editorial Excellence Award. In 2009, the NSCA named its annual award the "Terry J. Housh Young Investigator Award." Dr. Housh currently has over 25 former doctoral students teaching and conducting research in colleges and universities.

Glen O. Johnson, PhD, FACSM, (together with Dr. Bill Thorland) began the PhD program in Exercise Physiology at the University of Nebraska in the late 1970s and he taught Human Anatomy at UNL for 36 years. He received his BS and MS degrees from Winona State University and his PhD from the University of Iowa under Dr. Charles M. Tipton. He is a Distinguished Alumni of Winona State as well as a member of its Athletic Hall of Fame. He has co-authored over 250 peer-reviewed articles, been co-author or co-editor of six college textbooks and given numerous presentations at national conferences. Today, Dr. Johnson is a Professor Emeritus in the Department of Nutrition and Health Sciences at UNL.

About the Contributors

David I. Anderson, PhD, is a Professor in the Department of Kinesiology and the Director of the Marian Wright Edelman Institute for Study of Children, Youth, and Families at San Francisco State University. David has engaged in a wide range of service, teaching, and research activities, and has received significant funding for his research from the National Institutes of Health, the National Science Foundation, the Department of Education, and private foundations. His research centers on understanding how people of all ages acquire motor skills, how to promote the development of motor skills, and how motor activity influences psychological functioning and development. He is the former President of the North American Society for the Psychology of Sport and Physical Activity, the Co-founding President of the Federation of International Societies of Sport, Physical Activity, and Kinesiology, an Associate Editor for *Research Quarterly for Exercise and Sport*, a Section Editor for *Human Movement Science*, and serves on several editorial and advisory boards.

David J. Cornell, PT, DPT, PhD, CSCS, FACSM, is an Associate Professor in the Department of Physical Therapy and Kinesiology and serves as the Director of the Doctor of Physical Therapy Program and Co-Director of the Health Assessment Laboratory, at the University of Massachusetts-Lowell. He completed his BS in Exercise Science from Carroll University, and his MS in Kinesiology, PhD in Health Sciences, and Doctor of Physical Therapy degrees from the University of Wisconsin-Milwaukee. Dr. Cornell's interdisciplinary and community-engaged research agenda is concentrated on the optimization of health and human performance across various populations of interest, including tactical operators (e.g., firefighters, soldiers, etc.); elite athletes (e.g., professional athletes, collegiate student athletes, etc.); and various clinical populations. As a clinician-scientist, he is a licensed physical therapist (PT) and holds credentials as a Certified Exercise Physiologist (ACSM-EP), a Certified Strength and Conditioning Specialist (CSCS), and as a certified Tactical Strength and Conditioning Facilitator (TSAC-F). Dr. Cornell is a Fellow of the American College of Sports Medicine (FACSM) and is the recipient of the 2025 Sports Medicine and Rehabilitation Specialist of the Year Award from the National Strength and Conditioning Association (NSCA).

Joel T. Cramer, PhD, FACSM, FNSCA, FISSN, is the Interim Vice Provost for Faculty Excellence at the University of Central Florida. Joel earned a bachelor's degree in exercise science from Creighton University in 1997 and a master's and PhD in Exercise Physiology from the University of Nebraska–Lincoln in 2001 and 2003, respectively. Dr. Cramer has held tenure-track or tenured faculty positions at the University of Texas at Arlington, University of Oklahoma, Oklahoma State University, University of Nebraska–Lincoln, University of Texas at El Paso, and University of Central Florida. From 2003–2020, he managed a research lab that studied how human skeletal muscle adapts to exercise and nutrition interventions during clinical trials funded by industry, federal, and foundational sponsors. He has published over 200 peer-reviewed articles, nine book chapters, and a textbook, and has received honorific awards for his research and service. Dr. Cramer is passionate about using research as a teaching tool and has helped prepare eight doctoral students, nine master's students, 12 undergraduate honors students, and thousands of students in the classroom for successful careers in health-related professions. Since 2020, Joel has served in administrative roles dedicated to demonstrating the accountability, quality, and impact of higher education.

Kyle T. Ebersole, PhD, ATC, LAT, PES, is a Professor in the School of Rehabilitation Sciences and Technology and Director of the Human Performance and Sport Physiology Laboratory at the University of Wisconsin-Milwaukee. He completed his PhD in Exercise Physiology from the University of Nebraska-Lincoln in 2000. He currently teaches within the Physical Therapy and Athletic Training programs at the University of Wisconsin-Milwaukee. Dr. Ebersole was named as a Lubar Entrepreneur Teaching Fellow at the University of Wisconsin-Milwaukee in 2021. He has held a research and service partnership with the City of Milwaukee Fire Department since 2012 where he provides Athletic Training services as a Licensed Athletic Trainer (LAT) and serves as the Health and Fitness Coordinator for the department. His research focuses on the integrative contributions of movement efficiency, muscle function, and the autonomic nervous system to enhance work capacity for the health, fitness, and performance of cadets, recruits, and active-duty members.

Kelley G. Hammond, PhD, CSCS, is an Assistant Professor in the Department of Kinesiology and Exercise Science at the College of Saint Mary, in Omaha, where she teaches courses in human anatomy and exercise science. She earned her PhD in Rehabilitation Science from the University of Alabama at Birmingham and completed a postdoctoral fellowship at the University of Nevada Las Vegas. Her primary research focus is on the effects of exercise on skeletal muscle biology and physiology in Parkinson's disease and aging. Secondary interests include tactical strength and conditioning and nutrition. Dr. Hammond consistently publishes her findings in peer-reviewed journals and presents at national conferences.

Ashley A. Herda, PhD, is an Associate Professor in the Department of Health, Sport, and Exercise Sciences of the School of Education and Human Sciences at the University of Kansas. Dr. Herda earned her Master of Science and Doctor of Philosophy in Exercise Physiology degrees from the University of Oklahoma. Dr. Herda is currently the Director of both the Exercise and Human Performance Laboratory and the Metabolic and Body Composition Laboratory at the University of Kansas Edwards Campus. Dr. Herda's research interests include evaluation of exercise and functional performance outcomes across the lifespan with a specific interest in muscle and body composition following orthopedic surgery, rehabilitation, resistance training, or nutritional interventions.

G. Patrick Lambert, PhD, is Professor of Exercise Science and Pre-Health Professions at Creighton University. He has been teaching and conducting research for over 30 years.

His primary areas of teaching are Human Physiology and Human Nutrition. His research focuses on gastrointestinal function, heat stress, and hydration, and his publications have been cited over 3,000 times in other papers. He has written numerous book chapters and is a regular reviewer for physiology journals. Dr. Lambert is a long-time member of both the American College of Sports Medicine (ACSM) and the American Physiological Society (APS). He is Past-President of the Nebraska Physiological Society (former chapter of APS) and is an ACSM Certified Clinical Exercise Physiologist.

Aaron D. Likens, PhD, is an Associate Professor in the Department of Biomechanics and Director of the Quantitative Analysis Research Core at the University of Nebraska at Omaha. Dr. Likens is a quantitatively trained movement scientist with broad education and training in biomechanics, cognitive science, statistics, and motor control. His research focuses on describing statistical patterns that emerge in neural activity and human movement like those involved in gait, posture, and complex forms of behavior like driving. He also strives to understand how statistical patterns in gait and posture change over the natural course of aging, disease, and injury, and is developing new time series analyses for studying human movement and other forms of behavior.

Mitchel A. Magrini, PhD, CSCS(*D), NSCA-CPT(*D), is an Associate Professor in the Department of Exercise Science and Pre-Health Professions at Creighton University, where he teaches courses in Exercise Physiology and Human Anatomy. He earned his PhD in Health, Leisure, and Human Performance from Oklahoma State University and has spent the majority of his academic career investigating neuromuscular adaptations to different exercise protocols in older adult populations. Dr. Magrini has published widely in peer-reviewed journals and has presented his work at both national and international conferences. His research focuses on optimizing strength and power development to enhance physical function across the lifespan.

Anthony (Tony) M. Mayo, PhD, is a lecturer-faculty member in the Department of Kinesiology at San Francisco State University. He earned his PhD in Kinesiology from the University of Minnesota with an emphasis on motor learning and development. Dr. Mayo's research interests include the role of perceptual information in movement control, factors influencing skill development in sport, visually induced motion sickness (VIMS) in active virtual reality environments, and the effects of digital technology on physical activity. He regularly teaches undergraduate courses in motor development and motor learning and occasionally teaches neuromotor control.

Barbara B. Meyer, PhD, CMPC, is the Director of the Sport and Performance Psychology Laboratory at the University of Wisconsin-Milwaukee, which conducts research on health, performance, and recovery in the elite and occupational athlete. Her research focuses on identifying solutions to the real-life concerns of elite performers, with an emphasis on performance optimization, rest and recovery, and team science. Additionally, Dr. Meyer leads the Sport and Performance Psychology Department at the Olympic Winter Institute of Australia and serves as a mental performance consultant for elite and professional athletes, coaches, teams, and sport organizations worldwide. She has worked on the ground at five Olympic Games and provided off-site support at three others, and consulted with major professional sport teams at scouting combines and professional drafts. In addition to her work in elite sport, she also consults with tactical and corporate populations.

Nikolaos Stergiou, PhD, is a Professor and Founding Chair of the Department of Biomechanics, Distinguished Community Research Chair in Biomechanics, and Director of the Biomechanics Research Building at the University of Nebraska at Omaha. Dr. Stergiou's research focuses on understanding variability inherent in human movement. This research spans from infant development to older adult fallers and has impacted training techniques of surgeons and treatment and rehabilitation techniques of pathologies, such as peripheral arterial disease and multiple sclerosis.

Carly A. Wahl, PhD, CMPC, CSCS, is an Assistant Professor of Exercise Science at Eastern Illinois University, with an emphasis on teaching within the field of sport and performance psychology. In research and practice, she utilizes her dual training in performance psychology and exercise science to educate and implement holistic psychological, physical, and social recovery strategies to sport and tactical populations. Most recently, she has been awarded federal funding to research the psychophysiological recovery process utilized among firefighters. Dr. Wahl serves as the Certified Mental Performance Consultant for Eastern Illinois University Athletics.

Loree L. Weir, PhD, received her doctorate in Exercise Physiology from the University of Nebraska-Lincoln. She is an Assistant Teaching Professor and Graduate Program Director for Exercise Science in the Department of Health, Sport, and Exercise Science at the University of Kansas. Her interests include the impact of physical activity on metabolic function and its contribution to healthy aging with a focus on the role of resistance training in attenuating the loss of muscle mass and function due to age and chronic disease.

Tyler M. Wiles, PhD, is Dr. Aaron D. Likens' and Dr. Nikolaos Stergiou's most recently graduated doctoral student within the Department of Biomechanics at the University of Nebraska at Omaha. His research focuses on people's unique walking patterns that can be used for their identification, similar to the utilization of fingerprints to reveal a person's identity. He has been trained in biomechanics, motor control, dynamical systems, and physiology, and has additional academic interests in human movement variability, distance perception, and surfing.

Preface

Introduction to Exercise Science, Sixth Edition, is designed to introduce undergraduate students to key aspects of the field. The textbook introduces major areas of study, important technologies, certifications, professional organizations, and career opportunities in exercise science. It also helps students understand the history of the field and recognize current trends and future directions. Rather than offering in-depth discussions on individual subjects like anatomy, biomechanics, and exercise physiology, this book provides a broad overview and highlights important questions being explored in each area.

Each chapter includes helpful features, such as sample research abstracts, study questions, learning activities, suggested readings, and useful websites. Chapter 1 introduces the field of exercise science and describes its background, while Chapter 2 explains how to read and understand scientific research in the field. Chapters 3 through 10 focus on specific areas within exercise science. Each of these chapters offers a brief history, practical applications in health and sports, current technologies, educational paths, professional associations, career opportunities, and insights into the future of that specific area. A summary of each chapter is provided below.

CHAPTER 1, An Introduction to Exercise Science. This chapter opens by defining exercise science as the study of how and why the human body responds to physical activity. The chapter then explores the diverse academic areas that contribute to exercise science, offers a historical background of the field, and outlines typical components of exercise science degree programs. Students are also introduced to the foundational knowledge and practical experiences necessary for success in exercise science careers and provides a listing of career opportunities for exercise science graduates and certification options from professional organizations.

CHAPTER 2, Research in Exercise Science. This chapter provides a foundational overview of scientific inquiry in the field of exercise science, guiding students in the evaluation, location, and interpretation of scholarly research. Learners will begin by distinguishing scientific literature from non-scientific sources, such as popular media and social platforms, and will develop the ability to differentiate between primary and secondary sources. The chapter emphasizes the critical role of peer-reviewed literature in advancing evidence-based practice and encourages skepticism toward unverified information. Students will acquire practical skills for conducting literature searches using academic databases like PubMed, employing effective strategies involving keywords, author names, and publication dates.

Additionally, the chapter introduces core aspects of research design and methodology, including understanding the structure of scientific articles and recognizing distinctions between experimental and observational studies. A discussion on the peer review process highlights its importance in maintaining scientific integrity. The chapter concludes by exploring essential measurement and statistical concepts such as validity, reliability, levels of measurement, and the application of descriptive and inferential statistics. Together, these learning components equip students with the tools to critically evaluate research, make informed decisions, and apply scientific evidence in exercise science practice.

CHAPTER 3, Anatomy and Physiology. This chapter provides a foundational overview of human anatomy and physiology. Readers will be exposed to the basic structure and function of major body systems, including the musculoskeletal, cardiovascular, respiratory, and nervous systems. Key anatomical and directional terminology is introduced to build a framework for understanding movement, injury prevention, and performance enhancement. By establishing a strong anatomical and physiological foundation, this chapter equips students with the essential knowledge needed to analyze human movement and apply scientific principles throughout their studies in exercise science.

CHAPTER 4, Exercise and Sport Nutrition. Nutrition plays a vital role in maintaining health, supporting physical activity, and enhancing athletic performance. This chapter introduces the six classes of nutrients (carbohydrates, fats, protein, vitamins, minerals, and water) and explains how each contributes to energy production, recovery, and overall physiological function. Students will also explore key topics such as the glycemic index and glycemic load, consumer nutrition, and basic dietary concepts relevant to both general health and performance goals. The chapter also highlights educational pathways, career opportunities, emerging research tools, and future directions in the field. Understanding the relationship between nutrition, exercise performance, and long-term health provides exercise science majors with foundational knowledge to support clients, athletes, or their own personal goals through evidence-based dietary strategies.

CHAPTER 5, Exercise Physiology. This chapter defines exercise physiology, explains what exercise physiologists do, and delves into the field's roots in physical education and physiology, as well as the more recent incorporation of molecular biology and genetics into modern exercise physiology. The chapter relies on examples of research topics in health-related and sport-related aspects of exercise physiology (exercise snacks, sarcopenia, muscle growth, and plyometrics) to help the student gain an understanding of the breadth of topics in exercise physiology and how research can be applied to practice in the field. An overview of important technologies, including wearables, imaging, and "omics," is included. The chapter contains a practical discussion of possible career settings for exercise physiologists, including clinical, health/fitness, and sports performance environments, as well as an outline of pertinent educational requirements, professional organizations, and certifications for various career pathways.

CHAPTER 6, Exercise Prescription for Health and Sports Performance. Exercise prescription is utilized as a core tenant among health and fitness practitioners, human performance specialists, and allied health professionals. These professionals have different levels of education ranging from a high school diploma to a doctoral degree, and work in a variety of settings, including fitness centers, human performance labs, clinical environments, and tactical fields such as the military, fire service, and law enforcement. While the goals of exercise prescription vary depending on the population or context (e.g., general health promotion, sport performance, tactical readiness, rehabilitation), the underlying principles remain consistent across professions. This chapter explores the history and core principles of exercise prescription, as well as educational pathways, professional certifications, licensure requirements, and career opportunities in the field.

CHAPTER 7, Biomechanics. Biomechanics examines the forces acting on the human body and the effects they produce, aiming to deepen our understanding of the fundamental mechanisms that govern movement and the acquisition and control of motor skills. Professionals in this field contribute to a range of specialty areas, including developmental biomechanics, exercise and sport biomechanics, rehabilitative biomechanics, occupational biomechanics, and forensic biomechanics. Their work relies on diverse tools and technologies—such as sensors that measure muscle activation, high-speed motion-capture systems capable of tracking movements with millimeter precision, and instrumented treadmills that record ground-reaction forces. This chapter explores these applications in depth, while also providing an overview of the historical development of biomechanics, the educational pathways recommended for entering the profession, and emerging trends that are shaping the future of the field.

CHAPTER 8, Motor Behavior. This chapter provides an overview of the field of motor behavior, which incorporates the studies of motor control, motor learning, and motor development. Together, these three sub-disciplines address how skilled activity is controlled and how the capacity to engage in skilled activity is acquired. Although the modern field of motor behavior only emerged in the 1960s, the study of motor behavior has a rich history dating back to ancient civilizations. The field has witnessed remarkable advances over the last several decades in its understanding of the neurological substrates that contribute to motor control and motor disorders, the factors that influence the learning and development of new skills, and the factors that influence the relearning of skills lost through injury or disease. The study of motor behavior has almost limitless application to exercise science, although the most common applications occur in health and clinical-related settings and sport and performance-related settings. Many of the career opportunities related to motor behavior lie in teaching, coaching, and the allied health professions. The field of motor behavior will remain relevant because skill is a biological, social, and cultural necessity: a requisite for virtually every aspect of human life.

CHAPTER 9, Exercise and Sport Psychology. This chapter begins with a brief overview of the foundational moments in the history of exercise and sport psychology, as well as a detailed description of the discipline and its application to exercise science. A discussion of both the health-related and sport-related aspects of the discipline, along with cutting-edge research tools and technology (e.g., assessments, biofeedback, and virtual reality) provide the reader with the information necessary to explore the ways in which psychology is used to support both general health and athletic performance. Lastly, this chapter highlights the many career paths available in this growing field of study.

CHAPTER 10, Sports Injury Prevention and Rehabilitation. This chapter explores how active individuals and athletes recover from musculoskeletal injuries through rehabilitation techniques such as stretching, strengthening, and the restoration of cardiovascular fitness. It explains the importance of both injury prevention and post-injury rehabilitation. Injury care often involves a team of professionals (e.g., occupational therapists, sport psychologists, dietitians, personal trainers, strength and conditioning specialists, sports scientists, medical doctors, chiropractors). However, the management of the physical aspects of an injury, from prevention to rehabilitation, is typically associated with the role of an athletic trainer and physical therapist. This chapter concentrates on these two professions and discusses the educational pathways to each, along with the unique and shared practice roles, research tools and technology, and employment opportunities available to professionals in these important fields.

ABOUT THE WEBSITE AND EBOOK

The sixth edition of *Introduction to Exercise Science* is supported by a comprehensive instructor and student resources website. This resource offers students a variety of tools to reinforce their understanding of each chapter, including learning objectives, study questions, interactive learning activities, and curated lists of suggested reading and websites. These features are designed to enhance review and support active learning.

For instructors, the instructor and student resources website provides classroom activities/hands-on labs, that help apply key concepts, and customizable PowerPoint presentations summarizing essential chapter content. Additionally, a test bank of potential exam questions is included to assist with assessment development and instructional planning.

Overview of *Introduction to Exercise Science* (Sixth Edition)

NEW, EASY TO STUDY FORMAT

The sixth edition of *Introduction to Exercise Science* provides a clear and engaging overview of the main areas, or subdisciplines, of the field. Each chapter explores important topics such as the history of the subdiscipline, how it relates to both health and athletic performance, new technologies used in the field, and the certifications and professional organizations students can join. It also highlights a variety of exciting career paths in exercise science. Written by knowledgeable and experienced experts, this book gives students a strong, evidence-based foundation to help them explore and succeed in the field. The following areas and their importance to the field of exercise science are presented:

- research in exercise science
- anatomy and physiology
- exercise and sport nutrition
- exercise physiology
- exercise prescription
- biomechanics
- motor behavior
- exercise and sport psychology
- exercise and sport injury and rehabilitation

Using *Introduction to Exercise Science* (Sixth Edition)

A COMPLETE LEARNING RESOURCE FOR NEW STUDENTS

Introduction to Exercise Science is designed to help students actively engage with the subject. The book includes helpful learning tools such as sample research abstracts, study questions, learning activities, recommendations for further reading, and interesting websites to explore. It also comes with access to a companion website that features hands-on classroom activities/labs as well as helpful additional pedagogical support materials such as PowerPoint slides and a test question bank for each chapter. This makes it a great resource for both students and instructors alike. It is the perfect starting point for students interested in fields like biomechanics, kinesiology, exercise science, coaching, strength and conditioning, athletic training, physical therapy, sports medicine, and health and fitness. This textbook offers a solid and practical introduction to the key concepts in exercise science.

1 An Introduction to Exercise Science

Dona J. McCanlies

LEARNING OBJECTIVES

After studying this chapter, the student will be able to:

- define "exercise science"
- name and describe the roles of the scientific disciplines included under the umbrella of exercise science
- explain what exercise scientists study
- understand the historical development of exercise science
- explain why exercise science has become such a popular major in colleges and universities
- describe a typical undergraduate program in exercise science
- list potential careers in exercise science

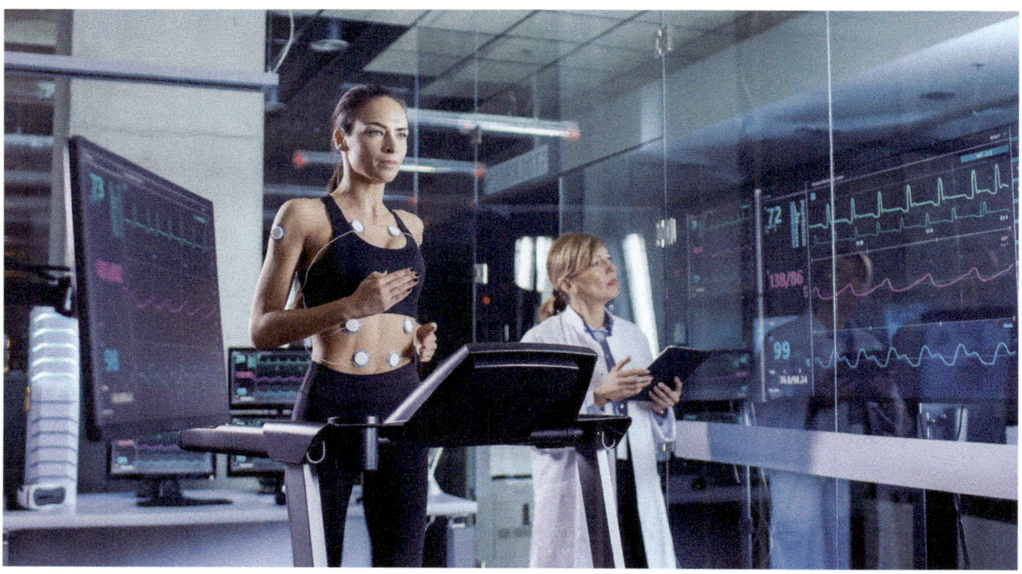

DOI: 10.4324/9781032697185-1

WHAT IS EXERCISE SCIENCE?

Exercise can be defined as "activity requiring physical effort, carried out to sustain or improve health and fitness" (Oxford University Press, n.d.a). **Science** is "the systematic study of the structure and behavior of the physical and natural world through observation, experimentation, and the testing of theories against the evidence obtained" (Oxford University Press, n.d.b). Therefore, **exercise science** is the systematic study of physical activity and its effects on the body. The field of exercise science is an umbrella term which encompasses a wide variety of scientific disciplines, including anatomy, physiology, nutrition, exercise physiology, performance enhancement, biomechanics, motor behavior, psychology, and rehabilitation. Exercise scientists utilize their in-depth understanding of these disciplines to study the effects of exercise on health, performance, and overall well-being. It is easy to see that the field of exercise science draws from a diverse range of disciplines, which allows exercise and its effects to be analyzed from many different perspectives. The following is a brief description of the way in which each of the key scientific disciplines within the field of exercise science plays a role:

Anatomy and Physiology examine the parts of the body (cells, tissues, organs, and organ systems) and how they work.

Nutrition explores the role of diet and nutrients in enhancing performance and recovery.

Exercise Physiology focuses on how body parts respond and adapt to exercise.

Exercise Prescription explores methods to improve both athletic performance and the performance of the activities of daily living through appropriate exercise prescription regimens.

Biomechanics examines the mechanical aspects of movement, including the relationships among the forces and motions that occur during physical activity.

Motor Behavior studies the various neural, anatomical, and experiential contributions to the development of motor skills.

Exercise and Sport Psychology investigates the mental and emotional aspects of exercise.

Sports Injury Prevention and Rehabilitation focuses on the use of exercise to recover from injuries or manage chronic conditions.

The principles of exercise science are not limited to humans but are also applied to nonhuman animals, such as racehorses, show horses, and racing dogs. These applications are particularly prominent in competitive animal sports, where understanding biomechanics, conditioning, and nutrition can enhance performance and reduce the risk of injury. For instance, exercise scientists may analyze a racehorse's gait to improve efficiency or study the effects of diet on a racing dog's endurance. Animal models are also valuable in research, as they can provide insights into physiological responses to exercise that are applicable to humans. Despite these applications, the primary focus of exercise science is on improving human health, fitness, and sports performance.

The diversity of exercise science is further highlighted when examining a simple activity such as walking. This single action can be explored from multiple perspectives within the field: an anatomist might describe the muscles involved, an exercise physiologist could study the body's cardiovascular and respiratory responses to the activity, and a biomechanist might assess the efficiency of each stride using the laws of physics. Similarly, an exercise psychologist might analyze what motivates individuals to walk, while a sports nutritionist could explain how the body converts food into energy to fuel the activity. This integration of the various areas within exercise science illustrates its complexity and interdisciplinary nature. While these subfields are often taught as standalone courses within academic programs, they collectively provide a comprehensive understanding of physical activity.

Exercise science integrates the knowledge derived from the study of the diverse sciences described above to enhance athletic performance, improve individual and population health, and guide evidence-based practices in fitness and rehabilitation. Because the various scientific disciplines involved in the study of exercise science are very intertwined, it is important to become knowledgeable in each and it is often important to study them in a particular order. A student of exercise science must first study the parts of the body (anatomy) and how those body parts work (physiology) to understand how the body responds and adapts to exercise (exercise physiology). In addition, an exercise science student may utilize their knowledge of anatomy, in addition to some knowledge of math and physics, to understand how forces act on the body to affect movement (biomechanics). General and neural anatomy, in addition to developmental biology, are important areas of study that are prerequisite to an understanding of motor behavior. A general knowledge of psychology is required prior to the application of psychological principles to exercise and sport psychology. Furthermore, a solid grasp of several subjects, including anatomy, physiology, nutrition, biomechanics, motor behavior, and psychology, is necessary for the proficient prescription of exercises to improve health and performance. Finally, an exercise science student must be able to skillfully read and interpret the scientific literature, as these are the skills required to understand the scientific studies that guide evidence-based practices in fitness and rehabilitation. Because humans are complex organisms and there are many aspects to consider when studying them and their responses to physical activity, integration of the various areas within exercise allows for a comprehensive understanding of the effects of exercise on health and performance.

Additionally, when examining the body's response to exercise, exercise scientists must evaluate both the immediate effects of a single exercise session (acute responses) and the long-term adaptations resulting from regular exercise (chronic responses). For instance, an exercise physiologist might observe that when an individual begins walking, their heart and respiratory systems adjust to meet the demands of the activity by increasing heart rate and breathing rate. These are acute responses. Over time, if the person adopts a routine of daily walking, their cardiovascular and pulmonary systems adapt by becoming more efficient, leading to lower resting heart and breathing rates. These changes exemplify chronic responses to exercise.

WHAT DO EXERCISE SCIENTISTS STUDY?

Exercise scientists focus on two main areas of inquiry: (1) the health-related benefits of physical activity (see Exhibit 1.1) and (2) sports performance (see Exhibit 1.2). Research in these areas offers critical insights into the connections among physical activity, health, and performance. For instance, exercise epidemiologists have found strong evidence that an active lifestyle, which includes appropriate exercise and diet, can lower the risk of diseases such as coronary heart disease (Wahid et al., 2016; Cheng et al., 2018) and certain types of cancer (Moore et al., 2016; Hojman et al., 2018; Matthews et al., 2020). Other research suggests that exercise can have an impact on the immune system and potentially alter the likelihood of developing infectious diseases (Chastin et al., 2021; Filgueira et al., 2021). However, significant gaps remain in determining the specific amounts and types of exercise required to reduce the risk of specific diseases. Another area of research, which is applicable to virtually every human, involves understanding how low to moderate

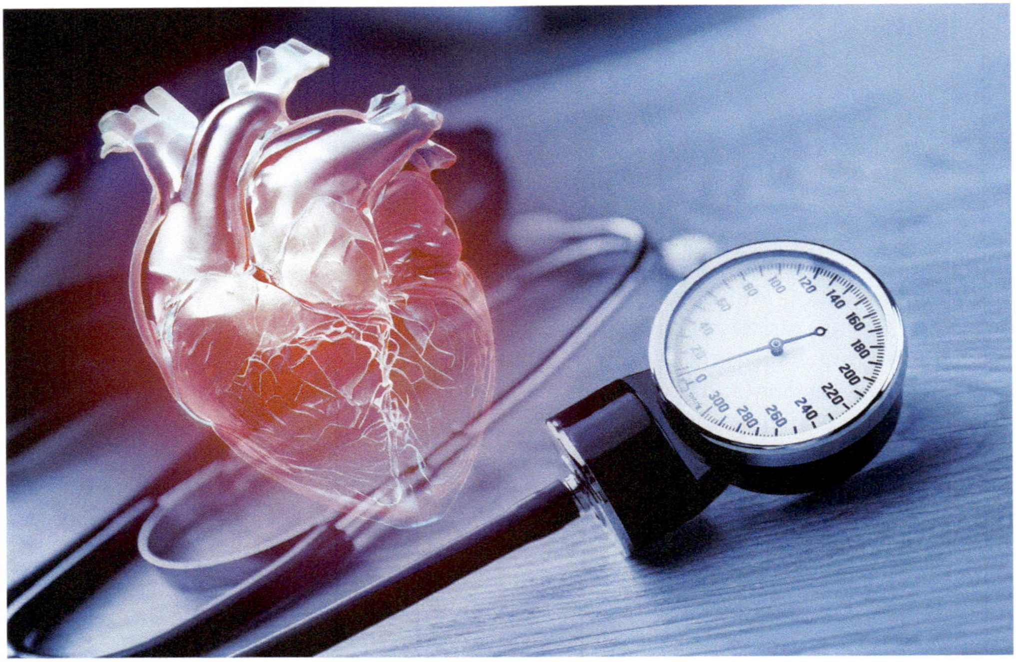

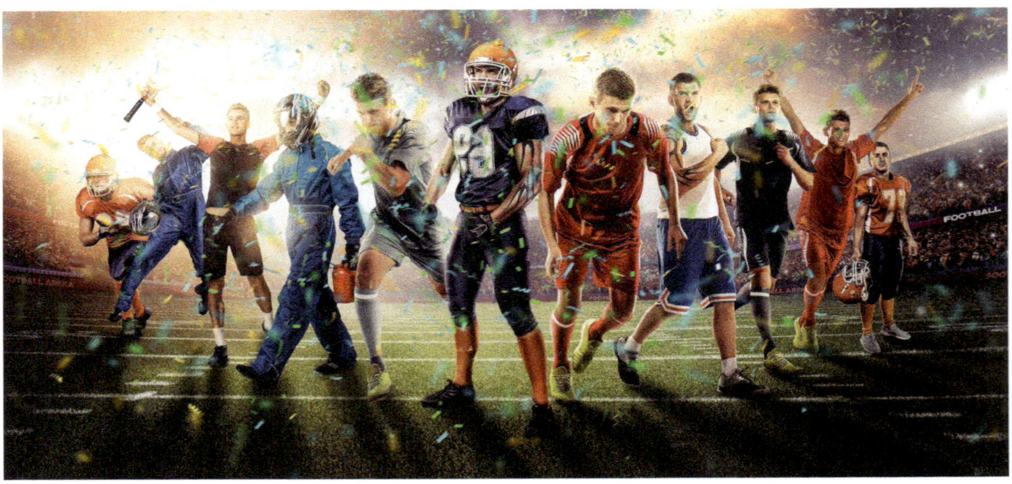

levels of exercise can enhance health and well-being across a person's lifespan (Milko et al., 2020; Lopez et al., 2022). Despite the great strides in scientific knowledge that have been made in recent years, the picture of the health-related benefits of physical activity remains incomplete and this lack of knowledge limits our ability to prescribe optimal exercise programs tailored to specific populations. Future generations of exercise scientists will continue to address these challenges and advance our understanding in this field.

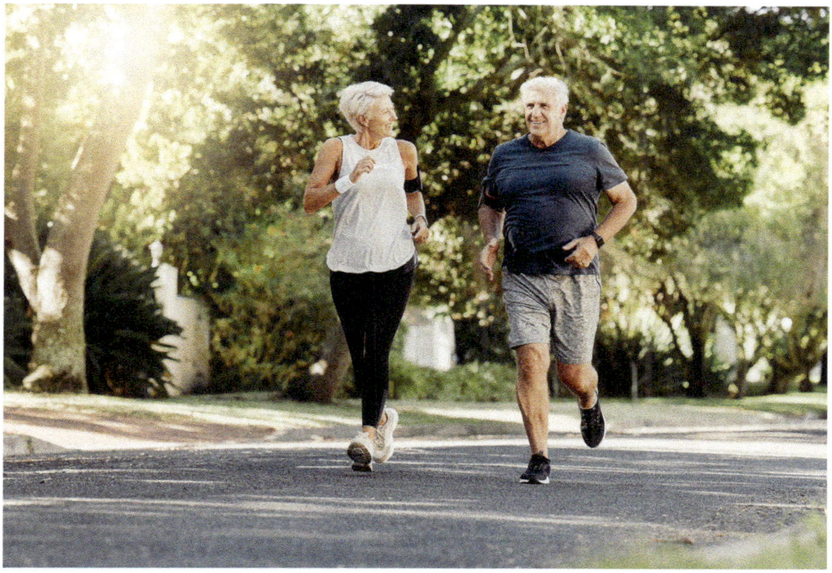

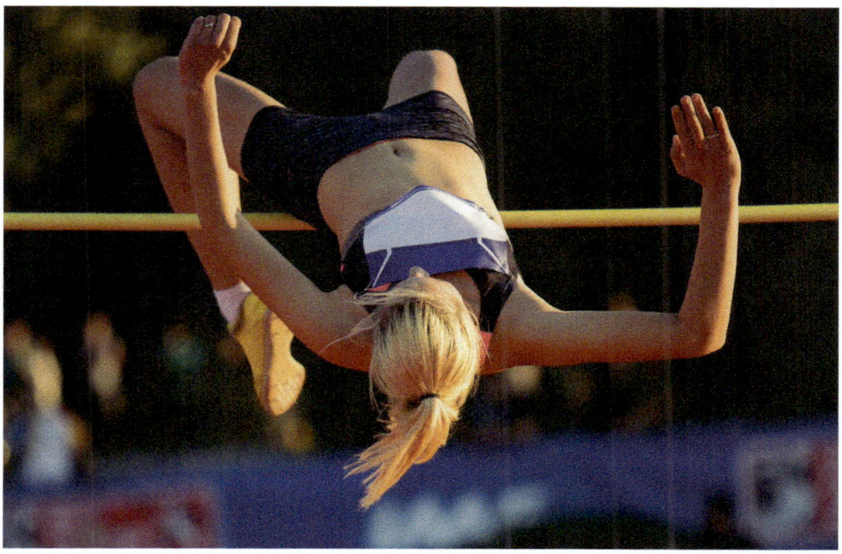

Exercise scientists, often referred to as sport scientists, also investigate factors that contribute to enhancing sports performance. This field encompasses a broad range of diverse topics that span across all ages. These include, but are not limited to, the growth and development of young athletes, the nutritional requirements of adult athletes, biomechanical analyses of elite competitors such as Olympic athletes, and the psychological traits of Master's-level athletes. A key focus for strength and conditioning coaches, particularly those affiliated with universities or professional teams, is applied research that involves developing and implementing effective training techniques for athletes (Kwok et al., 2021). Similarly, athletic trainers play a crucial role in exploring methods to prevent sports-related injuries and in devising strategies for the rehabilitation of athletes recovering from injuries sustained during competition or practice (Walters, Read, and Estes, 2018). The breadth of topics within sports performance highlights the vast opportunities available for exercise scientists to advance and apply knowledge in this dynamic field.

Exhibit 1.1 Research: health/clinical benefits of physical activity

Huang, J., Leng, L., Hu, M., Cui, X., Yan, X., Liu, Z., Wang, K., Wu, J., He, S., Deng, W., Li, P., Chen, Y., Gao, D., Wei, Y., and Huang, J. (2025). Comparative effects of different exercise types on cardiovascular health and executive function in sedentary young individuals. *Medicine and Science in Sports and Exercise*, 57(6), 1110–1122. https://doi.org/10.1249/MSS.0000000000003645

This study aimed to compare the impacts of different exercise types on cardiovascular health and executive function (EF) in sedentary young individuals, and to determine the associations between cardiovascular function and EF after exercise. Sixty-three sedentary participants were randomly divided into high-intensity interval training (HIIT), moderate-intensity continuous training (MICT), resistance exercise (RE), and control groups. Macro- and microvascular endothelial functions were assessed using brachial artery flow-mediated dilation and fingertip reactive hyperemia index, respectively. Arterial stiffness was evaluated through carotid-femoral pulse wave velocity, ankle-brachial index, and augmentation index. EF performance was evaluated using the Stroop and N-back tasks. Functional near-infrared spectroscopy was employed to measure cortical activation and real-time oxyhemoglobin concentration (Oxy-Hb) changes in different cerebral regions. Key circulating biomarkers for vascular and cognitive function, including brain-derived neurotrophic factor (BDNF), irisin, vascular endothelial growth factor, insulin-like growth factor 1 (IGF-1), and tumor necrosis factor-α, were measured using enzyme-linked immunosorbent assays. Eight weeks of HIIT, MICT, and RE effectively improved macro- and microvascular endothelial function while reducing arterial stiffness in sedentary young individuals. Furthermore, exercise-induced increase in BDNF level was correlated with enhanced macrovascular endothelial function, whereas an increase in IGF-1 level was associated with enhanced microvascular endothelial function and reduced arterial stiffness. Notably, both HIIT and MICT, but not RE, efficiently enhanced Oxy-Hb level in certain brain regions, such as the frontopolar area and dorsolateral prefrontal cortex, leading to the improvement in EF performance. Exercise-induced increase in Oxy-Hb level and EF performance were correlated with enhanced BDNF level and endothelial function and reduced arterial stiffness. Our study demonstrated that 8 weeks of HIIT, MICT, and RE effectively improved endothelial function in both macro- and micro-vessels, and arterial stiffness among sedentary young individuals. However, HIIT and MICT, but not RE, notably increased blood oxygen level in the frontopolar area and dorsolateral prefrontal cortex brain regions and improved EF performance. Due to the efficiency and time-saving features of HIIT, the present study highlights HIIT as an effective exercise prescription for promoting vascular function and EF in sedentary young individuals. Importantly, the observed improvements in cardiovascular function following exercise training are pivotal in improving EF, and elevated circulating levels of biomarkers like BDNF and IGF-1, induced by exercise, are involved in the regulatory mechanisms.

Exhibit 1.2 Research: sports/performance benefits of physical activity

Kamandulis, S., Dudėnienė, L., Snieckus, A., Kniubaite, A., Mickevicius, M., Lukonaitiene, I., Venckunas, T., Stasiule, L., and Stasiulis, A. (2024). Impact of anaerobic exercise integrated into regular training on experienced judo athletes: running vs. repetitive throws. *Journal of Strength and Conditioning Research*, *38*(9), e489–e495. https://doi.org/10.1519/JSC.0000000000004829

Anaerobic training in high-level athletes is of considerable interest to practitioners aiming to optimize performance. This study compared the impact of interval anaerobic training (IAT) sessions consisting of either high-intensity running or throwing that were performed twice a week together with regular judo training on the anaerobic and aerobic performance of experienced judo athletes. Employing a repeated-measures, counterbalancing research design, 12 national team judo athletes (7 women and 5 men; mean age, 20.4 ± 0.95 years; mean judo training experience, 13.4 ± 1.4 years; competitive level, black belt first and second Dan) performed each IAT modality for 6 weeks, for a full training cycle of 12 weeks. Assessments of their anaerobic fitness (Cunningham and Faulkner Anaerobic Treadmill Test), sport-specific anaerobic fitness (Special Judo Fitness Test [SJFT]), and aerobic capacity (maximal incremental treadmill running test) were performed before, after 6 weeks, and after 12 weeks of training. The uphill running performance improved by 13.1% over the 12-week period ($p = 0.047$). Simultaneously, there was a 9.0% improvement in the SJFT index and a 6.9% increase in the number of throws ($p = 0.011$ and $p = 0.017$, respectively). Although a trend for throwing drills being more effective than interval sprint running was observed, the interaction effect lacked statistical significance ($p = 0.074$). Moreover, no substantial changes were noted in aerobic endurance markers. In conclusion, this study suggests that incorporating specific and nonspecific high-intensity drills into a routine training regimen may enhance anaerobic capacity among well-trained judo athletes, potentially leading to favorable competitive outcomes.

THE HISTORY OF EXERCISE SCIENCE

The field of exercise science has a rich history that begins in ancient civilizations and extends to the modern era, reflecting the long-standing human desire to understand and optimize health and physical performance. Over time, exercise science has developed into a multidisciplinary field, which has enabled the modern-day exercise scientist to thoroughly examine the interactions among physical activity, health, and sports performance from many vantage points. The following section offers a brief description of the evolution of exercise science, which spans from the rudimentary realizations of early Greeks and Romans to the modern day, international, technologically advanced field of study it has become.

Early Civilizations

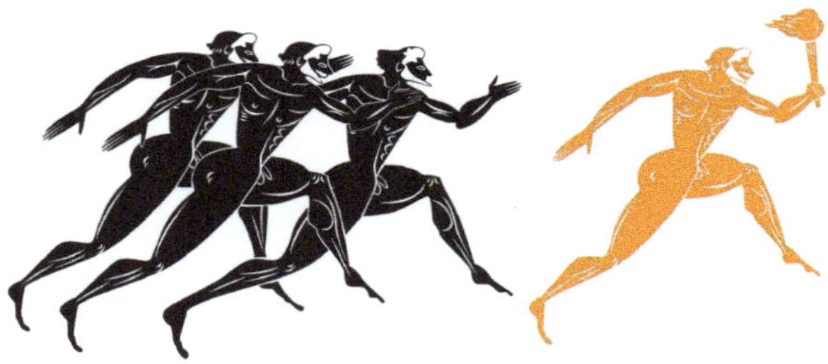

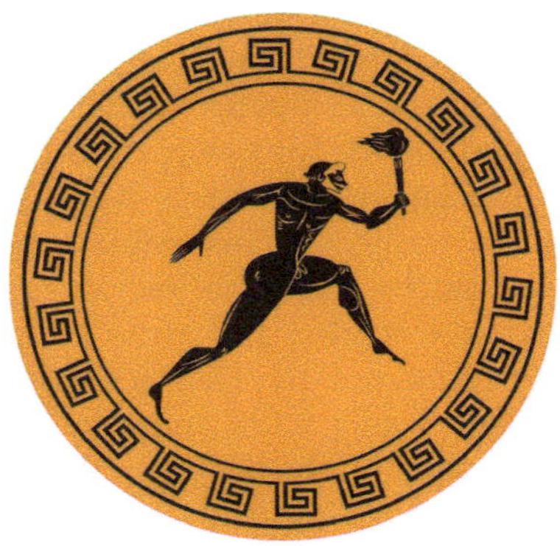

In ancient times, physical activity was necessary for survival. Early humans' daily activities, such as hunting, gathering, and other physical labor, naturally promoted physical fitness. The ancient Greeks, who were the progenitors of Olympic competition, were among the first to systematically study physical activity and its effects on the body. Hippocrates (460 BC–370 BC), often referred to as the "Father of Medicine," was a Greek physician and philosopher and one of the first to recognize the importance of not only exercise, but also the study of the effects of exercise on the human body, stating that "eating alone will not keep a man well. There must also be exercise, of which the effects must likewise be known" (Berryman, 2010; Sallis, 2009). The Greek philosophers Socrates (470 BC–399 BC), Plato (428 BC–347 BC), and Aristotle (384 BC–322 BC) also spoke of the importance of physical activity, with Aristotle describing "Excellence in Health and Fitness" as one of his "11 Excellences for Eudaimonia," which roughly translates to the 11 things he felt were necessary for "Living a Flourishing Life" (Broadie and Rowe, 2002; Rachels and Rachels, 2019). Greek athletes, such as those competing in the Olympic Games, trained by systematically following the teachings of these ancient scientists and philosophers. Galen (c. 129–216 AD), a Roman physician, expounded on the work of the early Greeks and wrote extensively about the role of exercise in developing and maintaining health, further laying the groundwork for viewing physical activity as essential to both physical and mental well-being (Berryman, 2003).

The Renaissance

The Renaissance was a historical period which occurred during the time span from the 14th to the 17th centuries. This era, driven by a renewed fascination with the human body, marked a pivotal point in the advancement of knowledge about anatomy and physiology. During this time, European scholars such as Leonardo da Vinci (1452–1519) and Andreas Vesalius (1514–1564) conducted detailed anatomical studies, providing a deeper understanding of the body's structure (Laurenza, 2012). In the 17th century, William Harvey (1578–1657), an English physician, discovered details of blood circulation, advancing the knowledge of the cardiovascular system and laying the foundation for modern exercise physiology (Ribatti, 2009).

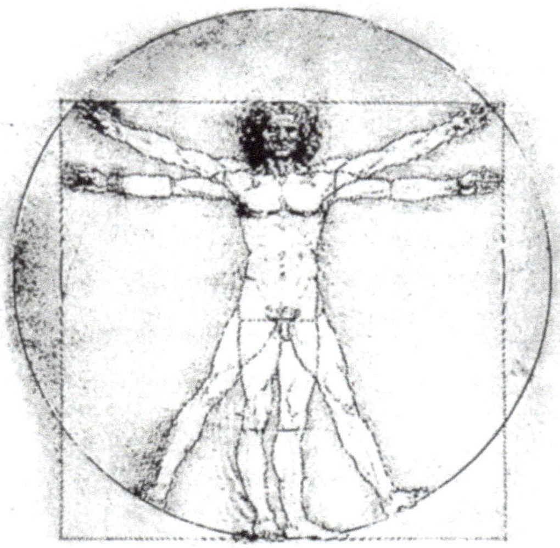

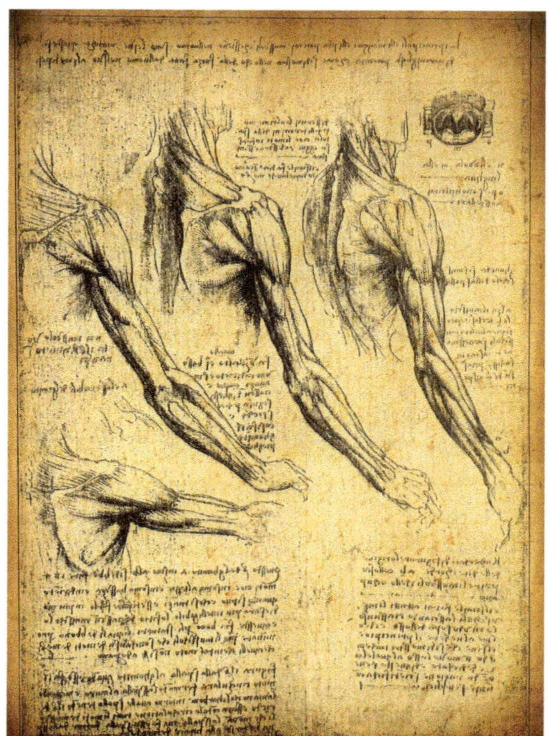

The Industrial Revolution

During the Industrial Revolution of the 18th and 19th centuries, advancements in technology drove a profound shift from an agrarian and craft-based society to one centered on machines and industrial manufacturing.

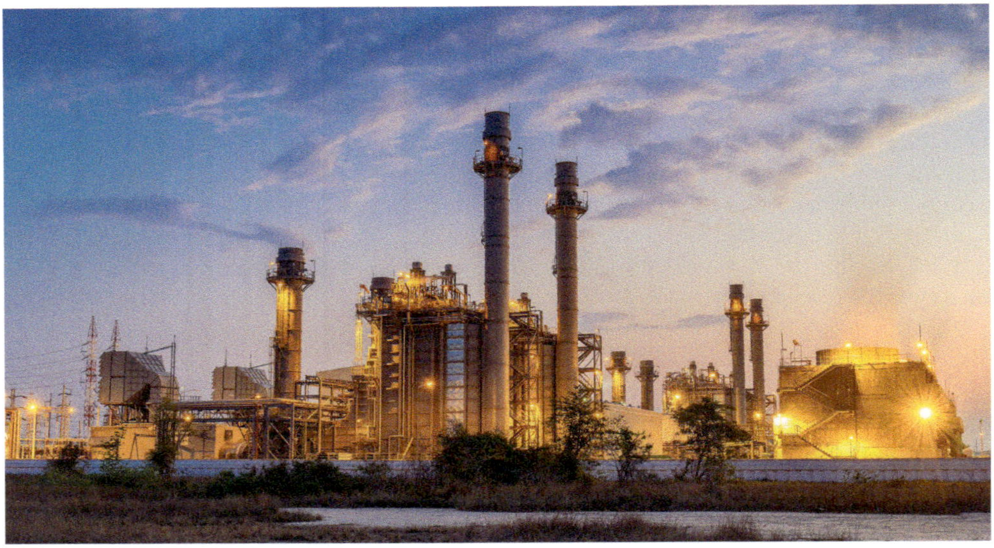

This transition reduced the reliance on traditional physical labor and opened the door to new forms of recreation, including the rise of organized sports. These societal changes sparked increased interest in physical training and athletic performance.

At the same time, progress in nutrition science, particularly the discovery of macronutrients and vitamins, began influencing dietary guidelines for athletes (Betts, 1953; Curry, 2015).

The 20th Century: Expansion of the Field

In the early 20th century, Dudley Sargent, a Yale-educated physician, educator, and fitness pioneer, began emphasizing the importance of physical activity not only for athletes but for all students. His efforts played a crucial role in the development of the discipline of physical education. Schools and universities, recognizing the value of structured physical activity for overall health and well-being, began offering physical education programs. Sargent further advanced the field by designing individualized exercise prescriptions aimed at improving health and performance, laying the groundwork for modern fitness and exercise science (Leonard, 1923; Sargent, 1928). This, in turn, fueled an interest in the scientific analysis of exercise and led to the numerous discoveries of this era, which included A.V. Hill's landmark work on VO_2 max and the critical role of oxygen in energy production in 1923 (Hill and Lupton, 1923; Burtscher, Millet, and Burtscher, 2023).

During World War II, driven by the need to assess the cardiovascular fitness of potential soldiers, the Harvard Step Test (Brouha, 1943) was developed by Lucien Brouha at the Harvard Fatigue Laboratory, followed by Per-Olof Astrand and Irma Rhyming's Cycle Ergometer Test (Astrand and Rhyming, 1954; Hoehn et al., 2015), which is used to estimate aerobic capacity. These tests provided valuable tools for assessing physical fitness and researchers began to link exercise to reduced risks of cardiovascular disease, diabetes, and obesity and to emphasize the health benefits of regular exercise. This period also saw an increased interest in rehabilitation following injury as soldiers returned from the battlefields. The emergence of sport psychology also occurred during this time, with researchers exploring the mental aspects of physical activity and the impact of motivation and goal setting.

In the 1950s and 1960s, the diverse areas of study within exercise science began to coalesce into a cohesive academic major in colleges and universities. Over time, as the field expanded and interests diverged, institutions began to recognize the need for separate majors that distinguished physical education from exercise science. This separation, which occurred during the mid- to late 1960s, helped to better address the unique focus and application of each major and fueled the development of exercise science as a rigorous scientific discipline, founded in research, and aimed at studying the body's response to physical activity. Such an evolution reflects the growing recognition of exercise science as a distinct and multidisciplinary field, which bridges the gap between scientific research and its practical application to health, human movement, and performance (Lewis, 2016).

The 21st Century: Technology and Personalization

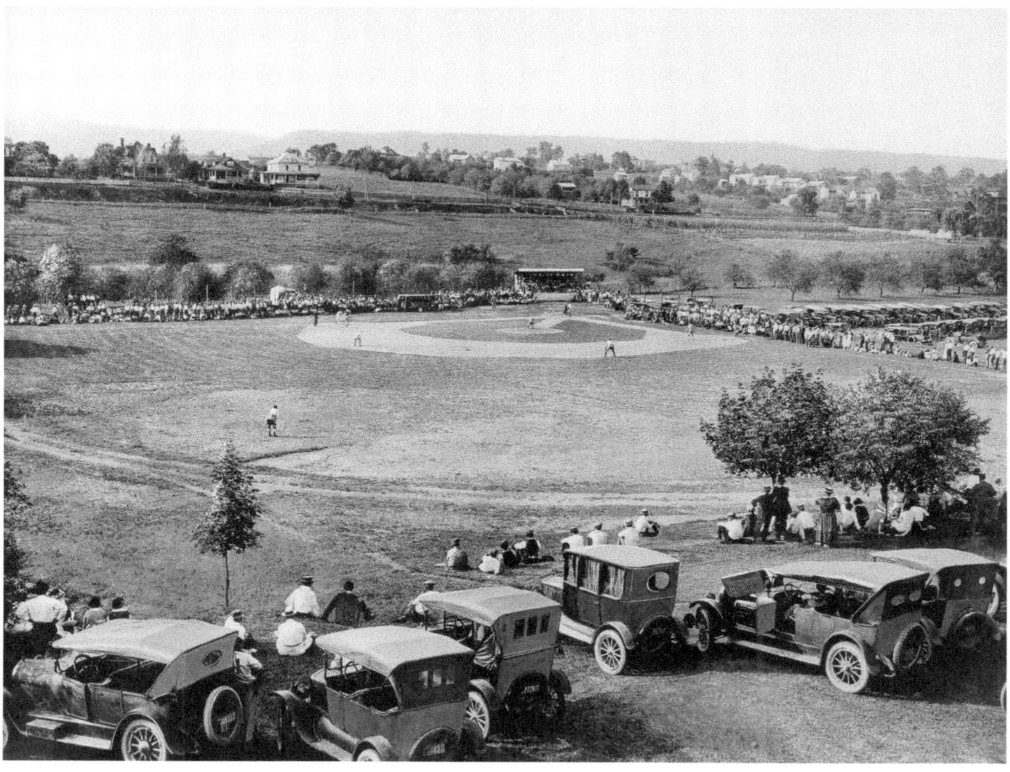

In recent decades, technology has transformed the field of exercise science. Wearable devices, advanced imaging techniques, biomechanical tools, and computer software technology are just a few of the modern-day advances that have played a role in achieving precise measurements of movement, energy expenditure, muscle activity, and countless other exercise related variables. Using these tools, researchers increasingly focus on personalized exercise prescriptions, tailoring recommendations to individual genetic, metabolic, and psychological factors.

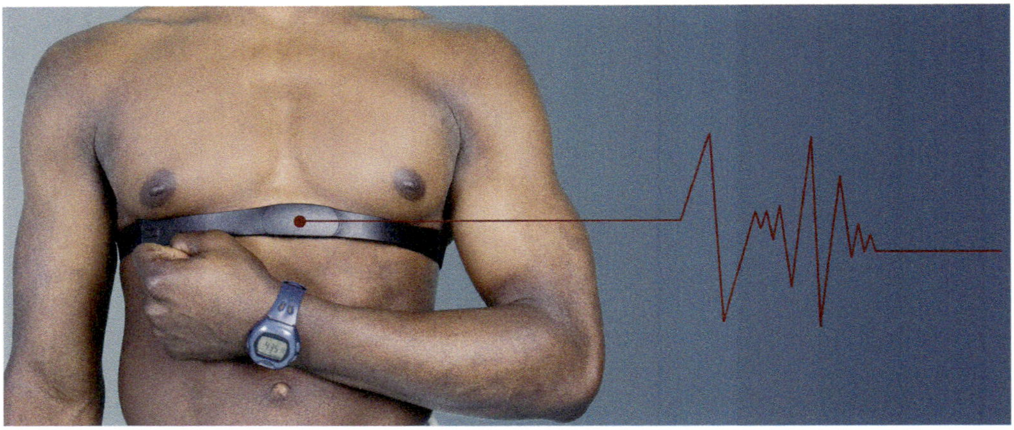

The integration of data science and artificial intelligence has revolutionized training and recovery strategies, enabling more efficient and effective performance optimization. In addition, the growing field of exercise immunology examines the role of physical activity in immune function and disease prevention, a focus that has gained urgency in the wake of global health challenges like the COVID-19 pandemic. Looking ahead, exercise science is poised to delve deeper into the role of physical activity in preventing and aiding recovery from a broad spectrum of diseases and conditions, including those that are yet to emerge. Advances in interdisciplinary research will likely uncover new pathways through which exercise influences health, guiding the development of targeted, evidence-based interventions for enhancing overall well-being.

Conclusion

The evolution of exercise science reflects humanity's ongoing efforts to understand and utilize the benefits of physical activity for health, performance, and rehabilitation. From ancient Greece to the digital age, advances in anatomy, physiology, nutrition, biomechanics, motor behavior, psychology, and rehabilitation have transformed the field into a multidisciplinary science with profound implications for improving both athletic performance and the quality of life across the lifespan. As the field continues to evolve, exercise scientists remain at the forefront of promoting health and enhancing human potential.

AMERICAN COLLEGE OF SPORTS MEDICINE

The historical development of exercise science reveals a strong connection to the field of medicine, which explains why many of its pioneers were trained as physicians. Their medical expertise provided a foundation for understanding the anatomical, physiological, and biomechanical principles underlying human movement, as well as the role of exercise in enhancing health, performance, and quality of life. In 1954, in recognition of the need to promote and integrate scientific research, education, and practical applications of sports medicine and exercise science, the American College of Sports Medicine (ACSM) was established by a small group of physicians and physical educators. Since its inception, the ACSM has served as a platform for collaboration among researchers, medical professionals, and educators, fostering advancements in exercise science and sports medicine and bridging the gap between theoretical research and practical application to health, fitness, and physical performance. The ACSM has grown substantially since its founding in 1954, reflecting the increasing recognition of the importance of exercise science and sports medicine. Established by a small group of 11 charter members, the organization has expanded its reach, now boasting over 50,000 members and certified professionals worldwide. This growth underscores the pivotal role ACSM plays in fostering multidisciplinary collaboration to promote fitness, health, and quality of life.

Members' interests span three primary areas:

1. **Basic and Applied Sciences**: focused on advancing the foundational and practical understanding of exercise science.
2. **Medicine**: concentrated on the role of physical activity in prevention, diagnosis, and treatment of medical conditions.
3. **Education and Allied Health**: emphasizing the dissemination of knowledge and integration of exercise science into various health-related professions.

ACADEMIC PROGRAMS IN EXERCISE SCIENCE

As previously described, the evolution of exercise science as a distinct academic field is deeply rooted in the broader discipline of physical education. During the mid-20th century, particularly in the 1960s, physical education emerged as an applied, professional discipline encompassing a wide range of topics related to sports, fitness, and physical activity. It focused on preparing individuals to promote physical well-being through structured activity, often in school-based settings. As societal interest in health, wellness, and athletic performance grew, academic programs began to branch out and specialize, leading to the development of exercise science as a unique area of study. Exercise science expanded to encompass scientific research on physical activity, integrating key biological sciences such as anatomy, physiology, biomechanics, and nutrition, among others. By the late 20th century, formal exercise science programs were appearing at colleges and universities, reflecting the increasing demand for professionals skilled in understanding the complex relationships between physical activity, health, and performance. Although closely intertwined, physical education and exercise science have emerged as two distinct entities, each with a unique focus. Today, physical education usually refers to the major that prepares students to teach in elementary and secondary schools, while exercise science typically refers to a non-teaching option.

The exercise science major is now one of the most popular undergraduate programs in fields related to health and human performance. The undergraduate major in exercise science attracts a diverse group of students, many of whom are initially drawn to the field by their personal experiences with athletic participation during childhood and adolescence. For these students, the opportunity to delve into the scientific principles underlying sport performance is particularly appealing. Studying areas such as exercise physiology, biomechanics, and sports nutrition allows them to connect academic learning with their own athletic endeavors, whether as competitive athletes or fitness enthusiasts. Beyond personal interest, many students find value in applying this scientific knowledge to practical settings, such as enhancing their own training regimens, supporting athletes in both performance and rehabilitation contexts, and assisting nonathletes in both clinical and nonclinical settings. These hands-on applications provide a strong sense of relevance and purpose, deepening their commitment to the field.

Curriculum

The typical undergraduate exercise science curriculum includes a solid foundation in the basic sciences, followed by a series of specialized courses related to exercise. While curricula may vary among institutions, they generally follow a similar structure. For example, the science core typically includes courses in anatomy, biology, chemistry, and physiology. Building on this base, the exercise-related courses often include biomechanics, exercise physiology, sports nutrition, exercise testing and prescription for healthy and special populations, first-aid and emergency care, leadership in exercise settings, computer proficiency, and practicum or internship experiences. A key strength of undergraduate exercise science programs is their integrated approach to knowledge. The exercise-related courses draw heavily on the concepts learned in the science core, enabling students to apply scientific principles to physical activity, health, and performance. This structured progression ensures that students develop both theoretical understanding and practical skills, preparing them for a variety of professional opportunities.

The philosophy underlying the undergraduate exercise science curriculum is that there is a knowledge base that all students should have. This foundation is essential for a range of specialized areas, including cardiac rehabilitation, corporate and agency fitness, physical therapy, and medicine. In addition to core courses, the curriculum encourages students to develop the skills and knowledge tailored to their specific area of interest. Specialization can be achieved through various avenues, such as elective courses, practicum experiences, volunteer activities, work experiences, and/or special training through professional certification programs. Many students further refine their expertise through postbaccalaureate experiences, including professional school (e.g., physical therapy, medicine, chiropractic) or graduate studies. To complement traditional exercise science programs, professional organizations have proposed more specialized curricula. The American Society of Exercise Physiologists (ASEP) has recommended programs for training undergraduate exercise physiologists, while the National Strength and Conditioning Association (NSCA) has developed guidelines for preparing strength and conditioning professionals. This combination of a broad foundational knowledge base and opportunities for specialization equips students to succeed in diverse and dynamic fields related to health, fitness, and human performance.

PROFESSIONAL STANDARDS FOR EXERCISE SCIENCE PROGRAMS

Several fitness-related organizations, including the American College of Sports Medicine (ACSM), American Council on Exercise (ACE), American Kinesiotherapy Association (AKTA), Cooper Institute for Longitudinal Studies (CILS), National Academy of Sports Medicine (NASM), and National Council on Strength and Fitness (NCSF) have adopted undergraduate academic standards and guidelines for exercise science programs. These standards and guidelines are based on recommendations from the Committee on Accreditation of the Exercise Sciences (CoAES), a specialized subcommittee established in 2004 under the Commission on Accreditation of Allied Health Education Programs (CAAHEP). The CoAES was created to address the need for accreditation standards specifically tailored to exercise science programs. Programs meeting these standards must integrate a comprehensive curriculum that includes classroom instruction, laboratory work, and clinical/practical activities. Programs that meet these criteria are eligible for CAAHEP accreditation. Currently, over 120 exercise science programs across 37 states hold CAAHEP accreditation. For information on academic standards and guidelines for exercise science programs visit www.acsm.org; www.akta.org; www.cooperinst.org; and www.ncsf.org. For more information on the accreditation of exercise science programs visit www.coaes.org and www.caahep.org.

CAREER AND EMPLOYMENT OPPORTUNITIES

The rapid expansion of exercise science programs at colleges and universities can be attributed to both students' initial interests and the increasing recognition of the field's relevance across multiple domains. The rising societal emphasis on health, fitness, and performance has created an abundance of opportunities for graduates, including careers in clinical and rehabilitative settings, consulting for athletes and sports teams, designing corporate wellness programs, and conducting research in human performance and preventative healthcare. One significant factor contributing to this growth is the expansion of corporate fitness facilities. Corporations are motivated not only by the desire to offer a valued fringe benefit for employees, but also by research indicating that maintaining a physically fit and active workforce can reduce health insurance costs and absenteeism, thereby benefiting the company financially (Wojcik, 2023). The need for qualified managers of these facilities has contributed to the development of exercise science majors at colleges and universities as well as certification programs through professional organizations such as the ACSM, the NSCA, the American Council on Exercise (ACE), and the International Society of Sports Nutrition (ISSN), among others (See Exhibit 1.3).

The combination of a degree in exercise science and certification from a reputable professional organization increases graduates' likelihood of success in the job market. Another career option for exercise science undergraduates is to attend graduate school. Graduate programs typically prepare students for advanced roles, such as corporate or agency fitness specialists, clinical professionals specializing in areas like cardiac rehabilitation, and researchers and educators in university settings.

Exhibit 1.3 Selected certifications in exercise science

Organization	*Certification(s)*
American College of Sports Medicine (ACSM) 6510 Telecom Drive Indianapolis, IN 46278 (317) 637–9200 www.acsm.org	ACSM Certified Group Exercise Instructor® (ACSM-GEI) This certification is for those who want to work in a group setting with clients who have no apparent medical conditions as well as clients with health challenges who are still able to exercise independently. Degree requirement: high school diploma ACSM Certified Personal Trainer® (ACSM-CPT) This certification is for those who want to work with apparently healthy clients and clients with health challenges who have been cleared to exercise independently. Degree requirement: high school diploma ACSM Certified Exercise Physiologist® (ACSM-EP) This certification is for those who want to work with healthy clients and those with medically controlled conditions to establish safe, healthy, and effective exercise and lifestyle behaviors. Degree requirement: bachelor's degree in exercise science ACSM Certified Clinical Exercise Physiologist® (ACSM-CEP) This certification is for those who want to use prescribed exercise and basic health behavior interventions to help clients with chronic diseases or conditions. Degree requirement: bachelor's degree in exercise science plus 1200 hours of hands-on experience or master's degree in clinical exercise physiology plus 600 hours of clinical experience
American Council on Exercise (ACE) 9444 Balboa Avenue Suite 290 San Diego, CA 92123-4901 (888-825-3636) www.acefitness.org	ACE Personal Trainer Certification This certification (ACE-PTC) is for those who want to design and apply unique exercise programs for clients with no medical conditions. Degree requirement: high school diploma ACE Group Fitness Instructor Certification This certification is for those who want to lead groups of individuals with no medical conditions. Degree requirement: high school diploma ACE Health Coach Certification (ACE-HCC) This certification is for those who want to design and implement dietary and exercise programs to reach clients' weight goals and improve overall health and wellness. Degree requirement: high school diploma ACE Medical Exercise Specialist Certification (ACE-MESC) This certification is for those who want to work with clients with health challenges, including exercise programming for special populations. Degree requirement: bachelor's degree in exercise science or related field

(*Continued*)

Exhibit 1.3 (Continued)

Organization	*Certification(s)*
American Society of Exercise Physiologists (ASEP) 1200 Kenwood Avenue Duluth, MN 55811 (218) 723–6297 www.asep.org	Exercise Physiologist Certified (EPC) This certification is for exercise physiologists who want to provide quality care in healthcare, fitness, and wellness settings. Degree requirement: bachelor's degree in exercise physiology or related field and specific course requirements
International Society of Sports Nutrition (ISSN) 785 SW Rustic Circle Stuart, FL 34997 (561) 239–1754 www.sportsnutritionsociety.org	Certified Sports Nutritionist (CISSN) This is a more advanced certification than the SNS (listed below) and is for health, fitness, and medical professionals who work with athletes or active individuals. Degree requirement: bachelor's degree in exercise science, nutrition, or related field Sports Nutrition Specialist (SNS) This is an entry level certification for health, fitness, and medical professionals who work with athletes or active individuals. Degree requirement: high school diploma
National Athletic Trainers' Association (NATA) 1620 Valwood Parkway Suite 115 Carrollton, TX 75006 (214) 637–6282 www.nata.org	Certified Athletic Trainer (ATC) This certification signifies that an athletic trainer (AT) is capable of performing all of the duties of an AT without being a threat to the public. Degree requirement: master's degree from an accredited athletic training program
National Strength and Conditioning Association (NSCA) 1885 Bob Johnson Drive Colorado Springs, CO 80906 (800) 815–6826 www.nsca.com	NSCA-Certified Personal Trainer (NSCA-CPT) This certification is for those who are interested in working with individuals or small groups to maintain or improve their physical capabilities and body composition. Degree requirement: high school diploma Certified Strength and Conditioning Specialist (NSCA-CSCS) This certification is for those who want to coach and train athletes for improvements specific to their sports. Degree requirement: bachelor's degree or currently enrolled college senior Certified Performance and Sports Specialist (NSCA-CPSS) This certification is for those who want to perform in-the-field research in the development of recommendations to improve the performance of athletes Degree requirement: 3 routes, each with its own degree requirement (bachelor's, master's and doctorate) Certified Special Populations Specialist (NSCA-CSPS) This certification is for those who want to work with individuals who have physical limitations, injuries, and health conditions. Degree requirement: bachelor's degree in exercise science or related field Tactical Strength and Conditioning Facilitator (TSAC-F) This certification is for those who want to train military, law enforcement, and fire and rescue personnel to maintain and improve their physical abilities. Degree requirement: high school diploma

In addition to its appeal to students who are looking to combine a passion for health, fitness, and science, the rigorous coursework in exercise science serves as a stepping stone to advanced education and diverse career paths. Exercise science programs often include foundational courses in anatomy, physiology, chemistry, and physics, creating a strong academic base for graduate studies in fields such as physical therapy, occupational therapy, chiropractic, dentistry, and medicine. The interdisciplinary nature of the major also offers pathways into corporate and agency fitness, personal training, strength and conditioning coaching, wellness programming, and exercise and sport science research. This combination of personal interest, academic rigor, and professional versatility makes exercise science one of the most dynamic and appealing majors for students seeking meaningful careers in health, fitness, and human performance (see Exhibit 1.4).

Exhibit 1.4 Careers in exercise science

Option	*Related Associations and Organizations*	*Selected Websites*	*Estimated Annual Salary Range**	*Average*
Agency and private sector fitness				
Health club fitness/wellness, personal training	American Council on Exercise (ACE) International Health, Racquet and Sportsclub Association (IHRSA) National Council for Certified Personal Trainers (NCCPT) National Council on Strength and Fitness (NCSF) National Strength and Conditioning Association (NSCA) American College of Sports Medicine (ACSM) Young Men's Christian Association (YMCA)	www.acefitness.org www.ncsf.org www.nsca.org www.acsm.org	$45,000–50,000	$46,000
Military fitness	Human Performance Resource Center	www.hprc-online.org	$46,000–80,000	$73,000
Corporate fitness and wellness	Health and Fitness Association IDEA Health and Fitness Association	www.healthandfitness.org www.ideafit.com	$83,000–110,000	$86,000
Ergonomics consulting	International Ergonomics Association (IEA) Human Factors and Ergonomics Society (HFES) Board of Certification in Professional Ergonomics (BCPE) American Society of Safety Professional (IASSP)	www.hfes.org	$64,000–107,000	$81,000
Strength and conditioning coach	NSCA	www.nsca.org	$69,000–116,000	$88,000

(*Continued*)

Exhibit 1.4 (Continued)

Option	*Related Associations and Organizations*	*Selected Websites*	*Estimated Annual Salary Range**	*Average*
Dietician	Academy of Nutrition and Dietetics	www.eatright.org	$64,000–75,000	$76,000
Occupational safety specialist	Occupational Health and Safety Administration (OSHA)	www.osha.gov	$69,000–99,000	$76,000
Health and fitness writer	American Medical Writers Association (AMWA)	www.amwancal.org	$42,000–136,000	$79,000
Clinical and rehabilitation				
Cardiac rehabilitation	American Association of Cardiovascular and Pulmonary Rehabilitation (AACVPR) American Heart Association (AHA) American College of Sports Medicine (ACSM)	www.aacvpr.org	$51,000–81,000	$64,000
Pulmonary rehabilitation	AACVPR American Lung Association (ALA)	www.aacvpr.org	$47,000–69,000	$57,000
Athletic training	National Athletic Trainers' Association (NATA) American College of Sports Medicine (ACSM) American Medical Society for Sports Medicine (AMSSM) American Orthopedic Society of Sports Medicine (AOSSM)	www.nata.org	$45,000–62,000	$55,000
Massage therapy	American Massage Therapy Association (AMTA) Associated Bodywork and Massage Professionals (ABMP) Massage Therapy Foundation (MTF)	www.amtamassage.org	$47,000–75,000	$58,000
Medical Technologist	American Medical Technologist (AMT) American Society for Clinical Laboratory Science (ASCLS)	www.americanmedtech.org	$47,000–124,000	$73,000
Professional schools				
Allopathic Medicine (M.D.)	American Medical Association (AMA) Association of American Medical College (AAMC)	www.ama-assn.org	$50,000–294,000	$160,000
Osteopathic Medicine (D.O.)	American Osteopathic Association (AOA) American Medical Association (AMA) American Association of College of Osteopathic Medicine (AACOM)	www.osteopathic.org	$188,000–243,000	$217,000

(*Continued*)

Exhibit 1.4 (Continued)

Option	*Related Associations and Organizations*	*Selected Websites*	*Estimated Annual Salary Range**	*Average*
Physician's Assistant (P.A.)	American Academy of Physician's Assistants (AAPA)	www.aapa.org	$105,000–122,000	$120,000
Dentistry (D.D.S.)	American Dental Association (ADA) Academy of General Dentistry (AGD) American Student Dental Association (ASDA)	www.ada.org	$131,000–300,000	$193,000
Physical Therapy (P.T.)	American Physical Therapy Association (APTA) Academy of Neurologic Physical Therapy (ANPT)	www.apta.org	$87,000–121,000	$104,000
Occupational Therapy (O.T.)	American Occupational Therapy Association (AOTA) American Occupational Therapy Foundation (AOTF)	www.aota.com	$77,000–94,000	$86,000
Chiropractic (D.C.)	International Chiropractors Association (ICA) American Chiropractic Association (ACA)	www.chiropractic.org	$98,000–165,000	$124,000
Optometry (O.D.)	American Optometric Association (AOA) American Academy of Optometry (AAO) National Optometric Association (NOA)	www.aoa.org	$130,000–15,000	$140,000
Nursing (R.N.)	American Nursing Association (ANA) National League for Nursing (NLN)	www.nursingworld.org	$70,000–110,000	$86,000
Teacher, researcher, and/or coach				
College/University Professor	American Association of University Professors (AAUP)	www.aaup.org	$65,000–157,000	$143,000
College/University strength and conditioning coach	NSCA	www.nsca.com	$49,000–67,000	$65,000
Athletic team coach	National Collegiate Athletic Association (NCAA)	www.ncaa.org	$53,000–80,000	$66,000

(*Continued*)

Exhibit 1.4 (Continued)

Option	*Related Associations and Organizations*	*Selected Websites*	*Estimated Annual Salary Range**	*Average*
Institutional research (e.g., Cooper Institute or Olympic Training Center)	American College of Sports Medicine (ACSM) NSCA Olympic Training Center Cooper Institute	www.acsm.org www.nsca.com www.teamusa.org www.cooperinstitute.org	$68,000–99,000	$84,000

Source: Bureau of Labor Statistics (2025); Indeed Editorial Team (2024).

SUMMARY

The evolution of exercise science as a formal academic discipline marks its transition from being a subset of physical education to becoming a distinct field rooted in scientific inquiry and practical application. While physical education focuses on teaching and curriculum design for school-aged populations, exercise science addresses a broader spectrum, preparing students for careers in health, fitness, wellness, and performance. This shift reflects society's growing demand for expertise in physical activity and health. The growth of exercise science as an academic field is evidenced by the increasing number of undergraduate and graduate programs available. At many institutions, enrollment in non-teaching exercise science programs now surpasses that of traditional physical education teacher preparation majors. This growth is driven by the diverse career opportunities available to exercise science graduates, including roles in corporate and agency fitness, personal training, clinical rehabilitation, allied health, private-sector consulting, and academia. In addition, the solid foundation in basic sciences associated with most undergraduate exercise science programs provides a solid foundation for students to meet the entrance requirements of a variety of professional schools. Complementing this scientific foundation, exercise science graduates gain practical experience through exercise-related courses, practicums, and internships. This combination ensures they are well-prepared to apply theoretical knowledge in real-world settings.

STUDY QUESTIONS

1. What is the primary focus of exercise science?

   a. The study of diet and nutrition
   b. The study of physical activity and its effects on the body
   c. The study of psychology and behavior
   d. The study of human evolution

2. Which of the following best describes motor behavior?

   a. It examines the development of motor skills
   b. It focuses on the mental and emotional aspects of exercise

c. It uses physics and the relationships among forces to examine the mechanics of movement
d. It explores the role of diet in health and performance

3. Which civilization is known for systematically studying physical activity and developing athletic training methods?

a. Ancient Rome
b. Ancient Egypt
c. Ancient Greece
d. Renaissance Italy

4. What major event in the 20th century increased interest in exercise science due to rehabilitation needs?

a. The Renaissance
b. World War I
c. World War II
d. The Great Depression

5. What is the difference between acute and chronic responses to exercise?

a. Acute responses happen immediately, while chronic responses occur over time
b. Chronic responses happen immediately, while acute responses occur over time
c. Acute responses are long-term adaptations to exercise
d. Chronic responses only occur in professional athletes

6. Exercise scientists study the effects of physical activity on health and sports performance. One of their primary goals is to:

a. Develop new diets for weight loss
b. Find ways to improve human performance
c. Eliminate the need for exercise
d. Promote a sedentary lifestyle

7. Which organization was founded in 1954 to promote research and education in exercise science?

a. National Strength and Conditioning Association (NSCA)
b. International Society of Sports Nutrition (ISSN)
c. American College of Sports Medicine (ACSM)
d. American Council on Exercise (ACE)

8. Exercise scientists can work in which of the following settings?

a. Corporate wellness programs
b. Hospitals and rehabilitation centers
c. Health clubs

   d. University research labs
   e. All of the above

9. What foundational subjects are typically included in an undergraduate exercise science curriculum?

   a. History, literature, and economics
   b. Anatomy, physiology, biomechanics, and nutrition
   c. Sociology, anthropology, and political science
   d. Marketing, finance, and accounting

10. Which accreditation body establishes academic standards for exercise science programs?

   a. The National Institutes of Health (NIH)
   b. The Commission on Accreditation of Allied Health Education Programs (CAAHEP)
   c. The American Medical Association (AMA)
   d. The International Olympic Committee (IOC)

Answers to Chapter 1 Study Questions

1. b
2. a
3. c
4. c
5. a
6. b
7. c
8. e
9. b
10. b

LEARNING ACTIVITIES

1. Visit the ACSM website (ACSM, n.d.). Under the "Membership" tab, choose "Join ACSM."

   a. Which ACSM membership should you apply for?
   b. What are the benefits of membership?
   c. How much does membership cost?

2. Visit the NSCA website (NSCA, n.d.). Under the "Membership" tab, choose "Membership Overview."

   a. Which NSCA membership should you apply for?
   b. How much does membership cost?
   c. What are the benefits of membership?

3. Explain how membership in ACSM and NSCA would fit your particular interests and situation.

4. Perform an online search for an exercise science topic of your choice.
   a. Find two sites that you find interesting
   b. Provide the URL for each site
   c. Provide a brief description of each and explain why you like these particular sites

5. Perform an online search on exercise science curricula.
   a. Choose two other universities, other than your own, with exercise science majors
   b. Compare the exercise science curricula of the two universities to the exercise science curriculum at your university

6. Perform an online search on an exercise science career opportunity that is of interest to you.
   a. What are the degree requirements for this career?
   b. What types of certifications are required?
   c. What is the setting for this career? Clinical (e.g., private practice, hospital), athletic/sport (e.g., collegiate, professional), agency (e.g., gym, military), educational (e.g., teacher, researcher, coach), etc.?

SUGGESTED READING AND WEBSITES

ACSM. (n.d.). American College of Sports Medicine. Available at: https://acsm.org (Accessed September 9, 2025).

Bushman, B.A. (2024). *Fitness professional's handbook* (8th ed.). Champaign, IL: Human Kinetics.

Chandler, T.J., Brown, L.E., Chandler, W.B, and Bishop, C. (2024). *Conditioning for strength and human performance* (4th ed.). New York: Routledge.

NSCA. (n.d.). National Strength and Conditioning Association. Available at: www.nsca.com (Accessed September 9, 2025).

Visit This Book's Instructor and Student Resources Website

Visit the Introduction to Exercise Science (IES) website. You may want to review and take notes on the Study Questions and Learning Activities. For additional "hands-on" learning, your instructor may want you to try out a Classroom Activity/Lab for each chapter. One of the Classroom Activities for this chapter, "An Introduction to Exercise Science" involves important forms, **Pre-participation Health Screening Questionnaire (Par-Q), Medical Clearance, and Informed Consent**, which must be completed prior to any investigation utilizing human subjects.

REFERENCES

ACSM. (n.d.). American College of Sports Medicine. Available at: https://acsm.org (Accessed September 9, 2025).

AKTA. (n.d.). American Kinesiotherapy Association. Available at: www.akta.org (Accessed September 9, 2025).

Astrand, P.O., and Rhyming, I. (1954). A nomogram for calculation of aerobic capacity (physical fitness) from pulse rate during submaximal work. *Journal of Applied Physiology*, 7(2), 218–221. https://doi.org/10.1152/jappl.1954.7.2.218

Berryman, J.W. (2003). Ancient and early influences. In C.M. Tipton (Ed.), *People and ideas: Exercise physiology* (pp. 1–38). Oxford: Oxford University Press. https://doi.org/10.1016/B978-019512527-6.50002-7

Berryman, J.W. (2010). Exercise is medicine: A historical perspective. *Current Sports Medicine Reports*, *9(4)*,195–201. https://doi.org/10.1249/JSR.0b013e3181e7d86d

Betts, J.R. (1953). The technological revolution and the rise of sport, 1850–1890. *The Mississippi Valley Historical Review,* 40(2), 231–256. https://doi.org/10.2307/1888926

Broadie, S. (Ed.) and Rowe, C. (Trans.) (2002). *Nicomachean ethics excellence of character: Selections from Books I and II* (pp. 95–122). Oxford: Oxford University Press. (Original work published 350 BCE.) https://doi.org/10.1017/S0034412502236203

Brouha, L. (1943). The step test: A simple method of measuring physical fitness for muscular work in young men. *Research Quarterly: American Association for Health, Physical Education, and Recreation*, 14(1), 31–37. https://doi.org/10.1080/10671188.1943.10621204

Bureau of Labor Statistics, U.S. Department of Labor. (2025, January 20). *Occupational Outlook Handbook, OOH data access and republishing information.* https://www.bls.gov/ooh/about/ooh/about/ooh-developer-info.htm (Accessed September 9, 2025).

Burtscher, J., Millet, G.P., and Burtscher, M. (2023). Celebrating 100 years of VO_2 max. *QJM: An International Journal of Medicine*, 116(9), 809. https://doi.org/10.1093/qjmed/hcad082

CAAHEP. (n.d.a.). Committee on Accreditation of the Exercise Sciences. Available at: https://www.caahep.org/committees-on-accreditation/exercise-science (Accessed September 9, 2025).

CAAHEP. (n.d.b). Commission on Accreditation of Allied Health Education Programs: About Us. Available at: https://www.caahep.org/about/about-us (Accessed September 9, 2025).

Chastin, S.F.M., Abaraogu, U., Bourgois, J.G., Dall, P.M., Darnborough, J., Duncan, E., Dumortier, J., Pavon, D.J., McParland, J., Roberts, N.J., and Hamer, M. (2021). Effects of regular physical activity on the immune system, vaccination and risk of community-acquired infectious disease in the general population: Systematic review and meta-analysis. *Sports Medicine*, 51(8), 1673–1686. https://doi.org/10.1007/s40279-021-01466-1

Cheng, W., Zhang, Z., Cheng, W., Yang, C., Diao, L., and Liu, W. (2018). Associations of leisure-time physical activity with cardiovascular mortality: A systematic review and meta-analysis of 44 prospective cohort studies. *European Journal of Preventive Cardiology,* 25(17), 1864–1872. https://doi.org/10.1177/2047487318795194

Curry, G. (2015). Making modern sport: The impact of the industrial revolution. *PE Review*, 11(1), 27–30.

Filgueira, T.O., Castoldi, A., Santos, L.E.R., de Amorim, G.J., de Sousa Fernandes, M.S., de Lima do Nascimento Anastacio, W., Campos, E.Z., Santos, T.M., and Souto, F.O. (2021). The relevance of a physically active lifestyle and physical fitness on immune defense: Mitigating disease burden, with focus on COVID-19 consequences. *Frontiers in Immunology,* 12: 587146. https://doi.org/10.3389/fimmu.2021.587146

Hill, A.V., and Lupton, H. (1923). Muscular exercise, lactic acid, and the supply and utilization of oxygen. *QJM: An International Journal of Medicine*, 16(62), 135–171. https://doi.org/10.1093/qjmed/os-16.62.135

Hojman, P., Gehl, J., Christiansen, J.F., and Pedersen, B.K. (2018). Molecular mechanisms linking exercise to cancer prevention and treatment. *Cell Metabolism*, 27(1), 10–21. https://doi.org/10.1016/j.cmet.2017.09.015

Hoehn, A.M., Mullenbach, M.J., and Fountaine, C.J. (2015). Actual versus predicted cardiovascular demands in submaximal ergometer testing. *International Journal of Exercise Science*, 8(1), 4–10. https://doi.org/10.70252/XFKJ1279

Indeed Editorial Team. (2024). *21 high-paying jobs in exercise science (with salaries)*. Indeed.com. https://www.indeed.com/career-advice/finding-a-job/high-paying-jobs-in-exercise-science (Accessed January 20, 2025).

Kenneth H. Cooper Institute. (n.d.). Kenneth H. Cooper Institute: About. Available at: https://www.cooperinstitute.org/about (Accessed September 9, 2025).

Kwok, Y., So, B.C.L., Tse, D.H.T., and Ng, S.S.M. (2021). A systematic review of meta-analysis: Biomechanical evaluation of the effectiveness of strength and conditioning training programs on front crawl swimming performance. *Journal of Sports Science and Medicine*, 20(4), 564–585. https://doi.org/10.52082/jssm.2021.564

Laurenza, D. (2012). Art and anatomy in Renaissance Italy: Images from a scientific revolution. *The Metropolitan Museum of Art Bulletin*, 69(3), 4–48. https://www.jstor.org/stable/23222979

Leonard, F.E. (1923). Physical education in American colleges and universities. In R.T. McKenzie (Ed.), *History of physical education* (pp. 279–289). Philadelphia: Lea and Febiger. http://www.archive.org/details/guidetohistoryofOOIeon

Lewis, J. (2016). Exercise science: A unique discipline comes of age. *Alumni Georgia*. https://alumni.uga.edu/2016/03/15/exercise-science-a-unique-discipline-comes-of-age/

Lopez, P., Traaffe, D.R., Galvão, D.A., Newton, R.U., Nonemacher, E.R., Wendt, V.M., Bassanesi, R.N., Turella, D.J.P., and Rech, A. (2022). Resistance training effectiveness on body composition and bodyweight and obesity across the lifespan: A systematic review and meta-analysis. *Obesity Reviews*, 23(5), e13428. https://doi.org/10.1111/obr.13428

Matthews, C.E., Moore, S.C., Arem, H., Cook, M.B., Trabert, B., Hakansson, N., Larsson, S.C., Wolk, A., Gapstur, S.M., Lynch, B.M., Milne, R.L., Reedman, N.D., Huang, W., Berrington de González, A., Kitahara, C.M., Linet, M.S., Shiroma, E.J., Sandin, S., Patel, A.V., and Lee, I. (2020). Amount and intensity of leisure-time physical activity and lower cancer risk. *Journal of Clinical Oncology*, 38(7), 686–697. https://doi.org/10.1200/JCO.19.02407

Milko, H., Zillmann, N., Ring-Dimitriou, S., Dorner, T.E., Titze, S., and Bauer, R. (2020). Effects of physical activity on health. *Gesundheitswesen*, 82(S 03), S184–S195. https://doi.org/10.1055/a-1217-0549

Moore, S.C., Lee, I., Weiderpass, E., Campbell, P.T., Sampson, J.N., Kitahara, C.M., et al. (2016). Association of leisure-time physical activity with risk of 26 types of cancer in 1.44 million adults. *JAMA Internal Medicine*, 176(6), 816–825. https://doi.org/10.1001/jamainternmed.2016.1548

Oxford University Press. (n.d.a). Exercise. In *Oxford English Dictionary*. https://panthersports-medicine.com/blog/dont-let-the-idea-of-exercise-stop-you-from-exercising/ (Accessed February 5, 2025).

Oxford University Press. (n.d.b). Science. In *Oxford English Dictionary*. https://oxfordreference.com/search?q=science (Accessed February 5, 2025).

NASM. (n.d.). National Academy of Sports Medicine. Available at: www.nasm.org (Accessed September 9, 2025).

NCSF. (n.d.). National Council on Strength and Fitness. Available at: www.ncsf.org (Accessed September 9, 2025).

Rachels, J., and Rachels, S. (2019). Virtue ethics. In *The elements of moral philosophy* (9th ed., pp. 169–185). New York: McGraw-Hill.

Ribatti, D. (2009). William Harvey and the discovery of the circulation of the blood. *Journal of Angiogenesis Research*, 1(3), 1–3. https://doi.org/10.1186/2040-2384-1-3

Sallis, R.E. (2009). Exercise is medicine and physicians need to prescribe it! *British Journal of Sports Medicine*, 43(1), 3–4. https://doi.org/10.1136/bjsm.2008.054825

Sargent, D.A. (1928). Dudley Allen Sargent: An autobiography. *JAMA*, 90(2), 141. https://doi.org/10.1001/jama.1928.02690290071040.

Wahid, A., Manek, N., Nichols, M., Kelly, P., Foster, C., Webster, P., Kaur, A., Friedemann Smith, C., Wilkins, E., Rayer, M., Roberts, N., and Scarborough, P. (2016). Quantifying the association between physical activity and cardiovascular disease and diabetes: A systematic review and meta-analysis. *Journal of the American Heart Association*, 5(9), e002495. https://doi.org/10.1161/JAHA.115.002495

Walters, B.K., Read, C.R., and Estes, A.R. (2018). The effects of resistance training, overtraining, and early specialization on youth athlete injury and development. *Journal of Sports Medicine and Physical Fitness*, 58(9), 1339–1348. https://doi.org/10.23736/S0022-4707.17.07409-6

Wojcik, J.R. (2023). Economic benefits of workplace wellness programs and changes since COVID-19. *American College of Sports Medicine (ACSM)*. https://acsm.org/workplace-wellness-programs-economic-benefit/ (Accessed April 3, 2025).

2 Research in Exercise Science

Ashley A. Herda and Joel T. Cramer

LEARNING OBJECTIVES

After studying this chapter, the student will be able to:

- distinguish between primary and secondary sources in exercise science
- recognize the differences between peer-reviewed scientific literature and non-scientific sources such as social media and popular magazines
- utilize academic databases (e.g., PubMed) to locate peer-reviewed research articles
- apply effective search strategies using keywords, author names, and publication years
- explain the key components of a scientific research article, including abstract, introduction, methods, results, discussion, and conclusion
- define key measurement concepts, including validity, reliability, and objectivity
- explain the significance of descriptive and inferential statistics in exercise science research

INTRODUCTION

Exercise science is a dynamic and evolving discipline that applies scientific principles to understand human movement, health, performance, and rehabilitation. Given the breadth and depth of the field, it is essential for students and professionals to become informed consumers of scientific literature. Research is the foundation of exercise science, shaping our understanding of human movement, health, performance, and rehabilitation. Unlike long-established fields such as chemistry, biology, and philosophy, which trace their roots back over 2,000 years to philosophers like Aristotle and Plato, exercise science has only recently emerged as a formal academic field. Its scientific foundation began to take shape in the early 20th century, with academic programs becoming more widespread in the mid-to-late 1960s (Henry, 1978). This relatively recent emergence has positioned exercise science as a field in scientific infancy, characterized by rapid growth and continuous innovation. Technological advancements and new research findings frequently challenge existing theories and open new avenues of inquiry.

As the field of exercise science evolves, the scope broadens and diversifies, which is evidenced by the breadth of this book. At its core, research in exercise science applies scientific principles to real-world challenges, ranging from optimizing athletic performance and preventing injury to managing chronic disease and promoting healthy behavior. The

DOI: 10.4324/9781032697185-2

research process follows a systematic approach: identifying a question, reviewing existing literature, designing a study, collecting and analyzing data, and drawing evidence-based conclusions (Kraemer, Fleck, and Deschenes, 2011; Shuttleworth, 2009). This structured method ensures that findings are not only valid but also applicable across subfields such as biomechanics, exercise physiology, motor behavior, sport and exercise psychology, strength and conditioning, clinical rehabilitation, and health promotion.

Understanding how to critically evaluate research, recognize credible evidence, and apply findings to practice is crucial, especially in an era where misinformation can spread rapidly through social media. Teaching and learning in exercise science are deeply rooted in current research, making it vital for educators and practitioners alike to stay engaged with the latest scientific developments. This chapter introduces key concepts in exercise science research, including a brief history of the scientific method, common research designs and methodologies, and the importance of peer-reviewed literature. Developing a solid understanding of the research process will help you see how evidence informs both theory and practice, and why research remains central to the progress and credibility of the field.

HISTORICAL PERSPECTIVES

The research process has evolved over many centuries, shaped by advancements in philosophy, science, and technology. The structured approach used today, focused on observation, experimentation, and analysis, can be traced back to ancient civilizations and has been refined over time. Early scientific thinking was mostly based on careful observation. Civilizations such as the Egyptians, Greeks, and Chinese recorded knowledge in areas such as medicine, astronomy, and physical health. Greek philosophers like Aristotle and Hippocrates emphasized logical reasoning and direct observations, although their methods lacked formal experimentation (Gower, 2012).

A more formal approach to science began during the Scientific Revolution in the 16th and 17th centuries. Figures like Francis Bacon, who supported learning through observation and experience (inductive reasoning), and René Descartes, who promoted drawing conclusions from general ideas (deductive reasoning), laid the foundation for modern scientific thinking. Scientists such as Galileo Galilei and Isaac Newton built on these ideas by conducting experiments and using mathematics to explain natural laws (Gower, 2012).

By the 19th century, scientific research became more structured, with greater emphasis on experimental design and hypothesis testing. Important breakthroughs, such as Charles Darwin's theory of evolution and Louis Pasteur's germ theory, showed how scientific methods could be applied to biology and medicine (Debré, 2022; Gower, 2012). These discoveries helped establish the modern research process that is now used in many fields, including exercise science.

In the 20th and 21st centuries, research has continued to evolve. Advances in statistical analysis, peer-reviewed publishing, and digital data collection have made research more precise and reliable. During this time, ethics in research also became a central concern, especially after the Belmont Report was published in 1979. The document highlighted important principles for conducting research with human participants, including respect for individuals, doing good (beneficence), and ensuring fairness (justice) (Nagai, Nakazawa, and Akabayashi, 2022).

Research in exercise science is rooted in a long history of scientific discovery and advancement. Whether investigating injury prevention, athletic performance, or long-term health outcomes, researchers apply systematic methods grounded in evidence and ethics. By understanding how the scientific method has developed over time, you can better evaluate scientific claims, think critically about research findings, and apply these principles in your own studies and future careers.

FUNDAMENTAL CONCEPTS

Literature Sources

The First Amendment of the US constitution allows people to write, disseminate, and sometimes publish just about anything. Supporting the growing excitement and interest in exercise science, social media outlets and the internet, in general, provide access to a vast amount of literature in the field. Sometimes social media presents high quality objective material; however, social media posts are subjective opinions that may lack research support and often include unsubstantiated claims. Thus, it is important to teach consumers of literature how to identify the quality and soundness of information. This may start with encouraging learners to simply read the original scientific literature source for themselves. Having first-hand knowledge of the original study empowers us to make up our own minds, rather than be influenced by someone else's interpretation. Ultimately, it is important to understand that *literature* in our field includes any written words related to exercise science that originates from both *scientific* and *non-scientific* sources.

Scientific Literature Sources

Typically, **scientific literature** undergoes a **peer-review process** whereas non-scientific literature is usually not reviewed (see Exhibit 2.1). When a scientific article or book chapter is submitted for publication, the document is reviewed by two or three **external reviewers** who are chosen because of their expertise in the content area. For example, when a manuscript is submitted to a journal, external reviewers assess whether the *research methods* are sound, the study design aligns with its *purpose*, that *statistical and data analyses* are appropriate, and that the study is valid in addressing the *research question*. They also evaluate the novelty or originality of the topic, recommend it for acceptance or rejection, and provide constructive feedback to the authors for improvement. Ultimately, the role of the external peer reviewer is to ensure scientific quality and rigor without oversaturation of any specific topic in the body of literature. It often takes several months to organize the review of a single manuscript. Based on the recommendations and comments from the external reviewers, the editor must decide whether to reject or accept the manuscript or request revisions from the author(s) before a decision regarding publication can be made. Typically, authors are given an opportunity to revise the manuscript and respond to the reviewers' comments. Once the revised manuscript and author responses are received, the editor either conducts a second review or makes the final decision regarding its publication status. Overall, the review process for most scientific literature is extensive and rigorous and demands higher standards than non-scientific, non-reviewed literature. There are two types of peer-reviewed scientific literature: *primary* and *secondary references*.

Exhibit 2.1 Examples of peer-reviewed research journals and non-peer-reviewed sources of information on exercise science

Peer-Reviewed Research Journals	*Non-peer-Reviewed Sources*
British Journal of Sports Medicine	TikTok, YouTube, WhatsApp, Snapchat, Instagram, X, Facebook, etc.
European Journal of Applied Physiology	Muscle & Fitness
American Journal of Sports Medicine	STRONG Fitness Magazine
Bone and Joint Journal	Runner's World
International Review of Sport and Exercise Psychology	Yoga Journal
Journal of Strength and Conditioning Research	Healthline.com

Primary References

In exercise science, primary references typically refer to original research articles published in scholarly journals that detail the purpose, methods, results, and conclusions of a scientific study. Reading and understanding primary references allows the reader to see, first hand, the results of a single study and draw conclusions based on those results and/or the author's interpretations. These *references provide* the most current information on topics in exercise science and expose the reader to the original report. The main drawback of primary sources is the vast amount of literature on a given topic, making it difficult to draw reliable conclusions from a single study. Therefore, readers must consider findings from multiple studies to develop a comprehensive understanding of the topic. The following represent two recent examples of primary literature in exercise science:

- Khanna, M.M., Guenther, C.L., Eckerson, J.M., Talamante, D., Yeh, M.E., Forby, M., Hopkins, K., Munger, E., Rauh, G., Chelluri, S., Schmidt, C., Walocha, I., and Sacco, M. (2025). Vigorous exercise enhances verbal fluency performance in healthy young adults. *Brain Sci.*, Jan 20; *15*(1), 96. doi: 10.3390/brainsci15010096. PMID: 39851463
- Perissiou, M., Saynor, Z.L., Feka, K., Edwards, C., James, T.J., Corbett, J., Mayes, H., Shute, J., Cummings, M., Black, M.I., Strain, W.D., Little, J.P., Shepherd, A.I. (2025). Ketone monoester ingestion improves cardiac function in adults with type 2 diabetes: a double-blind, placebo controlled, randomized, crossover trial. *J. Appl. Physiol.*, Feb 12; *138*(2), 546–558. doi: 10.1152/japplphysiol.00800.2024. PMID: 39818982

Secondary References

Secondary references include review articles and academic books or textbook chapters. These sources are still rigorously peer reviewed, but they often summarize and/or synthesize the results of many research studies which allow for a more inclusive understanding of the topic than any one research article. Consumers are not required to find and understand all of the primary references; rather, they can get the "big picture" all in one article review or book chapter. Secondary literature sources are also valuable for locating primary references that cannot be found using traditional literature searches. On the other hand, secondary references are often narrative reviews which are subjective interpretations by their nature (some literature reviews are objective—see the discussion on meta-analysis later in this chapter). Thus, the reader receives a secondhand interpretation of several primary sources. In addition, secondary references can be somewhat out-of-date at the time of publication. For example, a potential problem with book chapters is that they are often written one to three years in advance of their publication date and, therefore, may not include the most recent information. Below are citations for two recent articles and a book chapter as examples of secondary references.

- Stout, J.R., Kreider, R.B., Candow, D.G., Forbes, S.C., Rawson, E.S., Antonio, B., and Antonio, J. (2025). The birth of modern sports nutrition: tracing the path from muscle biopsies to creatine supplementation—A narrative review. *J. Intl. Soc. Sports Nutr.*, 22(sup1). https://doi.org/10.1080/15502783.2025.2463373
- Walden, T., Smith, N., Dempsey, A., Jonson, A.M., and Girard, O. Blood flow restricted walking: does the hypoxic environment compromise walking technique? *Front. Sports Act. Living*, Jan 9; 6: 1481315. doi: 10.3389/fspor.2024.1481315. PMID: 39850868; PMCID: PMC11754391
- Eckerson, J.M. Energy and the nutritional needs of the exercising female. In J.J. Forsyth and C.M. Roberts, Eds, *The Exercising Female: Science and Its Application* (pp. 44–65). Abingdon, OX, UK: Routledge, 2019.

Non-Scientific Literature Sources

Popular magazines, newspapers, websites, and many social media posts are published sources of *non-scientific* literature in exercise science. These are usually subjective, opinion-based articles or posts that have not been reviewed for credibility or content. For example, TikTok, YouTube, Instagram, *Muscle & Fitness, or Runner's World* (see Exhibit 2.1 for further examples) are sources that publish non-scientific content that have not been peer reviewed. However, non-scientific literature is not without value. Presented accurately, exercise science-related information disseminated to the lay public can increase awareness of critical issues in the field. For example, a newspaper article highlighting the benefits of balance training for older adults may help raise public awareness and reduce fall risk (O'Neill, 2024). In addition, non-scientific articles can be used as an impetus for conducting a scientific study. To illustrate, if an article in an online newspaper claims that dieting is more effective than exercise for weight loss (Carroll, 2015), this hypothesis can be tested by researchers in an experimental setting and published in a peer-reviewed journal (e.g., Donnelly et al., 2013). To summarize, non-scientific literature is not considered a legitimate source of information in exercise science; however, it may offer some value to society.

READING PRIMARY REFERENCES

As stated previously, a primary reference is an original study that is designed to answer a specific question. In most cases, published, original research investigations include seven sections: (1) Abstract; (2) Introduction; (3) Methods; (4) Results; (5) Discussion; (6) Conclusions; and (7) References.

Abstract

The purpose of the **abstract** is to provide a very brief overview of the purpose of the study, the methods used to collect and analyze the data, the results, and conclusions that can be drawn from the results. For many journals, the abstract is often restricted to 200 to 300 words in length. As shown in Exhibit 2.2, the abstract is a concise summary and does not contain detailed information regarding the study's experimental design and results. The abstract can usually be accessed free of charge on specialized websites allowing readers to determine within minutes whether or not they want to read the full-text article.

Exhibit 2.2 Example of an abstract and keywords from a primary research article

Herda, T.J., Holmes, E.A., Cleary, C.J., Minor, K.T., Thyfault, J.P., Shook, R.P., and Herda, A.A. (2024). Motor unit firing rates increase in prepubescent youth following linear periodization resistance exercise training. *Eur. J. Appl. Physiol.*, 124, 2675–2686. https://doi.org/10.1007/s00421-024-05455-w

Purpose: The purpose was to examine the effects of 8-weeks (3 days/week) of linear periodization resistance exercise training (RET) on neuromuscular function in prepubescent youth.

Methods: Twenty-five healthy prepubescent youth (11 males, 14 females, age=9.1±0.8 yrs) completed the RET (n=17) or served as controls (CON, n=8). Isometric maximal voluntary contractions (MVCs) and trapezoidal submaximal contractions at 35% and 60% MVC of the right leg extensors were performed with surface electromyography (EMG) recorded from the leg extensors (vastus lateralis [VL], rectus femoris, and vastus medialis) and flexors (biceps femoris and semitendinosus). EMG amplitude of the leg extensors and flexors was calculated during the MVCs. Motor unit (MU) action potential trains were decomposed from the surface EMG of the VL for the 35% and 60% MVCs. MU firing rates and action potential amplitudes were regressed against recruitment threshold with the y-intercepts and slopes calculated for each contraction. Total leg extensor muscle cross-sectional area (CSA) was collected using ultrasound images. ANOVA models were used to examine potential differences.

Results: Isometric strength increased post-RET (P=0.006) with no changes in leg extensor and flexor EMG amplitude. Furthermore, there were no changes in total CSA or the MU action potential amplitude versus recruitment threshold relationships. However, there were increases in the firing rates of the higher-threshold MUs post-RET as indicated with greater y-intercepts (P=0.003) from the 60% MVC and less negative slope (P=0.004) of the firing rates versus recruitment threshold relationships at 35% MVC.

Conclusions: MU adaptations contribute to strength increases following RET in prepubescent youth.

Keywords: children; cross-sectional area; hypertrophy; neural adaptations

Introduction

The **introduction** section of a research article has three primary functions: (1) to introduce the reader to important topics that are relevant to the manuscript; (2) to provide a purpose statement for the study; and (3) to propose one or more hypotheses regarding the studies outcome(s). Like the abstract, the introduction section is an important part of the research report because it introduces the reader to the question the investigators are trying to answer. Thus, most of the introduction section contains background information that informs the reader and provides justification for conducting the study. For example, if the purpose of a study is to examine the effect of an exercise program on muscle strength in children, the introduction section should contain information regarding the physiological mechanisms by which the exercise training could affect strength in youth and make an argument for why the current study was important to conduct (e.g., the authors may state that the training has not been previously studied in that population, or that the results from previous investigations resulted in conflicting findings).

After the background information has been presented, the introduction typically concludes with a *purpose statement* describing the specific research question that the study is designed to answer. Because most research questions usually cannot be answered conclusively with a single study, a common approach taken in exercise science laboratories is to conduct a series of related investigations that answer slightly different research questions by altering the methodology and/or studying different populations (e.g., young vs. older adults; males vs. females). The results from the series of studies are then interpreted as a whole, which allows the researchers to gain a more comprehensive understanding of the original research question and provide more credible and robust conclusions. Following the purpose statement, the author often proposes one or more hypotheses regarding the study outcomes. The hypotheses are usually based on background information presented earlier in the introduction and reflect what the author believes the study will show. Exhibit 2.3 shows an example of a purpose statement and hypothesis at the end of an Introduction section.

Exhibit 2.3 Example of purpose and hypothesis statements at the end of an Introduction section

Herda, T.J., Holmes, E.A., Cleary, C.J., Minor, K.T., Thyfault, J.P., Shook, R.P., and Herda, A.A. (2024). Motor unit firing rates increase in prepubescent youth following linear periodization resistance exercise training. *Eur. J. Appl. Physiol.*, 124, 2675–2686. https://doi.org/10.1007/s00421-024-05455-w

"**The purpose of the present study was to examine MU firing rates and action potential amplitudes relative to recruitment threshold of the VL following 8 weeks (24 sessions) of linear periodization RET in prepubescent youth in a similar manner performed in adults (Sterczala et al., 2020).** The strong positive relationship between MU action potential amplitude versus recruitment threshold relationships demonstrates that the later recruited higher-threshold MUs are larger than the earlier recruited lower-threshold MUs. Isometric maximal voluntary contractions (MVC) and trapezoidal muscle actions were performed at 35% and 60% of MVC. A weakness of previous RET research that includes MU recordings is not utilizing moderate- and higher-intensity contractions to isolate potential non-unform changes in firing rates (Herda, 2022). Furthermore, prepubescent youth had difficulties achieving 70% MVC or higher for the leg extensors in our previous research and, subsequently, 60% MVC was chosen for the present study. **We hypothesized that 8 weeks of RET would increase firing rates at 35% and 60% MVC and that this would be shown with higher y-intercepts from the MU firing rate vs. recruitment threshold relationships post-intervention. Thus, demonstrating increases in MU firing rates across recruitment thresholds contribute to greater isometric strength. Ultrasound images of the leg extensors (VL, rectus femoris [RF] and, vastus medialis [VM]) were taken to examine potential changes in CSA.** Previous research in adults indicates increases in action potential amplitudes of higher-threshold MUs as indicated by greater slopes in the MU action potential amplitude vs. recruitment threshold relationships. The greater slope from these relationships corresponds with increases in CSA of VL (Pope et al., 2016; Sterczala et al., 2020; Jenkins et al., 2020). Thus, we hypothesized the slopes from the MU action potential vs. recruitment threshold relationships and CSA will not increase in the prepubescent youth since we do not expect hypertrophy."

Methods

The **Methods** section provides detailed information regarding the characteristics of the study participants, the type of equipment used, and the tests performed, as well as the description of the experimental design including all independent and dependent variables. A **variable** is a characteristic of a person, place, or object that may assume more than one value. **Dependent variables** are the outcome measures, whereas **independent variables** are controlled by the researcher to measure their influence on the dependent variable(s). For example, if we want to determine how well skinfolds and bioelectrical impedance predict percent body fat, the independent variables are the two different techniques to assess body composition, and the dependent variable is percent body fat. The Methods section is useful to others who are interested in replicating the study or who wish to conduct a study with a similar experimental design. For example, a researcher who wants to replicate or slightly modify a study must have information regarding the equipment and procedures that were used to collect the data and how the data were analyzed. Thus, the Methods section is important for establishing the study's *external validity* (i.e., the degree to which the results of a study can be applied to a broader population or setting). The Methods section is also important when comparing the results from different studies. For example, when two studies with similar experimental designs report different results, the discrepancy could be due to differences in such factors as the type of study participants or the procedures used to collect the data. Exhibit 2.4 shows an excerpt from the Methods section of a research article.

Exhibit 2.4 Excerpt from the Methods section of a research article

Herda, T.J., Holmes, E.A., Cleary, C.J., Minor, K.T., Thyfault, J.P., Shook, R.P., and Herda, A.A. (2024). Motor unit firing rates increase in prepubescent youth following linear periodization resistance exercise training. *Eur. J. Appl. Physiol.*, 124, 2675–2686. https://doi.org/10.1007/s00421-024-05455-w

"*Study Design:* Prior to and following an 8-week intervention, longitudinal changes in maximal isometric leg extension and flexion torque along with CSA and subcutaneous fat thickness of the VL, RF, and VM were assessed. EMG amplitude of the VL, RF, VM, biceps femoris (BF), and semitendinosus (ST) muscles were recorded during the maximal isometric leg extensor and flexor MVCs. MU firing rates were recorded from the vastus lateralis during the 35% and 60% MVCs. Two visits were conducted during pre- and post-testing for a total of 4 testing visits. Standing and seated height, body mass, and ultrasound images were recorded along with participants practicing the isometric strength testing during visits 1 (pre) and 3 (post) with the experimental strength testing that included recordings of surface EMG signals occurring during visits 2 (pre) and 4 (post). The pre- and post-testing visits occurred within 1–5 days of each other.

"*Statistical Analysis*: Two-way mixed factorial ANOVAs (group [RET vs. CON] x time [pre- vs. post-intervention]) were used to measure potential changes in height, body mass, maturation offset, isometric leg extensor MVC strength, leg extensors and flexor peak EMG amplitude, total leg extensor CSA and sFAT. Three-way mixed factorial ANOVAs (group [RET vs. CON] x contraction intensity [35% vs. 60% MVC] x time [pre- vs. post-intervention]) were used to measure potential changes in the y-intercepts and slopes of the MFR- and $MUAP_{AMP}$-RT relationships. Alpha was set at $P < 0.05$ with partial eta-squared (η_p^2) and Cohen's *d* was calculated for the ANOVAs and follow-up statistical tests."

Results

Like the Methods section, the **Results** section is usually very detailed and presents the findings from the statistical analysis performed in the study. Thus, the Results section typically contains one or more figures and/or tables along with text that describes the results of the experiment. Although the Results section is typically written in technical and monotonous language, it provides essential, comprehensive information from the statistical analysis, which is crucial for examining the study's findings. For example, suppose several statistical analyses were performed but the author only chose to discuss what they believed to be the most interesting results or those most directly related to the research question. Some readers, however, may be interested in the results that are not directly related to the research question. Including all results ensures transparency, allows for a more comprehensive understanding of the data, and enables other researchers to explore alternative interpretations, replicate findings, or identify patterns that may have been overlooked. Additionally, full disclosure of all results helps prevent selective reporting, which can lead to biased conclusions and limit the study's overall contribution to the field. Another reason why the Results section must be comprehensive is because the findings from the statistical tests may be used in review articles, referred to as meta-analyses (see the Reviews section later in this chapter). Briefly, the meta-analysis is a review article in which the results from many studies are statistically combined. Therefore, if the

Results section of a particular study is not comprehensive, it may not be possible to use the data in the meta-analysis. Exhibit 2.5 shows an excerpt from the Results section of a research article.

Exhibit 2.5 Excerpt from the Results section of a research article

Herda, T.J., Holmes, E.A., Cleary, C.J., Minor, K.T., Thyfault, J.P., Shook, R.P., and Herda, A.A. (2024). Motor unit firing rates increase in prepubescent youth following linear periodization resistance exercise training. *Eur. J. Appl. Physiol.*, 124, 2675–2686. https://doi.org/10.1007/s00421-024-05455-w

"For isometric leg extension MVC strength, there was a significant two-way interaction ($P = 0.006$, $\eta_p^2 = 0.283$). There was no significant increase ($P = 0.742$, $d = 0.121$) pre- to post-CON, however, there was a significant increase ($P < 0.001$, $d = 0.285$) pre- to post-RET. There were no differences between RET and CON at pre- ($P = 0.213$, $d = 0.527$) or post-intervention ($P = 0.859$, $d = 0.077$). For leg extensor MVC EMG amplitude, there was no significant two-interaction ($P = 0.468$, $\eta_p^2 = 0.024$) or main effects for time ($P = 0.661$, $\eta_p^2 = 0.009$) and group ($P = 0.101$, $\eta_p^2 = 0.118$). There was a two-way interaction ($P = 0.048$, $\eta_p^2 = 0.166$) for peak EMG amplitude of the leg flexors during the leg extension MVCs. There were, however, no significant differences at pre- ($P = 0.399$, $d = 0.372$) and post-testing ($P = 0.504$, $d = 0.294$) between groups or changes pre- to post-RET ($P = 0.347$, $d = 0.243$) and CON ($P = 0.167$, $d = 0.545$) with the follow-up analyses."

Discussion

The **Discussion** section is one of the most important parts of a study because it connects the results to the information presented in the introduction and to findings from previous research.

It includes detailed information on how the results of the study align with the theory—that is, it provides a well-supported explanation of data that has been repeatedly confirmed through observation and experimentation and has gained general acceptance within the scientific community but has not yet been definitively proven. In most cases, the theory was developed in the Introduction section and provided a basis, or rationale, for conducting the study. The Discussion section usually contains information regarding the results from previous studies that have examined similar research questions and the findings from these investigations are then compared and contrasted with those from the current study. Hypotheses can then be proposed regarding why the experiment turned out the way that it did.

Another important part of the discussion section involves developing a basis for future studies. Because a particular research study is often a continuation of work done previously in the author's laboratory, the Discussion section may provide the basis for the next experiment planned by their research team. In fact, it is fairly common for scientists to spend their entire careers in one research area. Although extremely time-consuming, the process of conducting a sequence of slightly modified experiments helps researchers become very knowledgeable in a particular area, and the Discussion section is where they describe the results of their work. Exhibit 2.6 shows an excerpt from the Discussion section of a research article.

Exhibit 2.6 Excerpts from the Discussion section of a research article

Herda, T.J., Holmes, E.A., Cleary, C.J., Minor, K.T., Thyfault, J.P., Shook, R.P., and Herda, A.A. (2024). Motor unit firing rates increase in prepubescent youth following linear periodization resistance exercise training. *Eur. J. Appl. Physiol.*, 124, 2675–2686. https://doi.org/10.1007/s00421-024-05455-w

"The primary findings of the present study were that 8 weeks of RET increased RET in a non-uniform manner. Firing rates of the higher-threshold MUs increased, however, the lowest-threshold MUs measured during the 35% MVC did not. Total muscle CSA and slopes of the $MUAP_{AMPS}$ relative to RT did not increase with 8 weeks of RET suggesting there was no hypertrophy for higher-threshold MUs, a response that is different than previous studies in adults (Pope et al. 2016; Sterczala et al. 2020; Jenkins et al. 2020). Increases in isometric muscular strength in prepubescent youth who completed traditional linear periodization RET may be partially explained by changes in neural activation.

"It is still being determined if prepubescent youth experience similar relative increases in strength as those observed in adults (Faigenbaum et al. 2009), however, direct comparisons are lacking because RET programs and methods to analyze strength vary greatly across studies. In the present study, isometric leg extensor muscular strength increased by 16.2% and compares favorably to the increases (17.2%) reported for the same RET program and testing in young adults (Sterczala et al. 2020). Prepubescent youth may experience similar increases in isometric strength in comparison to adults when RET programs are matched."

Conclusions

The **Conclusions** section is typically presented either toward the end of the discussion or immediately thereafter. In the Conclusions section, the author briefly summarizes the most important findings from the study and whether or not the results support the hypotheses. In addition, the author may provide recommendations for future studies that help identify gaps in the current research, address limitations of the current study, and suggest new directions for further investigation. By highlighting unanswered questions or emerging trends, the author encourages continued exploration, which can lead to a deeper understanding of the topic and advancements in the field.

References

One of the most useful components of a journal article is the list of **references** used, which is presented at the end of the article. Specifically, the reference list provides all of the information necessary to locate the publications cited by the author(s) in the article. For example, for each journal article cited in the text, the author must provide the authors' names, the article's title, the name of the journal that published the article, the year of the publication, the volume and/or issue numbers, and the page numbers where the article can be found. Similar information must be provided for all books and book chapters cited. The reference list helps readers quickly locate groups of articles that address a particular topic, and it is not uncommon for a review article or book chapter to list 100 or more references. Because review articles and book chapters are comprehensive and written by experts in the field, they are an excellent starting point for beginning researchers or those interested in a particular topic to begin locating primary and secondary references. For example, delayed onset muscle soreness (DOMS) is one of the most researched topics in exercise science. Anyone interested in DOMS should acquire one of the many DOMS related review articles and begin collecting the articles, books, book chapters, and so on provided in the reference list. Although laborious, this is one of the quickest and most comprehensive methods for beginning research in a particular area.

READING SECONDARY REFERENCES

For many students, their first exposure to the literature comes from textbooks. However, as previously mentioned, textbooks represent only one of several types of secondary sources. Other valuable secondary sources in exercise science include review articles, meta-analyses, position statements from professional organizations, and systematic reviews, all of which synthesize and summarize primary research. These sources provide students with a broader understanding of key topics, highlight trends in the field, and offer evidence-based insights that can guide further study and research.

Textbooks

The purpose of textbooks in exercise science is to educate students and summarize the literature on various topics. A major advantage of textbooks is that they are usually written for teaching purposes; thus, the information may be presented at either an introductory or more advanced level. Most exercise science textbooks are very well organized with chapters that present fundamental concepts that should be mastered by beginning students. For example, an introductory exercise physiology textbook typically includes a chapter on muscle anatomy and physiology, while others address the cardiovascular response to exercise, bioenergetics, thermoregulation, and the endocrine response to exercise. Furthermore, the text's reference list is usually comprehensive, which allows interested readers to quickly access many literature sources on a particular topic.

Professional Books

Although exercise science is still a relatively new area of study, many comprehensive books have been written in the field on various specialized topics including *ACSM's Guidelines for Exercise Testing and Prescription* (Liguori, 2020) and the National Strength and Conditioning Association's book, *NCSA's Essentials of Training Special Populations* (Jacobs, 2018). The information presented in these types of books usually summarizes the results from several studies and may facilitate the development of future investigations. These types of books also often include a comprehensive reference list at the end of each chapter that serve as a useful resource for finding scientific literature.

Reviews

Review articles are similar to specialized professional books in that they are often comprehensive, usually written by experts in the field, and typically have an extensive reference list. However, review articles are even more focused than specialized books. For example, a specialized book may discuss DOMS, while a review article might address the factors that cause the cytoskeletal damage underlying DOMS.

Although review articles can be written in various forms, exercise science follows two primary types: **narrative reviews** and **meta-analytic reviews**. A narrative review summarizes the results for most, if not all, of the studies in a particular area and is usually written after a substantial number of studies have been conducted on a particular research topic. The primary purpose of a narrative review is to collectively discuss the results of several studies so that conclusions can be drawn, and future research ideas can be developed. Although narrative reviews are excellent starting points for beginning researchers, they are usually written at an advanced level and may be difficult to understand.

Unlike narrative reviews, meta-analytic reviews use statistical procedures to combine the results from several studies that address a similar research question. Briefly, the **meta-analysis** uses a standardized measure of effect size based on the quantitative results from related studies to determine the magnitude of difference between groups or the strength of a relationship between variables. The primary purpose of the meta-analysis is to use the results to draw general conclusions regarding a particular research question. Although the meta-analysis is a very useful statistical technique for quantitatively summarizing the results of several studies, a background in statistics is usually necessary to fully understand the results. Thus, meta-analyses are very helpful for researchers but may be difficult to understand for beginning exercise science students.

Using Scientific Literature in Decision Making

In addition to discussing the various types of primary and secondary references, it is important to consider how scientific literature translates into real-world decision making. In exercise science and allied health fields, professionals rely on research not just for knowledge but to guide practical applications. This approach is known as **evidence-based practice (EBP)**, which integrates the best available scientific evidence with clinical expertise, as well as individual client and/or patient needs, to help bridge the gap between research and practice. To illustrate, EBP ensures that exercise prescriptions, rehabilitation protocols, and performance strategies are grounded in reliable research rather than anecdotal experiences or outdated methods. This process involves critically evaluating primary and secondary sources, understanding study design and quality, and applying findings in a way that benefits individuals in diverse settings, ranging from clinical rehabilitation to high-performance athletics.

To help you differentiate between high- and low-quality evidence, recognize bias, and make informed decisions, the following sections outline the process for locating and allocating primary and secondary references; explain key components of measurement and research design; and provide a brief overview of common statistical analyses used in exercise science and related fields.

Locating References in Exercise Science

Perhaps the first and most common question from students and others who wish to find basic and applied scientific articles in exercise science is "Where do I look?" Government websites that host the PubMed database enable anyone with internet access to locate scientific articles published in exercise science and related fields.

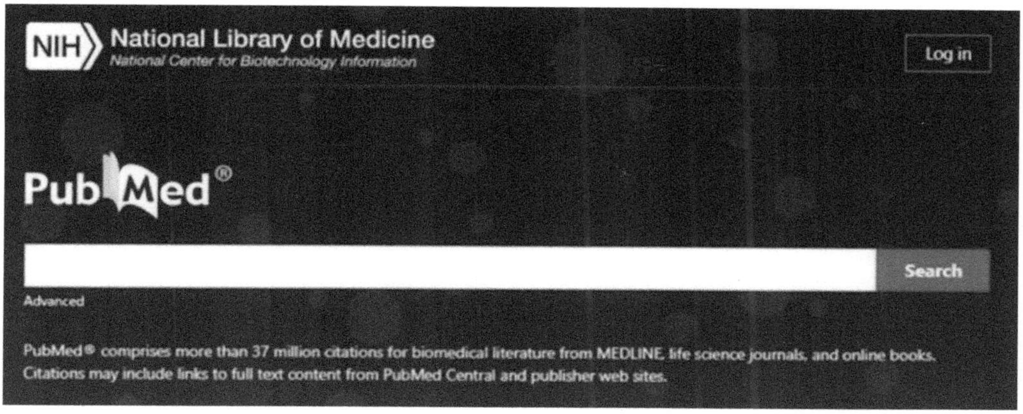

Exhibit 2.7 PubMed database for locating research literature in exercise science

The PubMed database in Exhibit 2.7 can be searched for references on specific topics; however, it may not provide the full-text article without an additional cost or paid subscription. Many times, conducting searches while on a college or university campus will allow free, full-text access to most articles, because most colleges/universities have subscriptions to these journals. Even if a full-text version is unavailable, online database searches yield the author(s) names, title, indexing information, and abstract. For example, Exhibit 2.8 shows the initial results of a PubMed search when the words "delayed onset muscle soreness (DOMS)" were used (Exhibit 2.8, a). There were 742 hits (b), or results, for this search. The initial search results provide the authors (d), title (c), and indexing information (e) for each hit (f), which allows the user to discern whether the article is of interest. In addition, much like other databases, each reference indexed by PubMed has a unique identification number called the PubMed Identification (PMID) number (e). This number is useful for quickly finding specific references in PubMed. Exhibit 2.9 shows the detailed information of the first article listed and two important benefits are that the user can read the article abstract (b) and a link to the full-text version of the article is provided (a).

Tips for Conducting Online Searches

Multiple strategies can be used to conduct online literature searches; however, the most common ways to search include using words in the title, the author's name, the year of publication, and **keywords**, which are word terms that describe the article's content but do not appear in the title. For example, the words "delayed onset muscle soreness (DOMS)" used in the search in Exhibit 2.8(a), constitute an example of a keyword search. The more specific the search terms, the smaller and more manageable the search results. For example, using the search terms "delayed onset muscle soreness" yields 742 hits (Exhibit 2.8, b), which is an impractical number to read. However, using the more specific search terms "strength training and delayed onset muscle soreness (DOMS) in female athletes" yields only 31 hits, which is a more manageable number.

Author searches are helpful for finding literature because there is usually a relatively small network of investigators who conduct research in a specific area. Therefore, if one

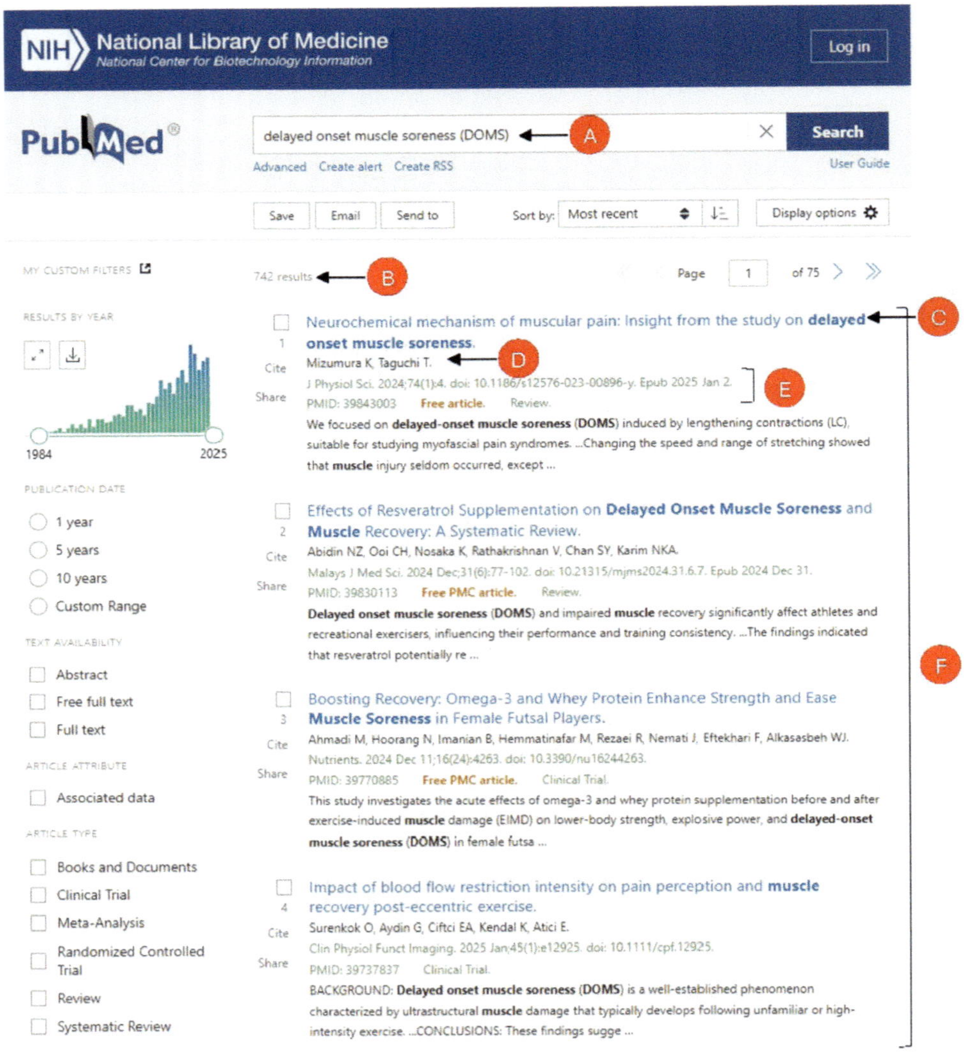

Exhibit 2.8 PubMed database search results in January 2025 for the terms "delayed onset muscle soreness (DOMS)" (a) Search terms; (b) Number of overall search results or hits; (c) Title; (d) Authors; (e) Indexing information including the journal name, year, issue, volume, page numbers, and PubMed identification number; F. First four hits for this search in order of most recent (Jan 2025)

is interested in finding articles authored by a particular individual (Exhibit 2.8, d), an author search can be conducted within a database. For example, searching for articles authored by Dr. Joan M. Eckerson (a co-editor of this textbook) in PubMed is done by using her last name and first two initials (i.e., Eckerson JM). The search may be narrowed by using the terms "Eckerson JM 2021" to retrieve the articles authored by Dr. Eckerson in the specified year. Using keywords, title phrases, authors' names, and other information to narrow an online search is necessary to obtain specific articles from a database.

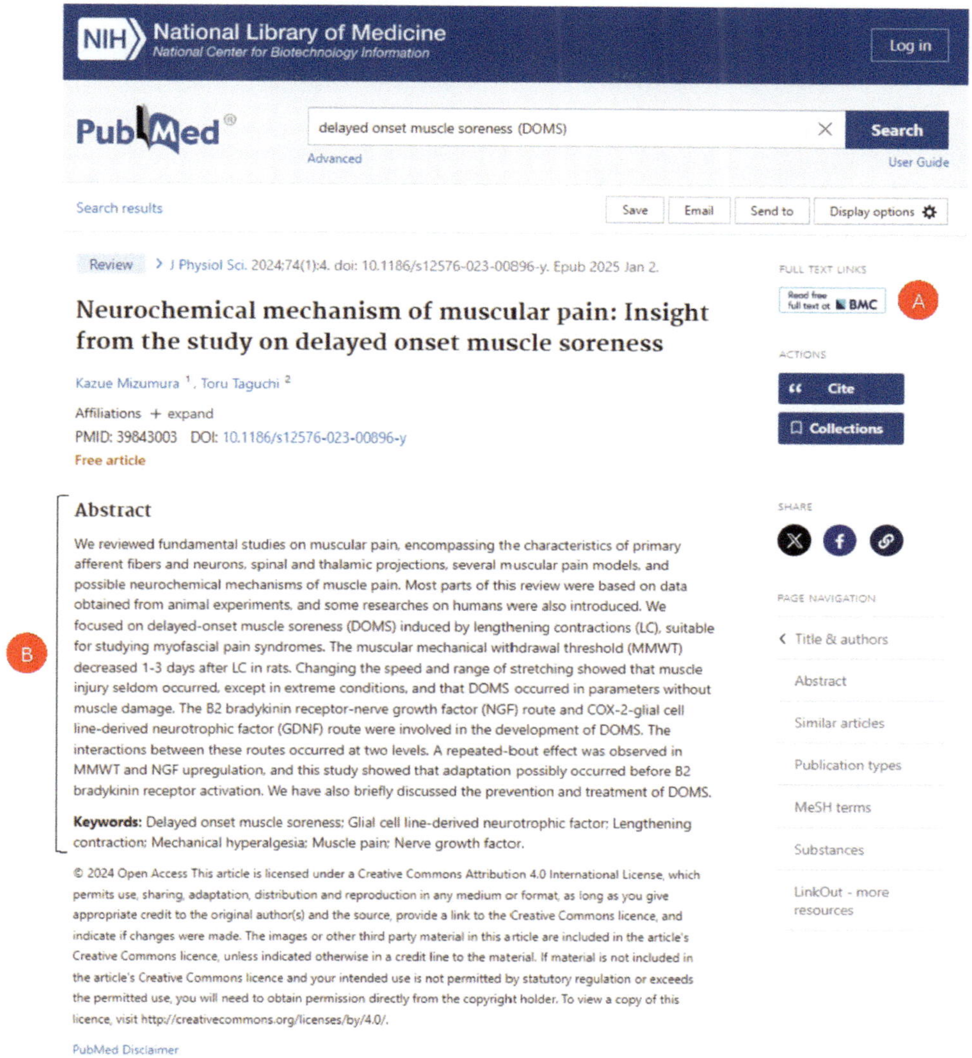
NIH National Library of Medicine
National Center for Biotechnology Information
Log in

PubMed®
delayed onset muscle soreness (DOMS)
Search
Advanced
User Guide

Search results
Save Email Send to Display options

Review > J Physiol Sci. 2024;74(1):4. doi: 10.1186/s12576-023-00896-y. Epub 2025 Jan 2.

Neurochemical mechanism of muscular pain: Insight from the study on delayed onset muscle soreness

Kazue Mizumura [1], Toru Taguchi [2]

Affiliations + expand

PMID: 39843003 DOI: 10.1186/s12576-023-00896-y

Free article

Abstract

We reviewed fundamental studies on muscular pain, encompassing the characteristics of primary afferent fibers and neurons, spinal and thalamic projections, several muscular pain models, and possible neurochemical mechanisms of muscle pain. Most parts of this review were based on data obtained from animal experiments, and some researches on humans were also introduced. We focused on delayed-onset muscle soreness (DOMS) induced by lengthening contractions (LC), suitable for studying myofascial pain syndromes. The muscular mechanical withdrawal threshold (MMWT) decreased 1-3 days after LC in rats. Changing the speed and range of stretching showed that muscle injury seldom occurred, except in extreme conditions, and that DOMS occurred in parameters without muscle damage. The B2 bradykinin receptor-nerve growth factor (NGF) route and COX-2-glial cell line-derived neurotrophic factor (GDNF) route were involved in the development of DOMS. The interactions between these routes occurred at two levels. A repeated-bout effect was observed in MMWT and NGF upregulation, and this study showed that adaptation possibly occurred before B2 bradykinin receptor activation. We have also briefly discussed the prevention and treatment of DOMS.

Keywords: Delayed onset muscle soreness; Glial cell line-derived neurotrophic factor; Lengthening contraction; Mechanical hyperalgesia; Muscle pain; Nerve growth factor.

© 2024 Open Access This article is licensed under a Creative Commons Attribution 4.0 International License, which permits use, sharing, adaptation, distribution and reproduction in any medium or format, as long as you give appropriate credit to the original author(s) and the source, provide a link to the Creative Commons licence, and indicate if changes were made. The images or other third party material in this article are included in the article's Creative Commons licence, unless indicated otherwise in a credit line to the material. If material is not included in the article's Creative Commons licence and your intended use is not permitted by statutory regulation or exceeds the permitted use, you will need to obtain permission directly from the copyright holder. To view a copy of this licence, visit http://creativecommons.org/licenses/by/4.0/.

PubMed Disclaimer

FULL TEXT LINKS
Read free full text at BMC
A
ACTIONS
Cite
Collections
SHARE
PAGE NAVIGATION
Title & authors
Abstract
Similar articles
Publication types
MeSH terms
Substances
LinkOut - more resources
B

Exhibit 2.9 The detailed search results information that is displayed on the first article listed in Exhibit 2.8; (a) Link to the full-text version of the article; (b) Article's abstract

Accessing the Full-Text Article

Although more and more journals are beginning to allow online access (Exhibit 2.9, a) to full-text article versions, there may be a cost involved. As mentioned above, students conducting online searches while on a university or college campus (or through proxy servers connected through the university) may access the full-text version of an article using the university's library subscription information. If the university or college does not subscribe to a specific journal, students are encouraged to use library resources. Advances in library technology and services provide substantial resources for students and faculty across college and university campuses. For more information about specific library services, contact your local librarian.

Using Scientific Literature to Locate Graduate Programs in Exercise Science

An often overlooked, yet extremely valuable tool for undergraduate and master's-level students is the ability to use sources of research literature to locate graduate programs and faculty mentors. One particularly effective strategy is to study the literature and determine where most of the research is being conducted. For example, if a student is interested in neuromuscular adaptations to resistance training, there are many primary references in this area authored by Dr. Trent J. Herda at the University of Kansas. Thus, studying these articles is an excellent way to begin focusing on a particular graduate program. Because the author's contact information is usually listed in the article or book, students can contact these individuals to inquire about potential graduate school openings. This is perhaps the most direct way of aligning the students' interests with the expertise of those capable of training graduate students.

INTRODUCTION TO MEASUREMENT AND STATISTICS IN EXERCISE SCIENCE

To apply research findings to EBP, it is important to have a basic understanding of measurement and statistics. Being an informed consumer of scientific literature does not require advanced expertise in math or statistics, but rather a working knowledge of key concepts. This foundational understanding helps students critically read, evaluate, and apply research effectively. As students gain experience with these topics, they often develop valuable skills in data interpretation and scientific reasoning.

Definitions of Measurement

All disciplines rely on accurate measurement of variables of interest. As intuitive as this statement may be, it is sometimes overlooked in the process of proposing new ways to accomplish goals or designing research projects. For example, if we think that exposure to a particular exercise regimen will improve a specific attribute of a group of individuals (e.g., physical fitness, attitude toward activity, or knowledge about heart rates), how do we determine whether our belief is true or not? To make such a determination we must be able to accurately assess the amount of the specific attribute individuals possess. Measurement is a critical component of scientific inquiry that involves developing, evaluating, and refining methods used to assess variables relevant to exercise science.

Measurement Versus Evaluation

In exercise science, the typical meaning of the word **measurement** refers to the act of assigning a symbol (most often a number) to each member of a group of individuals or objects based on the amount of a specific attribute each possesses. **Evaluation**, on the other hand, is a statement of quality, goodness, value, or merit about what was measured. The act of evaluation involves judgment and decision making, and the decision is usually based partially on measurements and partially on a knowledge of normative data (Weir and Vincent, 2021). For example, if you use a stopwatch to determine the amount of time it takes an individual to run the 40-yard dash, you are making a measurement. When you comment to the individual, "Wow, that was fast," you are making an evaluation. Notice that the same measurement can be evaluated differently. For example, in the case of a 10-year-old girl, you would evaluate a time of 7.5 seconds as "fast," but you would evaluate the same measurement for a 15-year-old boy as "slow."

Measurement Accuracy

Measurement accuracy is influenced by the clarity of the attribute's definition. For example, response time, defined as the time elapsed between the presentation of a stimulus and the completion of the required movement, is relatively straightforward to measure. In contrast, despite increased attention to physical fitness in recent years, exercise scientists continue to debate its specific attributes. Generally, characteristics that can be measured directly (e.g., time to run a 40-yard dash) are assessed with greater precision than those measured indirectly (e.g., percentage of body weight composed of fat).

The two most fundamental questions to be answered regarding the accuracy of the measurement process are whether it actually measures what it is intended to measure (**validity**) and whether it does so consistently (**reliability**). Validity, then, is the degree of truthfulness in a measurement, and reliability is the consistency or repeatability of a measurement (Weir and Vincent, 2021). This section also includes a discussion of the concept of objectivity, which is a subset of reliability.

Validity

As mentioned above, validity refers to the truthfulness of a measurement (i.e., does the measurement reflect the amount of the characteristic you are trying to measure). It is rather easy to see, for example, that weight in pounds is probably not a very good (valid) measure of flexibility. Sometimes, a measurement's invalidity is not so obvious. Consider a device to measure forearm flexion strength consisting of a bar held in front of the body with both hands at a 90° angle to the elbows. Assume the bar is attached to a dynamometer anchored in the floor that records the force when the individual attempts to pull up on the bar. At first inspection, this apparatus would seem to measure forearm flexion strength, but what about those individuals who are unable to keep their hands extended? Perhaps their biceps strength scores would be lower than they could achieve if the test did not also rely on hand and wrist strength.

There are several methods to evaluate the validity of a measurement depending upon the situation. The following discusses three types of validity (content, criterion, and construct) and the kinds of evidence used to support each type.

Content Validity

Content validity considers the degree to which the sample of tasks or items on a test represents the actual content to be assessed. For example, you might examine the questions on a written examination to determine how well they assess the material to be tested. As another example, some might question the content validity of selecting offensive linemen for a football team based on their time to run a 40-yard dash, a task they seldom perform in the game. Thus, content validity primarily depends on a judgment of how closely the measurement process reflects the characteristic being assessed (Weir and Vincent, 2021).

Criterion Validity

Criterion validity is determined by examining how well the measurement correlates with a criterion measure believed to be a true assessment of the characteristic of interest. For example, maximal oxygen consumption (VO_2 max) measured from a graded exercise test to exhaustion on a treadmill is considered to be an accurate index of an individual's cardiovascular fitness. However, the test requires expensive equipment, a great deal of time, trained personnel to administer, and a maximal effort by the participant. Because VO_2 max has been shown to be highly correlated to running performance, field tests, such as the Cooper 12-minute run test or a 20-meter shuttle test, provide a reasonably valid measure of cardiovascular fitness.

The situation described above is an example of *concurrent validity*, which is the degree to which a new test or measurement correlates with an established and validated test, when both measures are taken at the same time, to demonstrate how well the new test (e.g., a distance run test) agrees with an established "gold standard" (e.g., maximal graded exercise test) for assessing the same measure (VO_2 max). In contrast, *predictive validity* refers to the degree to which a test or measurement accurately predicts future behavior, performance, or outcomes (Weir and Vincent, 2021). For example, low grip strength is a strong predictor of future fall risk in older adults. As a high school student, you may have taken the SAT or ACT, which university admissions committees use to predict your future success in college.

Construct Validity

Construct validity refers to the degree to which a test measures an intangible quality or attribute (a construct). For example, the concept of IQ is a construct. It is not tangible. The typical procedure for collecting construct validity evidence is to conduct experiments using the hypothesis that a particular construct does exist. For example, is it possible that some individuals possess a higher degree of kinesthetic awareness than others? If so, and if a test of jumping forward while blindfolded to land at a certain spot on the floor actually measures the construct of kinesthetic awareness, it might be hypothesized that divers and gymnasts should perform better on the test than non-athletes. If this is confirmed, it provides evidence (not conclusive) that the test measured the construct.

Reliability

Typically, a measurement is made by using some test, device, or procedure to assign a numerical score that reflects the amount of some characteristic possessed by an individual. Unfortunately, no matter how carefully this is done, it is possible to introduce error into the process. For example, we could misread the scale, record an incorrect number, or fail to record the individual's best effort. A measurement is perfectly reliable only in the absence of error, and is a condition that is rarely, if ever, achieved. As the amount of error increases, the reliability of the measurement decreases. Therefore, to reduce measurement error and improve reliability, it is important to use high quality, calibrated instrumentation, develop standardized procedures for obtaining the measures, ensure that individuals taking the measurements are well trained, control the environmental conditions, and recheck the data. For readers interested in learning more, one of the most highly cited research articles on test-retest reliability is available from Weir (2005).

Importance of Validity and Reliability

It is important to note that a measurement does not possess validity or reliability. The validity and reliability of a measurement are situation specific and relative. For example, one tester might produce very reliable skinfold measurements, and another might not. A shuttle run test designed to validly measure *agility* of athletes may not measure this characteristic at all for inactive adults. It is important to understand the concepts of validity and reliability to evaluate the worth of any measurement process.

Objectivity

Objectivity is a subset of reliability. It assesses differences in test administrators, a very important potential source of error. Suppose an examiner administered a pull-up test to a group of athletes one day, and a different examiner administered the pull-up test to the same group of athletes a few days later. If all conditions under which the tests were administered were the same, we would expect the resulting two sets of scores to be reasonably similar (thus, reliable). However, if one examiner was very strict in administering the test (e.g., allowed no kipping action, made certain the chin was fully over the bar and that the arms were fully extended at the bottom of the exercise, did not permit any resting) and the other examiner was not as diligent, the two scores for each individual might differ considerably. If the athletes' scores varied under the two test administrators, not because they possessed differing amounts of arm strength and endurance but because the administrators applied the measurement differently, the test would be considered low in objectivity and, thus, demonstrate low reliability. Tests that have standardized procedures that are carefully applied during their administration tend to be more objective than tests that involve subjectivity in their administration or scoring procedures. It is important to administer tests carefully and according to their instructions to increase their objectivity.

Measurement Levels

Measurements may be classified based on the type and amount of information they yield. For example, it is possible to rank a group of individuals in height either by inspection or by using a measuring tape and recording the height in inches or centimeters. The type of information obtained from each procedure is different. In the inspection procedure, the results permit only statements such as "Sally is shorter than Betty," but in the measuring procedure, it is possible to determine how much shorter Sally is than Betty. Measurements can be placed into four categories—nominal, ordinal, interval, and ratio—based on the information they provide (Weir and Vincent, 2021).

Nominal Measurement

Nominal measurement conveys a minimal amount of information. It permits only the assessment of equality or difference. Nominal measurement often uses word descriptors to classify people or objects into categories. For example, a person may be classified as a letter winner, a girl, having brown hair, and so on. Occasionally, numerals are used in a nominal way. Baseball players, for example, are identified by numerals on their uniforms, but this is simply for identification. The numerals possess no measurement properties.

Ordinal Measurement

Ordinal measurement permits the ranking of the people or objects measured. Information regarding greater than or less than becomes relevant with ordinal measurement. For example, individuals' ability in handball may be ranked at the completion of a round-robin tournament. The ranking identifies one object greater or less than another but does not indicate the distance between the absolute values of the object's score.

Interval Measurement

Interval measurement allows comparisons based on equal distances between values. Temperature is an example of an interval measurement. The same distance exists on the Fahrenheit scale between 0° and 40° as exists between 40° and 80°. However, it is not appropriate to say that 80° is twice as hot as 40°, because the zero point on the Fahrenheit scale is an arbitrary point and does not really indicate an absence of heat. Likewise, a fifth-grade boy who can do four chin-ups is not twice as strong as another fifth-grade boy who can do only two chin-ups, because doing zero chin-ups does not indicate the absolute lack of any upper-arm strength.

Ratio Measurement

Ratio measurement permits statements of comparison such as twice as much or one-third as much. To achieve this level of measurement, an absolute zero point is necessary. It is possible to say, for example, that a high jump of 6 feet is twice as high as a high jump of 3 feet.

Basic Statistics

Statistics is the science of collecting, analyzing, interpreting, and presenting data. It helps us make informed decisions based on data patterns and trends. Data are collected from either a population or a sample. A **population** is the entire group you're interested in studying. For example, all athletes in a university. A **sample** is a subset of the population. For example, 40 athletes selected from the university.

Descriptive statistics are simple, common measures for summarizing and organizing data that include the:

- **mean:** the average value
- **median:** the middle value when data is ordered
- **mode:** The most frequently occurring value
- **standard deviation:** A measure of variability or how spread out the values are

As an example, Exhibit 2.10 is a normal distribution with the locations of the mean and standard deviations. This type of graph is called a **histogram** or **frequency distribution.** A practical example would be a sports science study that measures the 100 m dash times of athletes (shown in red text on Exhibit 2.10). If the mean 100 m dash time is 11.50 seconds with a standard deviation of 0.50 seconds, we can say that most athletes' 100 m dash times are between 11.00 and 12.00 seconds. This is commonly written in the research literature as 11.50 ± 0.50 seconds (mean ± standard deviation).

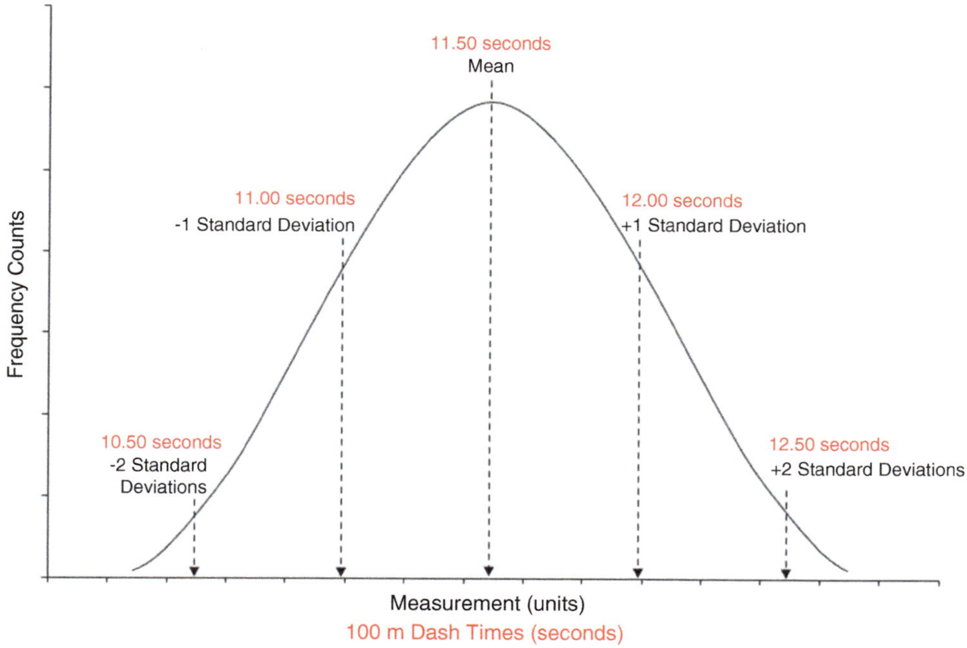

Exhibit 2.10 Histogram showing a normal distribution, mean, and standard deviations

Inferential statistics are slightly more complex methods that allow us to draw conclusions or inferences about a population based on a sample. When measuring the entire population is not realistic, inferential statistics can infer the results from a sample about the entire population. This includes **hypothesis testing, comparing means,** and **correlation/regression analyses.**

For example, suppose you want to determine if a new sprint training program improves 100 m dash times in rugby players. You could compare the average 100 m times of a sample of athletes before and after the training program using a paired t-test. See the Group 2 data in Exhibit 2.11.

Hypothesis testing is used to determine whether there is enough evidence to support a specific claim or hypothesis. For example, researchers might hypothesize that a new strength training program leads to greater muscle gains compared to a traditional program. By collecting data from a sample of participants and performing statistical hypothesis tests, such as t-tests or analysis of variance (ANOVA) (described below), the researchers can assess whether the observed differences in muscle gains are statistically significant or not. If the t-test or ANOVA show that the differences are significant, they can be confident that the differences are not due to random chance. Likewise, if the outcome is not significant, any differences that may exist are likely due to random chance. This process helps exercise scientists make data-driven decisions and advance the field with EBP.

Using data in Exhibit 2.11, sports science researchers would hypothesize that the 12-week sprint training program performed by the rugby players will improve (decrease) sprint times. Based on the outcome, does the data support their hypothesis?

Player No.	Group 1	Player No.	Group 2 (Pre-test)	Group 2 (Post-test)
1	12.89	21	11.88	11.40
2	13.54	22	12.38	11.80
3	12.34	23	11.88	11.40
4	12.30	24	11.93	11.44
5	13.10	25	11.72	11.28
6	12.80	26	11.76	11.32
7	12.39	27	12.00	11.70
8	12.57	28	12.04	11.60
9	12.70	29	11.30	10.81
10	13.41	30	12.27	11.72
11	12.85	31	11.31	10.93
12	13.03	32	12.29	11.76
13	12.05	33	11.77	11.32
14	13.04	34	11.55	11.14
15	12.55	35	12.79	12.13
16	13.19	36	11.05	10.73
17	12.70	37	12.54	12.04
18	13.79	38	12.16	11.63
19	12.99	39	11.88	11.40
20	13.10	40	11.49	11.09

Exhibit 2.11 Hypothetical, but physiologically realistic data representing 100 m dash times of n=40 individual athletes with player numbers assigned to each. For the purpose of demonstration, players 1 – 20 were basketball players measured once in the 100 m dash (Group 1) during the off-season. Players 21 – 40 were rugby players measured twice in the 100 m dash during the off-season, before (Group 2 Pre-test) and after (Group 2 Post-test) a sprint training program. Sprint times are measured in seconds

Comparing means or average values is a fundamental aspect of statistics in many fields, including exercise science. Two common methods for comparing means are **t-tests** and **ANOVA**. A t-test is used to compare the means of two groups to determine if they are significantly different from each other. There are two types of t-tests: **independent t-tests** for comparing two separate groups and **paired t-tests** for comparing two related groups. ANOVA, on the other hand, is used when comparing the means of three or more groups. It helps determine if at least one group mean is **significantly different** from the others.

Using data in Exhibit 2.11 and the histograms plotted in Exhibit 2.12a and 2.12b, sports science researchers could test their hypothesis by performing a paired t-test to compare the means of Group 2 (pre-test) and Group 2 (post-test). On average, there was an improvement in sprint times by 0.47 seconds. Is that a sufficient change to conclude that the 12-week sprint training program should be recommended to other rugby players?

T-tests are very common statistical procedures that can be completed in most spreadsheet software programs or online using various free websites. The outcome of the paired t-test shows that there was a significant improvement with a low probability of error, often written as $p \leq 0.05$. This simply means that the researchers can be 95% confident that the 12-week sprint program does, indeed, improve sprint performance in rugby players.

Again, using the data from Exhibit 2.11, sports scientists could also hypothesize that there is no difference between 100 m dash times in off-season basketball and rugby players. To test this hypothesis, sports scientists would perform an independent t-test to compare

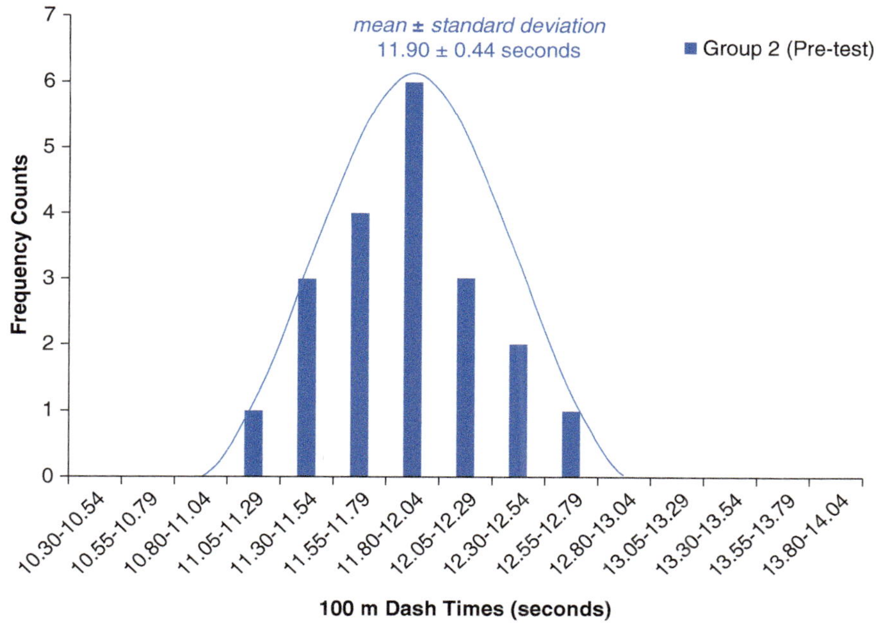

Exhibit 2.12a Pre-test data from one group in Exhibit 2.11, plotted as a histogram

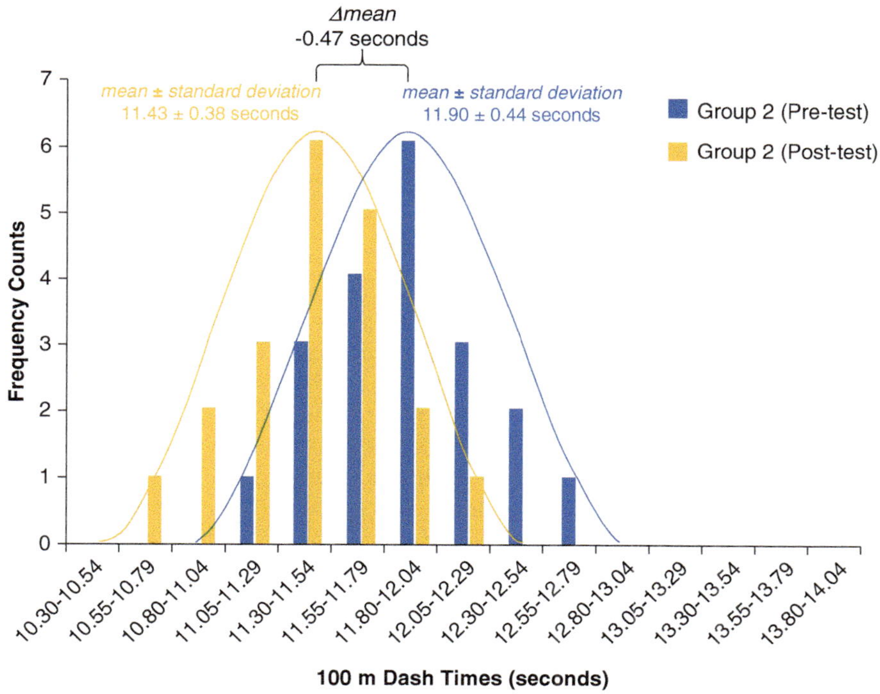

Exhibit 2.12b Pre-test and post-test data from one group in Exhibit 2.11, plotted as histograms

the means of Group 1 and Group 2 (pre-test). Exhibit 2.12c shows similar histograms of those group data. Are there sufficient differences between the 100 m dash times of the basketball players (Group 1) and rugby players (Group 2, pre-test) during their off seasons?

The outcome of the independent t-test shows that there was a significant difference with a low probability of error, $p \leq 0.05$. This means that the researchers can be 95% confident that basketball players are not as fast in the 100 m dash as rugby players during the off season.

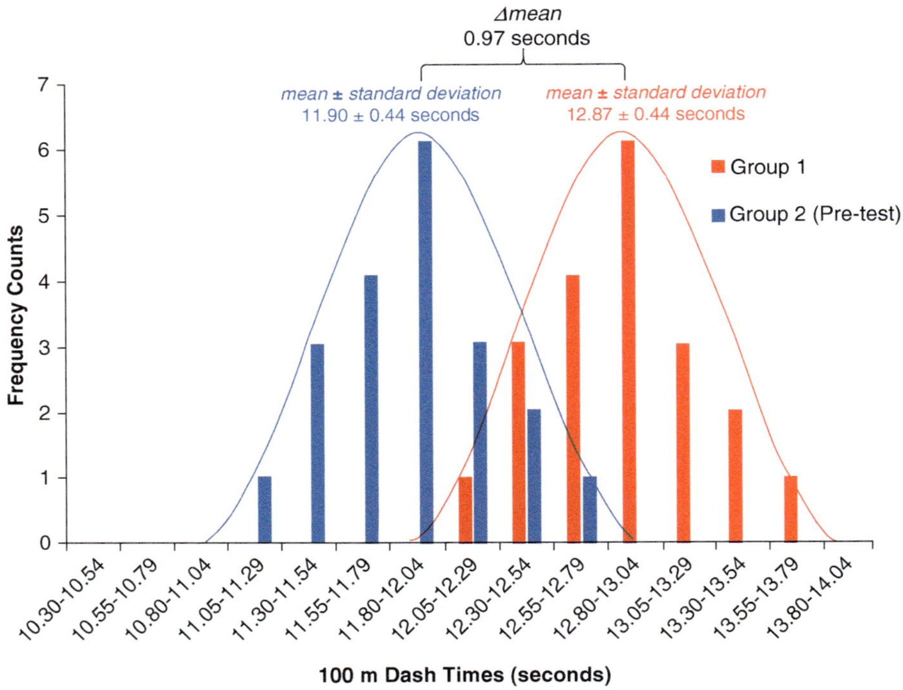

Exhibit 2.12c Pre-test data from two groups in Exhibit 2.11, plotted as histograms

Correlation and regression analyses are also commonly used in exercise science research. **Correlation** measures the strength and direction of the relationship between two variables. Correlation coefficients (represented as **r-values**) are easily calculated in most spreadsheet software programs and various free online tools. When the coefficient is a positive number, that means the two variables being correlated are directly related. That is, as one goes up, the other increases in similar fashion. Correlation coefficients greater than 0.75 are generally considered "strong." A coefficient of zero or near zero indicates no linear relationship between the two variables. Correlation r-values range between -1.00 and +1.00, each of which demonstrates a perfect, indirect relationship and a perfect, direct relationship between two variables, respectively (Weir and Vincent, 2021).

Correlation coefficients, while simple to calculate, have limitations. Specifically, correlation does not imply causation. That is, just because two variables are correlated, does not mean that one causes the other. A common example is the correlation between shoe size and IQ. It is common that as shoe size increases, a person's IQ also increases, but that does not mean that increases in foot size necessarily causes improvements in cognitive ability.

Using the data in Exhibit 2.11, correlations can be calculated between Group 1 and Group 2 (pre-test). Would a sports scientist expect a relationship between the 100 m dash times of basketball and rugby players? As demonstrated in Exhibit 2.13a, the results show a correlation coefficient of r = 0.03, which is a weak and almost negligible relationship between these groups. This would be expected, because these are two separate

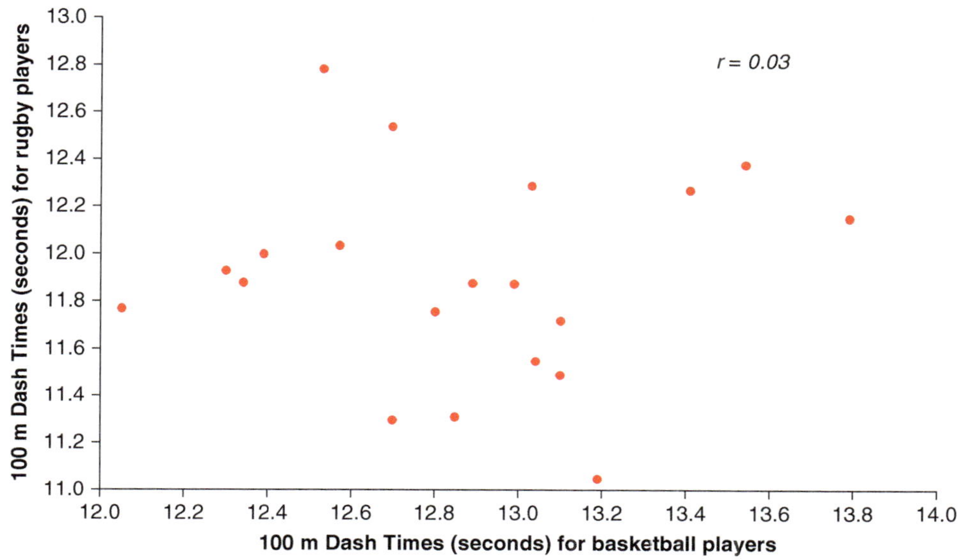

Exhibit 2.13a Scatterplot showing the lack of relationship between two groups in Exhibit 2.11

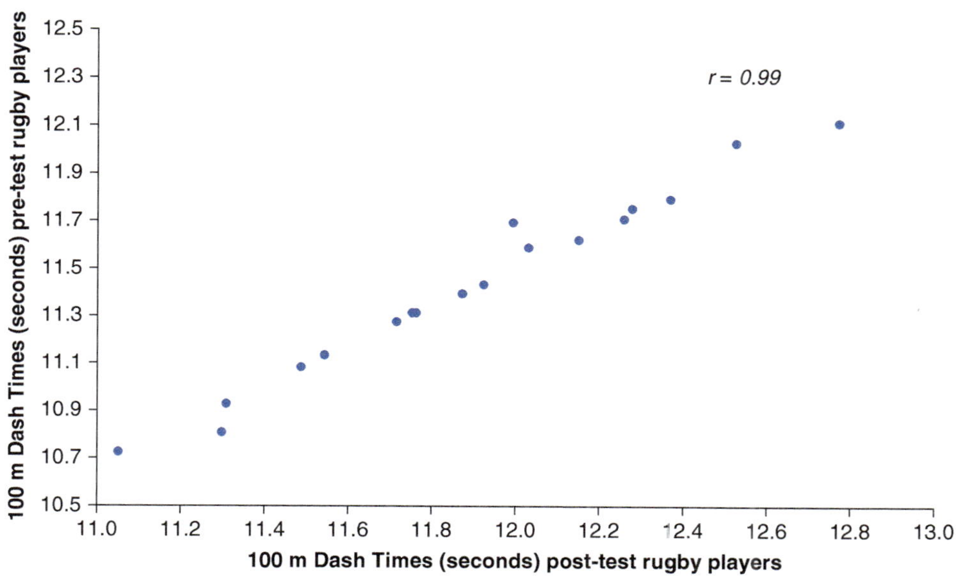

Exhibit 2.13b Scatterplot showing a strong, direct, linear relationship the same group measured twice in Exhibit 2.11

groups of athletes with nothing physiologically linking them. Not surprisingly, this also explains why the t-test comparing these groups is *independent*.

In another related question, would a sports scientist expect a relationship between the pre- and post-test scores for rugby players? As demonstrated in Exhibit 2.13b, the results show a correlation coefficient of $r = 0.99$, which is a strong, direct, linear relationship between these variables. This would be expected, because these are the same athletes being tested twice, separated only by a 12-week sprint training program. This is also why the t-test comparing the pre- and post-test measurements is *paired*.

Regression is used to predict the value of one variable based on another. Regression starts with correlation. If there is a weak relationship between two variables, one will not be able to accurately predict the other. However, if there is a strong relationship, an exercise scientist could use the regression equation ($y = mx + b$, where m is the slope and b is the y-intercept of the linear trendline) to predict the y-axis variable from the x-axis variable. Regression is difficult, because prediction requires validation and cross-validation to understand the accuracy of prediction. Nevertheless, being able to predict an outcome in exercise science is valuable.

A basic understanding of statistics is helpful for exercise science students, because it enables them to analyze data effectively and make informed decisions. Whether you're measuring the impact of a new training program or studying the relationship between diet and performance, statistical methods provide the tools needed to draw meaningful conclusions.

TECHNOLOGY AND RESEARCH TOOLS

Technology plays an important role in the design and execution of research in exercise science. Software programs such as the Statistical Package for the Social Sciences (SPSS), R (The R Project for Statistical Computing), and Microsoft Excel are commonly used to organize data, perform statistical analyses, and interpret results. Online tools for survey development and data collection, such as Qualtrics, RedCAP, or Google Forms, are also frequently used, especially in studies involving human participants. These resources support key steps in the research process, from selecting an appropriate design to analyzing findings. Tools specific to individual subdisciplines are introduced throughout this textbook, but the technologies described above are fundamental to research across the field.

CAREER AND EMPLOYMENT OPPORTUNITIES

Understanding research design and statistics can open the door to a variety of career paths in exercise science and related fields. Students who develop these skills may work as research assistants, data analysts, or clinical study coordinators in hospitals, universities, or private research labs. Others may find roles in public health, corporate wellness, or sports performance settings, where collecting and interpreting data helps improve health programs or athletic outcomes. As students gain more experience, they may also contribute to grant writing, program evaluation, or policy development. These skills are highly valued across many professions and provide a strong foundation for graduate study in fields such as physical therapy, athletic training, public health, and medicine.

EDUCATION REQUIREMENTS

Research Assistants

A research assistant typically holds a bachelor's degree in exercise science, biology, psychology, or a related field. These entry-level positions often involve helping faculty or clinical researchers with data collection, managing equipment, or coordinating participants. Some students may begin gaining experience in this role through part-time or work-study opportunities during their undergraduate studies.

Clinical Coordinator

A clinical study coordinator usually has a bachelor's degree, though additional training or certification is often preferred. These professionals manage the daily operations of clinical research studies, including participant enrollment, scheduling, and data management. Many employers prefer or require certification through organizations such as the Association of Clinical Research Professionals (ACRP) or the Society of Clinical Research Associates (SOCRA).

Data Analyst

A data analyst generally needs at least a bachelor's degree for entry-level positions, although a master's degree is often preferred for more advanced roles. Data analysts work with software such as Excel, SPSS, or R to analyze and interpret data in healthcare, sports performance, or academic research settings.

Public Health Evaluator/Policy Assistant

Similarly, a public health program evaluator or policy assistant typically holds a bachelor's degree for assistant-level roles, but a master's degree is usually required for higher-level positions. One common graduate degree for these roles is the Master of Public Health (MPH). These professionals assess the effectiveness of health programs and may contribute to policy development or community health initiatives. A strong background in research methods and statistics is essential, and undergraduate internships can provide valuable experience.

Corporate Wellness Specialist

A corporate wellness specialist, particularly one focused on program evaluation, usually holds a bachelor's degree in exercise science, health promotion, or public health. These specialists often collect and analyze data related to employee health programs and outcomes. Earning certification as a Certified Health Education Specialist (CHES) or Clinical Exercise Physiologist (CEP) can enhance employment opportunities.

Sports Performance Analyst

A performance and sports scientist or performance analyst often has a bachelor's degree in exercise science, kinesiology, or a related field. However, a master's degree is commonly preferred for advanced performance analysis roles. These positions involve collecting, analyzing, and interpreting athlete performance data to guide training programs and reduce injury risk. A strong understanding of research design and data interpretation is crucial for success in this field.

PROFESSIONAL ORGANIZATIONS

Several professional organizations support research-related careers in exercise science and its related disciplines. These organizations play an important role in advancing the field by promoting high-quality research, setting professional standards, and fostering collaboration among scientists, clinicians, and educators. For students and early-career professionals, membership can provide valuable opportunities to present research, apply for student grants, attend conferences, and stay up to date with the latest scientific findings through peer-reviewed journals. Involvement in these organizations also helps build a professional network and can support long-term career development in both academic and applied settings. The following organizations represent key sub-disciplines within exercise science, including biomechanics, strength and conditioning, sport and exercise psychology, and public health.

American College of Sports Medicine (ACSM)

One of the leading organizations in exercise science, ACSM supports research across a range of areas including physiology, biomechanics, and clinical exercise. It hosts annual scientific meetings, publishes multiple peer-reviewed journals (e.g., *Medicine & Science in Sports & Exercise*), and provides student research awards and networking opportunities.

National Strength and Conditioning Association (NSCA)

While NSCA is best known for strength and conditioning certifications, it also supports research through its journals (e.g., *Journal of Strength and Conditioning Research, Strength and Conditioning Journal*) and grants. It offers opportunities for students and professionals interested in performance, injury prevention, and data-driven training methods.

American Society of Biomechanics (ASB)

ASB promotes the study of biomechanics, often with a strong focus on research design and quantitative analysis. It supports student research, annual meetings, and collaborations across engineering, kinesiology, and clinical sciences.

North American Society for the Psychology of Sport and Physical Activity (NASPSPA)

This organization supports research in motor behavior, sport psychology, and exercise psychology. It's an excellent resource for those interested in behavioral research methods and statistical analysis in physical activity settings.

Society for Health and Physical Educators (SHAPE America)

SHAPE America supports professionals in health and physical education and is involved in research that informs public health, policy, and education. It is particularly relevant for those interested in school-based or community health evaluation and program design.

American Public Health Association (APHA)

For students interested in applying research skills to public health, APHA offers access to the latest health research, policy discussions, and job boards. Its Physical Activity Section often overlaps with exercise science.

JOURNALS

While the other chapters in this textbook will highlight journals specific to anatomy, physiology, sports nutrition, exercise physiology, exercise prescription, biomechanics, motor behavior, sport psychology, and injury prevention and rehabilitation, it is also important to recognize journals that focus on research design, testing and measurement, and statistical methods. The journals listed below regularly publish studies on new research methods, instrument validation, data analysis techniques, and innovations in study design.

Measurement in Physical Education and Exercise Science

This publication focuses on the development and evaluation of measurement tools, testing protocols, and statistical techniques in physical activity and health-related research.

Research Quarterly for Exercise and Sport (RQES)

Although broader in scope, RQES regularly features articles on research methodology, statistical applications, and study design relevant to physical activity, sport, and health research.

Journal of Quantitative Analysis in Sports

Dedicated to the application of quantitative methods and statistical modeling in sports science, this journal's topics often include performance analysis, predictive modeling, and experimental design.

Journal of Statistical Software

Relevant for students or professionals using software tools like R, SPSS, or Python, the *Journal of Statistical Software* features papers that explain new statistical methods and how to apply them using open-source tools.

FUTURE DIRECTIONS

As exercise science continues to grow, new tools and technologies are changing how research is designed, measured, and analyzed. Wearable devices and mobile apps (discussed in several chapters throughout this textbook) now allow researchers to collect real-time data in everyday settings, making studies more practical and accurate. The rise of big data and machine learning helps researchers find patterns, predict outcomes, and improve performance or health interventions. Artificial intelligence (AI) is also becoming more common in the research process. Tools like ChatGPT, Elicit, and AI-powered features in programs like SPSS and Excel can help researchers summarize studies, extract data, and even generate research questions. For example, Elicit is designed to assist with literature reviews by identifying relevant studies and organizing key findings. However, as with any AI-based tool, it is important to critically evaluate the outputs. AI can be helpful, but it may sometimes misinterpret information or miss important details. That is why researchers still need to review sources carefully and apply their own judgment. As these technologies continue to evolve, gaining experience with them can give students an edge and prepare them to contribute to high-quality, evidence-based research.

SUMMARY

The rapid growth of exercise science over the past 50 years has led to the development of a broad and diverse body of literature encompassing disciplines such as anatomy and physiology, sports medicine, biomechanics, exercise epidemiology, exercise physiology, sports nutrition, sport sciences, exercise and sport psychology, motor behavior, and strength and conditioning. As in many scientific fields, the literature in exercise science is categorized as either scientific or non-scientific. Scientific sources include peer-reviewed research articles, systematic reviews, books, textbooks, and book chapters, while non-scientific sources typically consist of social media, popular magazines, and websites. It is essential for students to distinguish between these sources and critically evaluate the credibility and applicability of the information they provide. Additionally, understanding sound research design and basic statistical procedures is crucial for interpreting and evaluating the scientific literature. A strong foundation in these areas enables students to assess the validity of research findings, identify potential biases, and apply evidence-based knowledge in professional practice. One valuable resource for accessing research articles in allied health and exercise science fields is PubMed (n.d.), a government database that provides free access to a vast collection of scientific studies. Developing proficiency using databases and critically analyzing research will enhance students' ability to stay informed and make evidence-based decisions in their future careers.

STUDY QUESTIONS

1. What are the key differences between primary, secondary, and non-scientific literature sources, and why is it important for exercise science professionals to be able to distinguish between them?
2. Explain the purpose of each section in a scientific research article (i.e., Abstract, Introduction, Methods, Results, Discussion, Conclusion, and References). How do these sections help readers evaluate the credibility and findings of the study?
3. Define the terms validity, reliability, and objectivity as they apply to measurement in exercise science. Provide a real-world example of how each might influence research outcomes.
4. What is the difference between descriptive and inferential statistics? How would an exercise scientist use each type when analyzing data from a training intervention study?
5. Describe the concept of evidence-based practice (EBP). How can exercise science professionals apply EBP in designing training programs or health interventions?
6. How can undergraduate students use research databases like PubMed to explore exercise science topics or identify potential graduate programs and mentors?

LEARNING ACTIVITIES

1. Divide into small groups. Each group will be given a topic to search on Google Scholar or PubMed (e.g., "effects of resistance training on older adults"). Each group should find one **primary peer-reviewed article**, one **secondary source** (e.g., a review article or textbook chapter), and one **non-scientific source** (e.g., a blog post or magazine article). Then, each group should present: the source type and how they identified it, the credibility of the source, and a brief summary of the findings.
2. Using a primary research article provided by your instructor, interpret the structure and content of the article. Each student should break down the article sections, or if working in a small group; each student will choose a section (e.g., Abstract, Introduction, Methods, Results, Discussion). For each section, summarize the information, identify key elements (e.g., hypothesis, variables, statistical methods), and explain how the section contributes to the overall study. Discuss each article as a class or larger group.

SUGGESTED READING AND RELATED WEBSITES

A History of the Scientific Revolution. (2022) Available at: https://socialsci.libretexts.org/@go/page/132401?pdf (Accessed September 9, 2025).

Amonette, W.E., English, K.L., and Kraemer, W.J. (2016). *Evidence-based practice in exercise science: the six-step approach*. Champaign, IL: Human Kinetics.

Weir, J.P. (2005). Quantifying test-retest reliability using the intraclass correlation coefficient and the SEM. *Journal of Strength and Conditioning Research*, *19*(1), 231–240. https://doi.org/10.1519/15184.1

REFERENCES

Carroll, A.E. (2015, June 15). To lose weight, eating less is far more important than exercising more. *The New York Times*. Available at: https://www.nytimes.com/2015/06/16/upshot/to-lose-weight-eating-less-is-far-more-important-than-exercising-more.html (Accessed September 9, 2025).

Debré, P. (2022). Pasteur at the Academy of Medicine: from hygiene to germ theory. *Comptes Rendus Biologies*, *345*(3), 83–92.

Donnelly, J.E., Honas, J.J., Smith, B.K., Mayo, M.S., Gibson, C.A., Sullivan, D.K., Lee, J., Herrmann, S.D., Lambourne, K., and Washburn, R.A. (2013). Aerobic exercise alone results in clinically significant weight loss for men and women: Midwest exercise trial 2. *Obesity*, *21*(3), E219–E228. https://doi.org/10.1002/oby.20145

Gower, B. (2012). *Scientific method: a historical and philosophical introduction*. Routledge. https://doi.org/10.4324/9780203046128

Henry, F.M. (1978). The academic discipline of physical education. *Quest*, *29*(1), 13–29.

Jacobs, P.L. (2018). *NSCA's essentials of training special populations* (1st ed.). Champaign, IL: Human Kinetics. Available at: https://us.humankinetics.com/products/nscas-essentials-of-training-special-populations (Accessed September 9, 2025).

Kraemer, W.J., Fleck, S.J., and Deschenes, M.R. (2011). *Exercise physiology: integrating theory and application*. Philadelphia, PA: Lippincott Williams & Wilkins.

Liguori, G. (2020). *ACSM's guidelines for exercise testing and prescription*. Philadelphia, PA: Lippincott Williams & Wilkins.

Nagai, H., Nakazawa, E., and Akabayashi, A. (2022). The creation of the Belmont Report and its effect on ethical principles: a historical study. *Monash Bioethics Review*, *40*(2), 157–170. https://doi.org/10.1007/s40592-022-00165-5

O'Neill, M. (2024, November 7). A 30-second balance test can indicate how well you're aging, study shows. *Verywellhealth*. Available: https://www.verywellhealth.com/balance-test-for-longevity-8738090 (Accessed 9 September 2025).

PubMed. (n.d.). PubMed. Available at: www.pubmed.gov (Accessed 9 September 2025).

Shuttleworth, M. (2009, August 18). *History of the scientific method*. Available at: https://explorable.com/history-of-the-scientific-method (September 9, 2025).

Weir, J.P. (2005). Quantifying test-retest reliability using the intraclass correlation coefficient and the SEM. *Journal of Strength and Conditioning Research*, *19*(1), 231–240. https://doi.org/10.1519/15184.1

Weir, J.P. and Vincent, W.J. (2021). Statistics in Kinesiology (5th ed.). Champaign, IL: Human Kinetics.

3 Anatomy and Physiology

Mitchel A. Magrini and Kelley G. Hammond

LEARNING OBJECTIVES

After studying this chapter, the student will be able to:

- identify key anatomical structures, including bones, joints, and skeletal muscles, and describe their roles in movement
- explain the mechanics of muscle contraction and relaxation, and how muscles generate movement
- describe the structure and function of the cardiovascular system, including the heart, blood vessels, and blood
- understand the cardiac cycle and the conduction system of the heart
- identify the components of the respiratory system and explain the processes of gas exchange, oxygen (O_2) delivery, and carbon dioxide (CO_2) removal
- explain the organization and function of the nervous system, including neural control of movement and sensory feedback

INTRODUCTION

Anatomy and physiology form the foundation of exercise science. Understanding the structure and function of the human body is essential for students as they prepare for advanced topics such as exercise physiology, biomechanics, motor behavior, and exercise prescription, all of which are introduced later in this textbook. **Anatomy** is the study of body structures, including bones, muscles, nerves, and organs, and their relationships to one another. **Physiology** focuses on how these systems function, with emphasis on processes that produce movement, maintain homeostasis, and support physical activity.

This chapter introduces the body systems most relevant to exercise: the muscular, skeletal, cardiovascular, respiratory, and nervous systems. These systems work together to produce and control movement, support posture, and meet the physical demands of activity. For example, during exercise, the cardiovascular and respiratory systems work together to deliver oxygen to active muscles, while the nervous system coordinates movement and processes, and integrates sensory input. Physiology explains how these processes occur by exploring topics such as oxygen transport, energy production, nerve transmission, and recovery, all of which are essential to physical performance.

By exploring how these systems interact during physical activity, students will gain a foundational understanding of how the body moves, adapts, and improves with training. This knowledge is essential for understanding human performance and designing effective and safe exercise programs.

DOI: 10.4324/9781032697185-3

HISTORICAL PERSPECTIVES

Anatomy and physiology have evolved together over centuries, shaping our understanding of the structure and function of the human body. Ancient civilizations, including the Egyptians, Greeks, and Chinese, began studying the human body for spiritual and practical purposes, laying the groundwork for later scientific inquiry. Early Egyptian practices, like mummification, led to basic anatomical knowledge of organs, while early Greek thinkers such as Hippocrates and Aristotle introduced systematic observation and began attributing disease to natural rather than supernatural causes. This marked a critical step toward a more scientific approach to understanding anatomy and physiology (Conti and Paternostro, 2019).

In the Roman Empire, Galen of Pergamon made significant contributions to both fields through animal dissections, since human dissection was forbidden. His discoveries about bones, muscles, nerves, and the circulatory system were foundational in shaping medical knowledge of the human body in Europe and the Islamic world for centuries (Conti and Paternostro, 2019). During the Islamic Golden Age, scholars such as Avicenna and Al-Razi expanded upon Galenic teachings, integrating them with experimental practices and setting the stage for future advancements (Lakhtakia, 2014).

The Renaissance brought renewed interest in human anatomy marked by Andreas Vesalius's influential work *De humani corporis fabrica* (*On the Fabric of the Human Body*) in 1543 (Denkler and Norman, 2012). Vesalius challenged longstanding anatomical beliefs by conducting human dissections, which provided more accurate illustrations of the human anatomy. In the 17th century, William Harvey's discovery of blood circulation revolutionized physiology by explaining the heart's role as a pump, fundamentally changing the understanding of how bodily functions sustain life (Friedland, 2009). Prior to Harvey, the prevailing thought was that blood was produced in the liver and used by organs, but not actively circulated.

Advances in microscopy in the 17th century by Robert Hooke and Antonie van Leeuwenhoek allowed scientists to observe cells for the first time, bridging anatomy and cellular physiology (Ford, 1991). As knowledge expanded, researchers like Luigi Galvani and Claude Bernard made groundbreaking discoveries in bioelectricity and homeostasis, highlighting the body's self-regulating systems and mechanisms of muscle contraction and nerve function (Piccolino, 1997; Davies, 2016).

The 19th and 20th centuries witnessed the rapid development of physiology as a distinct scientific discipline, with discoveries about metabolic processes, nerve impulses, and cellular functions. This era also introduced the publication of several anatomical texts, including *Gray's Anatomy* in 1858 (Chien and Gargus, 1987), which is still used today. The development of X-rays, magnetic resonance imaging (MRI), and computer tomography (CT) scans in the 20th century allowed for non-invasive visualization of internal structures, further enhancing anatomical studies. Physiological research was also transformed by technological advancements, that allowed for deeper insights into molecular biology and genetics that explain the body's adaptations and responses to stimuli (Chien and Gargus, 1987).

Today, anatomy and physiology remain essential to the health sciences, supported by advances in digital imaging, 3D modeling, and molecular research (Li et al., 2017; Rühli, van Schaik, and Henneberg, 2016). These fields form the foundation of exercise science by helping professionals understand movement, design effective training programs, and promote optimal health and performance. From early dissections to modern technology, each era has deepened our understanding of the body's structure and function, making anatomy and physiology core areas of study for anyone preparing for a career in health or exercise science.

FUNDAMENTAL CONCEPTS

Anatomical Directional Terms, Regions, and Planes

Before discussing the major systems of the body, it is important to become familiar with the body's regions and directional terms used to describe the relationship of anatomical structures, as shown in Exhibit 3.1. In anatomy, there is universal agreement that descriptions of any region or body part assume that the body is in **anatomical position,** in which the person is standing upright, facing forward, feet flat on the floor, arms at the sides, and palms facing forward (i.e., forearms supinated).

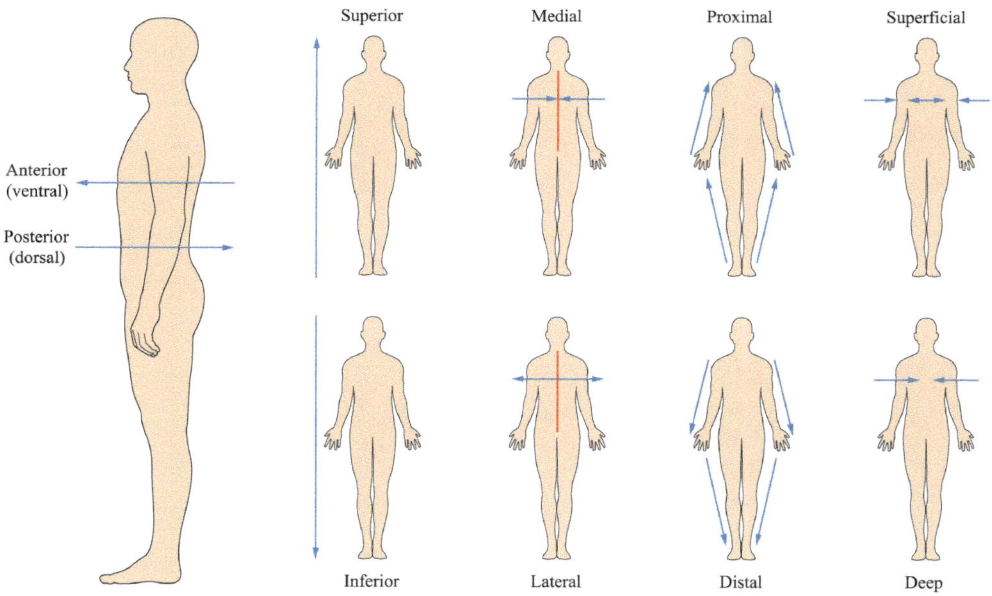

Exhibit 3.1 Anatomical directional terms

Directional term	*Definition*	*Example*
Superior	Toward the head or upper part of a structure; above	The head is superior to the chest.
Inferior (caudal)	Away from the head or toward the lower part of a structure; below	The stomach is inferior to the heart.
Anterior (ventral)	Toward or at the front of the body; in front of	The sternum is anterior to the heart.
Posterior (dorsal)	Toward or at the back of the body; behind	The spine is posterior to the lungs.
Medial	Toward or at the midline of the body; on the inner side	The nose is medial to the eyes.

(*Continued*)

Exhibit 3.1 (Continued)

Directional term	*Definition*	*Example*
Lateral	Away from the midline of the body; on the outer side	The arms are lateral to the chest.
Intermediate	Between a more medial and a more lateral structure	The collarbone is intermediate between the breastbone and the shoulder.
Proximal	Closer to the origin of the body part or the point of attachment of a limb to the body trunk	The elbow is proximal to the wrist.
Distal	Farther from the origin of a body part or the point of attachment of a limb to the body trunk	The fingers are distal to the elbow.
Superficial (external)	Toward or at the body surface	The skin is superficial to the muscles.
Deep (internal)	Away from the body surface; more internal	The lungs are deep to the rib cage.
Ipsilateral	On the same side of the body	The right hand is ipsilateral to the right foot.
Contralateral	On the opposite side of the body	The left hand is contralateral to the right hand.
Supine	Lying face upward	During a physical examination, the patient was in a supine position.
Prone	Lying face downward	For a back massage, the patient was in a prone position.

The body may also be studied in terms of anatomical planes, imaginary flat surfaces that divide it into sections. The **sagittal plane** divides the body into left and right sides; the **frontal** or **coronal plane** divides the body into anterior (ventral) and posterior (dorsal) portions; and the **transverse plane** divides the body into superior and inferior portions. Body movements occur parallel to the anatomical planes. For example, flexion and extension of the elbow when performing a biceps curl occur in the sagittal plane, while a jumping jack, which involves abduction and adduction of the upper and lower extremities, occurs in the frontal/coronal plane.

The Musculoskeletal System

Although the muscular and skeletal systems are two separate systems, because they work together to generate movement, they are commonly grouped together and referred to as the musculoskeletal system. The skeleton serves as the framework of the body and stores important minerals such as calcium and phosphorus, protects vital organs, and serves as levers for movement. Skeletal muscles attach to bones through tendons and generate the force needed to produce movement.

The Skeletal System

The skeleton is an organ composed of various tissues including bone, cartilage, blood vessels, nerves, and connective tissue (Marieb and Hoehn, 2022). **Bone** tissue is composed of three major cell types that build, maintain, and remodel bone. **Osteoprogenitor cells** are stem cells that can differentiate into many types of cells including **osteoblasts**, which build bone, **fibroblasts** that make tendons and ligaments, **adipocytes** (i.e., fat cells), and **chondroblasts,** which make cartilage.

Osteoblasts mature into **osteocytes**, which no longer build bone, but maintain the health of bone tissue. Calcium is deposited into bone by osteoblast activity. In contrast, **osteoclasts**, which are also derived from osteoprogenitor cells, are involved in bone resorption, which is the process of bone tissue breakdown leading to demineralization of bone matrix, and the release of calcium into the blood. Bone health and calcium homeostasis in the blood are primarily maintained by a balance of osteoblast and osteoclast activity. As humans age, osteoclast activity becomes greater than osteoblast activity, leading to low bone density, and can result in osteoporosis (*osteo* = bone; *porosis* = porous) (Marieb and Hoehn, 2022).

Bone tissue is classified into two main types: compact and trabecular bone. **Compact bone** is the dense superficial layer of bone that contains passageways for blood vessels, lymph vessels, and nerves. This layer provides rigid strength, support, and protection for the underlying trabecular bone. Compact bone consists of tightly packed **osteons** that are arranged in concentric circles around a **central canal,** which serves as a passageway for the blood vessels, lymph vessels, and nerves that provide the tissue with nutrients and sensory information. Compact bone provides strength and resistance to compressive and tensile forces for long bones while supporting load (i.e., body weight and, sometimes, external loads) during movement (Wingerd, 2014).

Trabecular bone is found primarily at the ends of long bones (i.e., humerus, radius, femur, tibia), where it makes up most of the **epiphyses** (i.e., ends of long bones), and is also sandwiched between thin outer layers of compact bone in flat bones, like the ribs and sternum. Trabecular bone, which is also referred to as cancellous or spongy bone, is composed of bony "spikes" called **trabeculae**, which resemble a honeycomb or lattice-like structure that is filled with red bone marrow. The lattice-like structure of spongy bone helps to distribute forces evenly across the bone during weight-bearing activities and contributes to the tremendous load capacity of long bones. One critical function of red bone marrow is the production of red blood cells, white blood cells, and platelets (i.e., hemopoiesis) that are essential for numerous functions including immune system support, oxygen transport, and blood clotting. Yellow marrow is found in the shaft, or **diaphysis**, of long bones, in a hollow passageway called the medullary cavity. It provides a local site for fat storage (McKinley, O'Loughlin, and Pennefather-O'Brien, 2020).

The human skeleton consists of 206 bones that are typically classified into five different types: flat, short, long, irregular, and sesamoid bones (Exhibit 3.2) (Marieb and Hoehn, 2022). The shape and structure of the different bone types vary to optimize movement and support of the body. **Flat bones** are thin, flattened, and sometimes curved. As mentioned above, flat bones have two thin outer layers of compact bone separated by a layer of trabecular bone, called **diploë**. **Short bones** are cube-like with a trabecular bone core surrounded by compact bone. Short bones provide support and stability during weightbearing movements (i.e., bones of the ankle, or tarsals) and help facilitate fine motor movements (i.e., bones of the wrist, or carpals). Most of the bones in the body are **long bones**, which are characterized by their elongated shape (i.e., longer than they are wide). As mentioned above, a typical long bone has a shaft, called the diaphysis, and two enlarged ends called the epiphyses. Long bones provide structure, support, and act as levers for muscles to pull on to produce movement. **Irregular bones** have peculiar shapes that do not fit into the other classifications. They are diverse in appearance and have a variable amount of compact and trabecular bone. Irregular bones uniquely provide support, protection, and stability for specific regions of the body (e.g., vertebrae, facial bones, and hyoid) (Wingerd, 2014). Finally, **sesamoid**, or "floating" **bones** are small, round bones that are embedded in tendons or muscles near joints to help reduce friction and pressure and, as the name implies, are shaped like sesame seeds. Sesamoid bones located in the hands and feet vary in number and location from person to person,

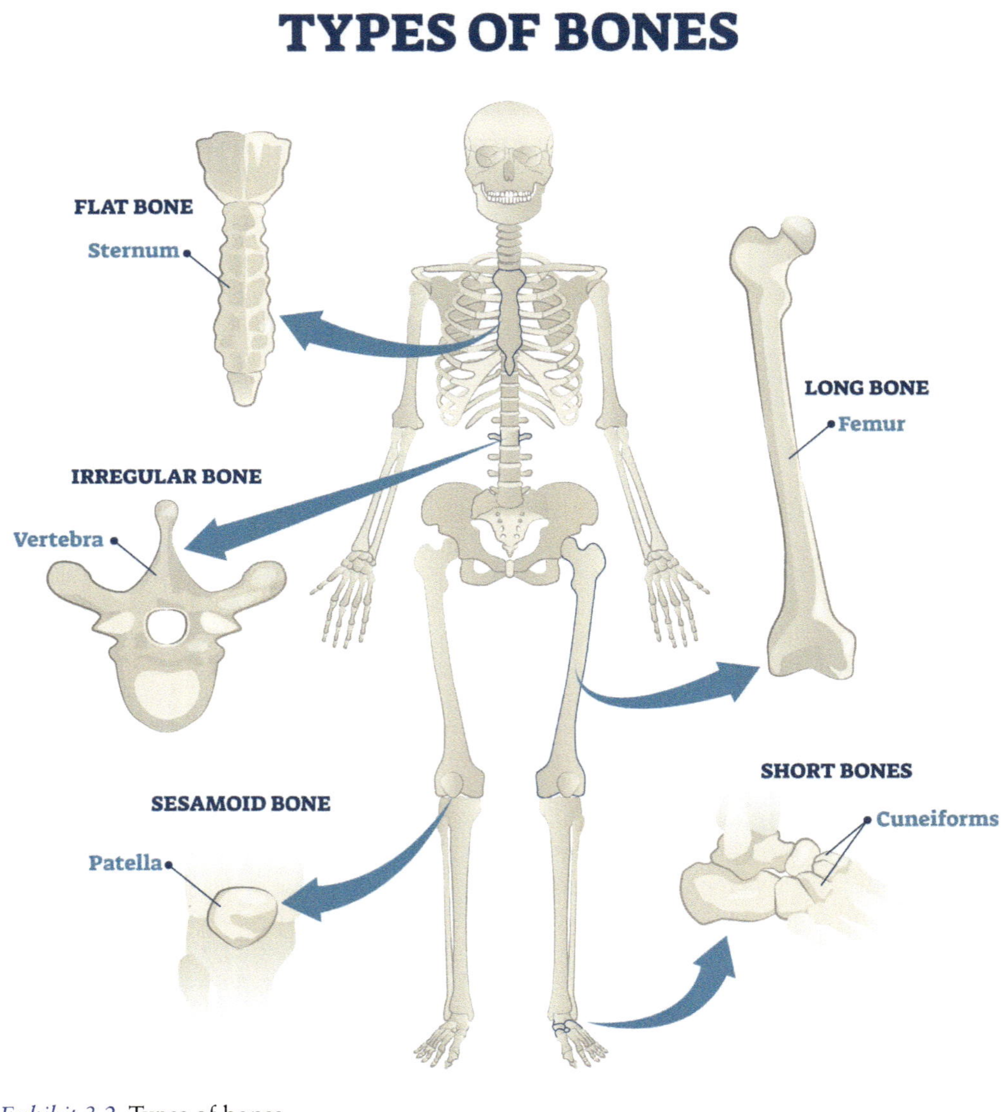

Exhibit 3.2 Types of bones

but the patella (kneecap) is present in virtually everyone (McKinley, O'Loughlin, and Pennefather-O'Brien, 2020).

The Axial and Appendicular Skeleton

The skeleton is grouped into two divisions: the axial and appendicular skeletons. The **axial skeleton** forms the vertical axis of the body, providing protection for the underlying organs, and consists of 80 bones, including the skull, vertebral column, and thoracic cage (Marieb and Hoehn, 2022). The head and neck consist of the bones of the skull and seven cervical vertebrae. The atlanto-occipital and atlanto-axial joints connect the head and neck and allow for movement of the head (see Exhibit 3.3). The thoracic cage (see Exhibit 3.4) is formed by the 12 pairs of ribs, which form joints with the 12 thoracic vertebrae posteriorly and with the sternum anteriorly, with the exception of ribs 11 and 12, which have no anterior attachment (floating ribs).

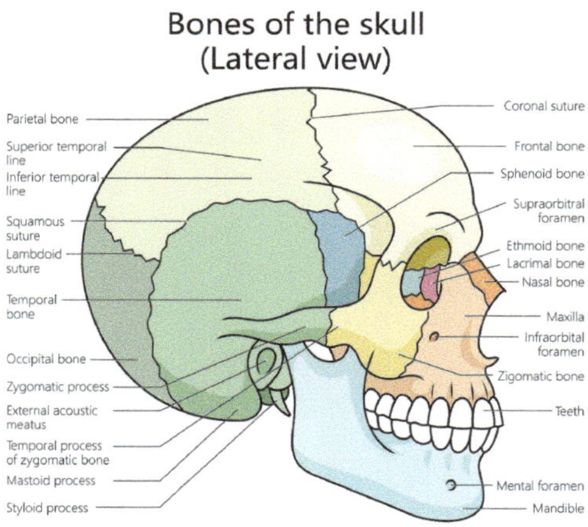

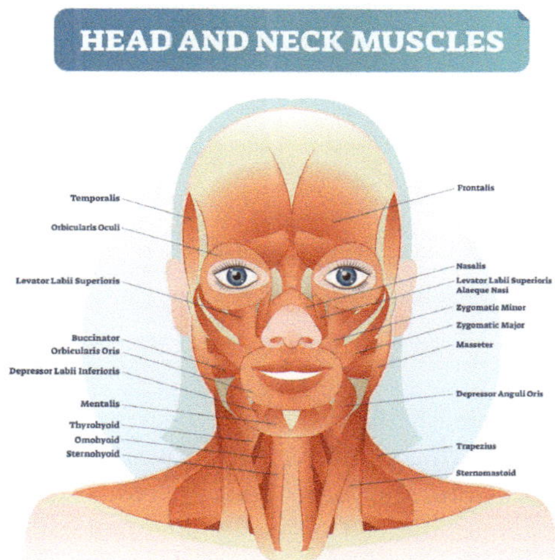

Exhibit 3.3 Head and neck

Component	*Structure/Feature*	*Description/Function*
Bones	Frontal, Parietal, Occipital, Temporal, Mandible, Maxilla, Zygomatic	Form skull and facial structure
Joints	Atlanto-occipital (condyloid), Atlantoaxial (pivot)	Allow nodding (flexion/extension) and rotation of the head
Muscles	Sternocleidomastoid, Splenius capitis	Sternocleidomastoid: neck flexion, rotation Splenius: head extension, rotation
Movements	Flexion, Extension, Rotation, Lateral flexion	Movements of the head and upper cervical spine

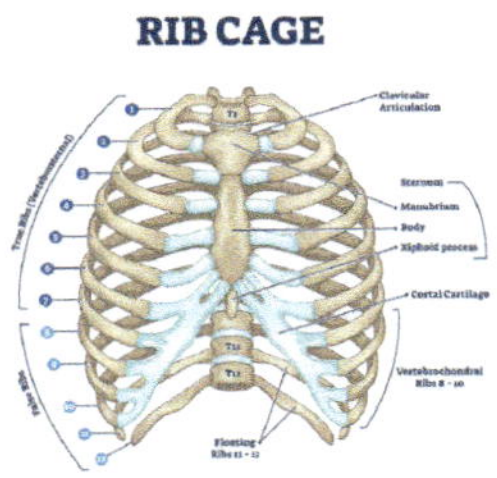

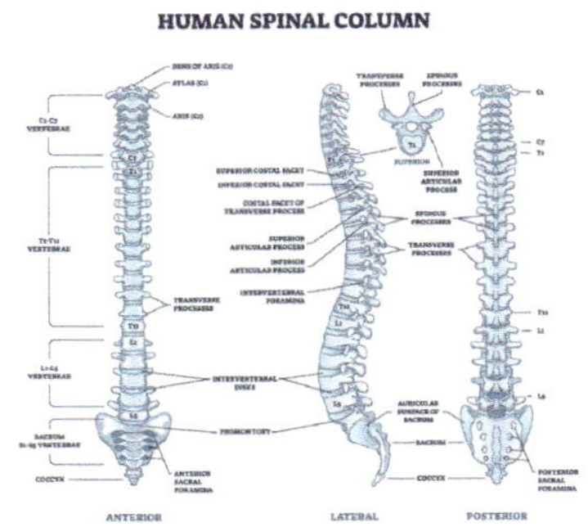

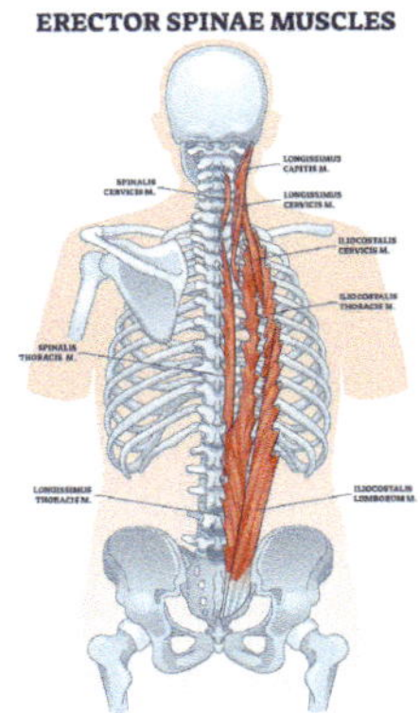

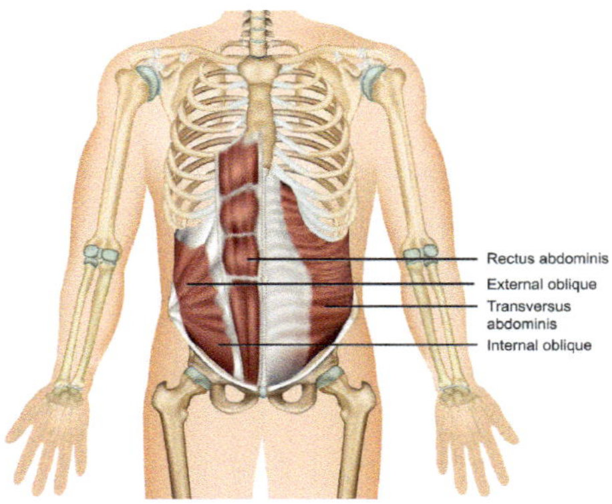

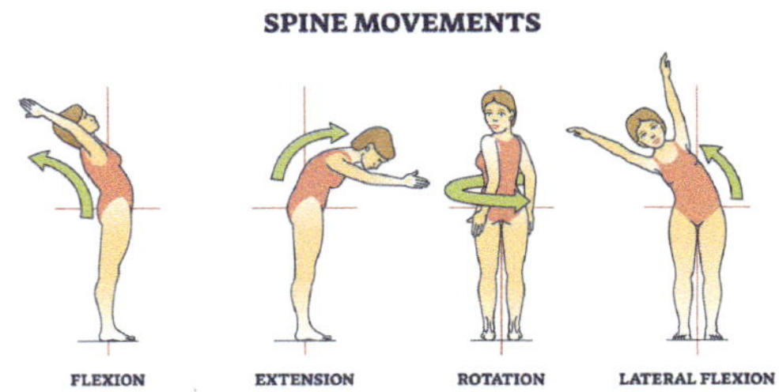

The **appendicular skeleton** consists of 126 bones and includes the upper and lower extremities and the bones that form the shoulder (pectoral) and hip (pelvic) girdles, which connect the extremities to the axial skeleton. Although the bones of the upper and lower extremities are organized similarly, they have different functions (Marieb and Hoehn, 2022).

The Pectoral Girdle and Upper Extremity

The right and left upper extremities (see Exhibit 3.5) consist of the humerus, radius, ulna, and the bones of the wrist and hand (carpals, metacarpals, and phalanges). The clavicle and scapula form the pectoral girdle that connects the upper extremity to the axial skeleton. The clavicle, or "collarbone," is located on the anterior aspect of the body and articulates medially with the manubrium of the sternum at the sternoclavicular joint and laterally at the acromion process of the scapula at the acromioclavicular joint. The clavicle allows for the pectoral girdle to be oriented laterally while allowing for movement of the arm and transmission of forces from the upper extremities to the axial skeleton. The scapula, commonly known as the "shoulder blade," is located on the posterior aspect of the body, superficial to the thoracic cage. The scapula is classified as a flat bone, and it has a triangular shape. The scapula has distinct landmarks such as the body (main flat portion), acromion process (clavicle articulation site), coracoid process (attachment site for muscles and ligaments of the shoulder), spine (a raised ridge on the posterior portion of the scapula), and the glenoid fossa. The glenoid fossa forms the socket that articulates with the head of the humerus to form the shoulder or glenohumeral joint, which is a type of ball-and-socket joint. Because the glenoid fossa is shallow and the head of the humerus is nearly twice its size, the shoulder joint allows for a wide range of motion but has limited inherent stability. To help compensate, several soft tissue structures reinforce the joint. These include the **glenoid labrum**, a ring of fibrocartilage that deepens the socket; a fibrous joint capsule; supporting ligaments; and the **rotator cuff**. Together, these structures enhance stability while preserving the joint's wide range of motion (McKinley, O'Loughlin, and Pennefather-O'Brien, 2020).

The Hip Girdle and Lower Extremity

The hip girdle, or pelvic girdle, is formed by two hip bones (also called coxal bones or os coxae) (see Exhibit 3.8). Each hip bone consists of three fused bones: the ilium, ischium, and pubis (i.e., pubic bone). The two hip bones are separated posteriorly by the sacrum and are joined anteriorly at the pubic symphysis. The primary function of the hip girdle is to connect the lower extremities to the axial skeleton. The hip joint is a ball-and-socket joint formed by the articulation of the head of the femur with the acetabulum of the pelvis. Because joints are typically named after the bones that form them, the hip joint is also referred to as the acetabulofemoral joint. The bones of the lower extremity include the femur, patella, tibia, fibula, and the bones of the ankle and foot (tarsals, metatarsals, and phalanges). The femur is the strongest and largest bone of the human body, is the only bone in the thigh, and receives the load of the trunk and upper body when standing or walking/running.

Cartilage

Cartilage is a type of connective tissue that contributes to body structure and support and is found in close proximity to the skeleton. Connective tissue cells called **chondroblasts** produce three major types of cartilage: hyaline, elastic, and fibrocartilage. **Hyaline cartilage** is the most common type and is moderately flexible and contains a high density of collagen fibers. It is found on surfaces that provide structural support, such as the ends of long bones (also called **articular cartilage**) and the costal cartilage at the anterior end of the ribs. Hyaline cartilage on the ends of long bones creates articular surfaces at the joints to reduce friction during movement. **Elastic cartilage** contains a high number of elastic fibers that provide the tissue with greater flexibility and elasticity compared to hyaline cartilage and allows a tissue to return to its original state after being deformed or stretched. Elastic cartilage is found in the external ear, tip of the nose, and epiglottis. Finally, **fibrocartilage**

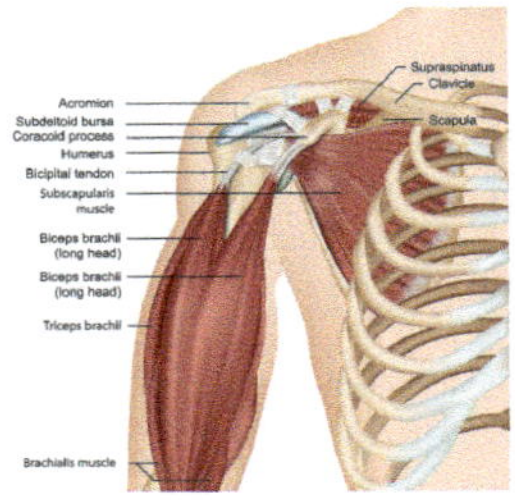

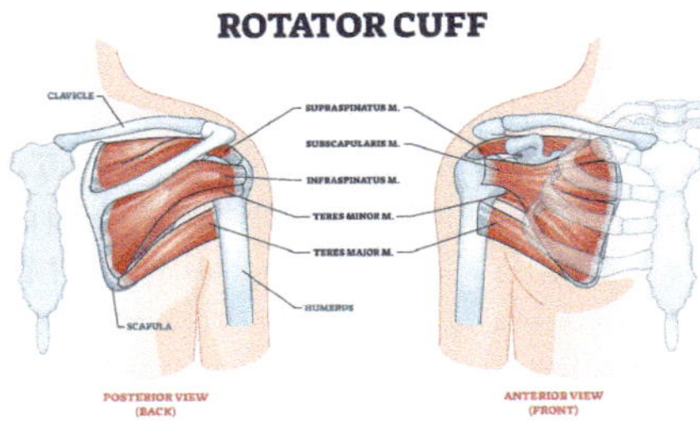

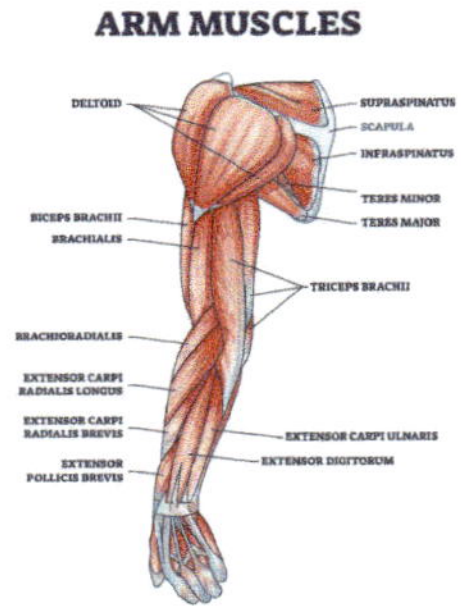

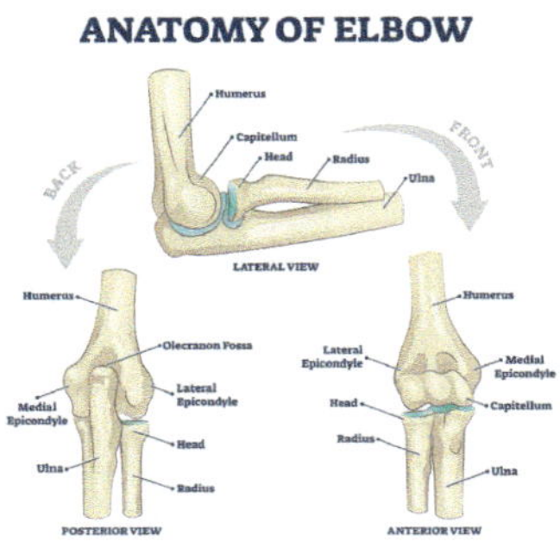

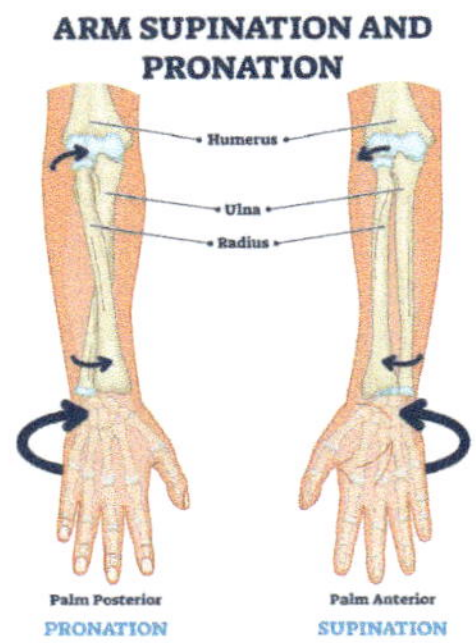

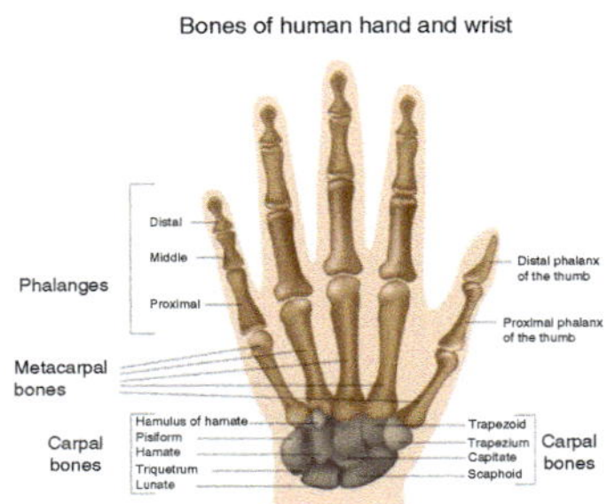

Exhibit 3.4 Regional table: trunk, spine, and ribs

Component	*Structure/Feature*	*Description/Function*
Bones	Vertebrae (C1–C7, T1–T12, L1–L5), Sacrum, Coccyx, Ribs, Sternum	Provide axial support, protect the spinal cord, and thoracic organs
Joints	Intervertebral (cartilaginous), Costovertebral, Sternocostal	Allow spinal movement and thoracic expansion
Muscles	Erector spinae, Rectus abdominis, External/Internal obliques, Transversus abdominis	Enable trunk extension, flexion, rotation, and stabilization
Movements	Flexion, Extension, Lateral flexion, Rotation	Enable bending forward/ backward, side bending, and trunk twisting

contains a high percentage of collagen fibers compared to hyaline and elastic cartilage that provide the tissue with tensile strength, support, and resilience. Fibrocartilage serves as a "shock absorber" and is found in locations throughout the body that experience repetitive high mechanical compression and tension, such as between the vertebrae in the form of

Exhibit 3.5 Regional table: upper appendage (including shoulder)

Component	*Structure/Feature*	*Description/Function*
Bones	Clavicle, Scapula, Humerus, Radius, Ulna, Carpals, Metacarpals, Phalanges	Form shoulder girdle, arm, forearm, and hand
Joints	Glenohumeral (ball-and-socket), Elbow (hinge), Radioulnar (pivot), Wrist (condyloid)	Enable full range of upper limb motion
Muscles	Serratus Anterior, Trapezius, Levator Scapulae, Serratus Anterior, Deltoid, Biceps brachii, Triceps brachii, Flexor/extensor forearm groups, Rotator cuff	Control shoulder girdle, upper limb, elbow, wrist, and hand movement
Movements	Shoulder: Flexion, Extension, Abduction, Adduction, Rotation, Circumduction; Elbow: Flexion, Extension; Forearm: Supination, Pronation; Wrist: Flexion, Extension, Abduction, Adduction	Provide functional reach, lift, grip, and fine motor control

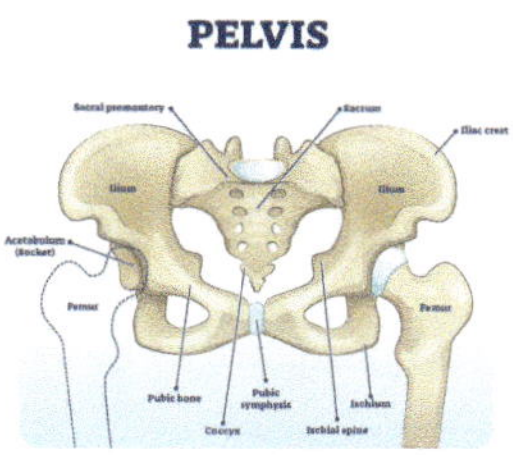

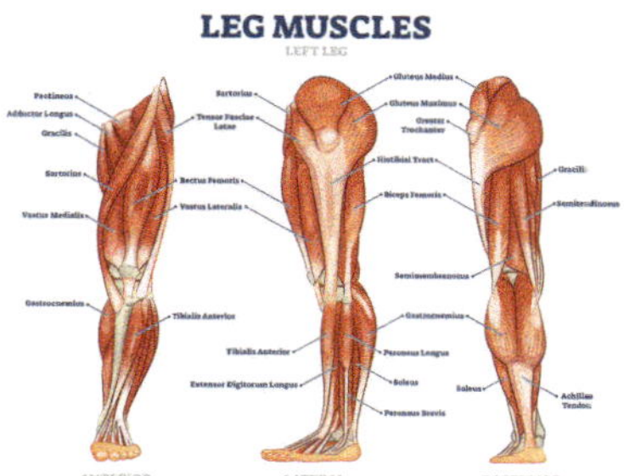

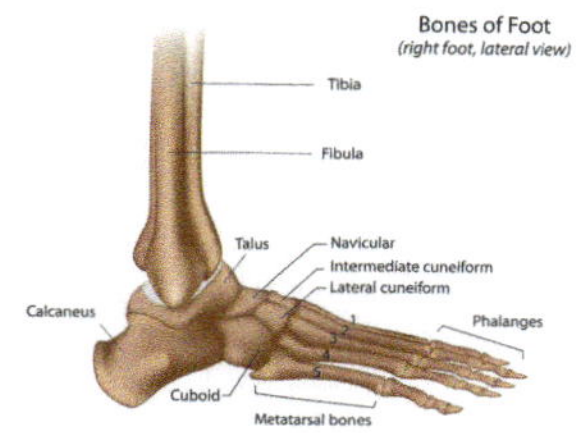

Exhibit 3.6 Regional table: lower appendage (including hip)

Component	*Structure/Feature*	*Description/Function*
Bones	Pelvis (Ilium, Ischium, Pubis), Femur, Patella, Tibia, Fibula, Tarsals, Metatarsals, Phalanges	Support body weight and locomotion
Joints	Hip (ball-and-socket), Knee (hinge), Ankle (hinge), Subtalar (gliding)	Enable lower limb stability and mobility
Muscles	Gluteals, Hamstrings, Quadriceps, Adductors, Gastrocnemius, Soleus, Tibialis anterior	Produce hip, knee, and foot movements
Movements	**Hip:** Flexion, Extension, Abduction, Adduction, Internal/External Rotation; **Knee:** Flexion, Extension; **Ankle:** Plantarflexion, Dorsiflexion, Inversion, Eversion	Enable standing, walking, balance, and propulsion

intervertebral discs, within ball-and-socket joints in the form of ring-like structures called labrums, and between the two pubis (or pubic) bones on the anterior side of the body at the pubic symphysis. The lateral and medial menisci found within the knee joint are also examples of fibrocartilage (McKinley, O'Loughlin, and Pennefather-O'Brien, 2020).

Skeletal Muscle Structure and Function

The three main types of **muscle** in the body are skeletal, cardiac, and smooth, and each type has specific characteristics and unique functions in the body. This chapter specifically focuses on skeletal muscle tissue.

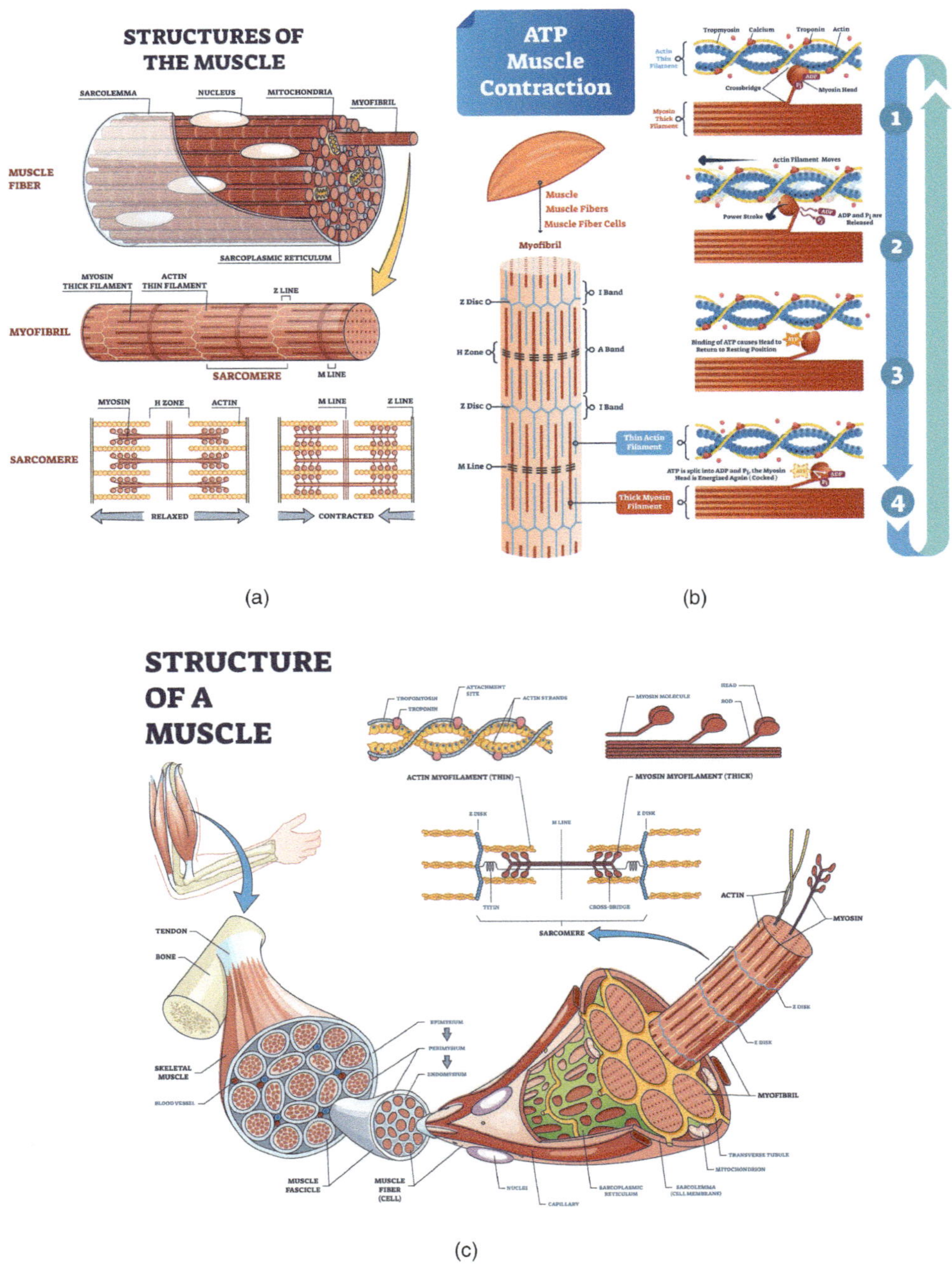

Exhibit 3.7 Anatomy of skeletal muscle

Skeletal muscles are attached to bones by tendons to produce movement and are composed of specialized cells called muscle fibers. Muscle fibers are long and cylindrical and are arranged in tightly packed bundles called fascicles. Each muscle fiber is surrounded by a plasma membrane called the sarcolemma (*sarco* = flesh; *lemma* = sheath) and has a dense connective tissue covering called the endomysium, and each fascicle has a dense connective tissue covering called the perimysium. The entire muscle, made up of tightly packed fascicles, is surrounded by a dense connective tissue covering called the epimysium. Each of the connective tissue coverings acts as a sort of shrink wrap keeping the muscle fibers and fascicles packed together in a particular orientation based upon the movement the muscle generates. (Exhibit 3.7 c).

The functional units of the muscle fiber that are responsible for contraction are called **sarcomeres**, which are made up of contractile proteins (mainly **actin** and **myosin filaments**) that either overlap or are separated from each other giving the muscle a striated or "striped" appearance. A typical muscle fiber contains several thousand sarcomeres that are separated by z-discs (or z-lines), which serve as anchor points for actin (thin filaments) and form the boundaries of each sarcomere. When a muscle contracts, these z-discs move closer together, shortening the sarcomere and generating force to create movement (Franzini-Armstrong, 2018). The I band is located between two adjacent sarcomeres and consists of actin filaments and no thick filaments (myosin). When the muscle contracts, the I band gets shorter because the actin filaments are pulled closer together. The A band is the darker, central part of the sarcomere characterized by the length of the myosin. Actin and myosin overlap in the A band, which is essential for muscle contraction, and the length remains the same whether the muscle is contracting or relaxed. The H band is located in the middle of the A band and is characterized by myosin only, with no overlap of the actin filaments. The H band becomes smaller as the muscle contracts and the actin filaments "slide" toward the center of the sarcomere (Exhibit 3.7 a) (Marieb and Hoehn, 2022).

The **sliding filament theory** describes the complex physiological processes underlying muscle contraction (Exhibit 3.7b). To summarize briefly, during contraction, the thin actin filaments slide over the thicker myosin filaments bringing the Z lines closer together. This action shortens the sarcomere which, in turn, shortens the entire muscle fiber, producing the force needed for movement. Skeletal muscle contraction is under voluntary control, initiated by signals from the brain. The strength and duration of contractions can vary, ranging from brief twitches to sustained tetanic contractions, depending on the frequency of electrical impulses or "action potentials" transmitted to the muscle fibers (Franzini-Armstrong, 2018).

Muscle Attachments, Shapes, and Fiber Arrangements

Skeletal muscles are often named based on characteristics such as their shape, fiber arrangement, origin, insertion, and action. The tendon of **origin** of a muscle attaches to the more stationary/non-movable bone and is closer to the torso, or **proximal**, whereas the tendon of **insertion** is attached to the more moveable bone, and is typically further away, or **distal**, to the center of the body. When skeletal muscles contract, they shorten, which creates a pull on the moveable bone and brings the insertion closer to the origin, resulting in movements such as extension, flexion, abduction, adduction, and rotation depending upon the type of joint they cross.

Skeletal muscles can also be described by shape and orientation such as parallel, fusiform, pennate, convergent, circular, flat, and quadrate (Exhibit 3.8). **Parallel muscles** are oriented such that muscle fibers run parallel to the long axis of the muscle. Two examples are the rectus abdominus and sartorius. A **fusiform muscle**, such as the biceps brachii or gastrocnemius, is a type of parallel muscle that has a wider muscle belly and tapers on the ends toward the tendons of origin and insertion. Most of the muscles are classified as **pennate muscles**, which have three different types of fiber arrangement: unipennate, bipennate, and multipennate. The fibers in a pennate muscle extend from a central tendon and are arranged diagonally toward the direction of pull, which allows for an increased number of muscle fibers and, thus, a greater cross-sectional area compared to parallel or fusiform fiber arrangement types. **Unipennate** muscles have fibers extending at an angle from one side of the central tendon, and examples include the tibialis anterior and extensor digitorum muscles. **Bipennate** muscles have muscle fibers extending from both sides of the central tendon resembling a feather (e.g., rectus femoris). Finally, the fiber arrangement in **multipennate** muscles resemble feathers placed side by side, and the central tendon may branch into two or more tendons. This type of arrangement allows for a high density of muscle fibers, which increases the force the muscle can generate. The deltoid,

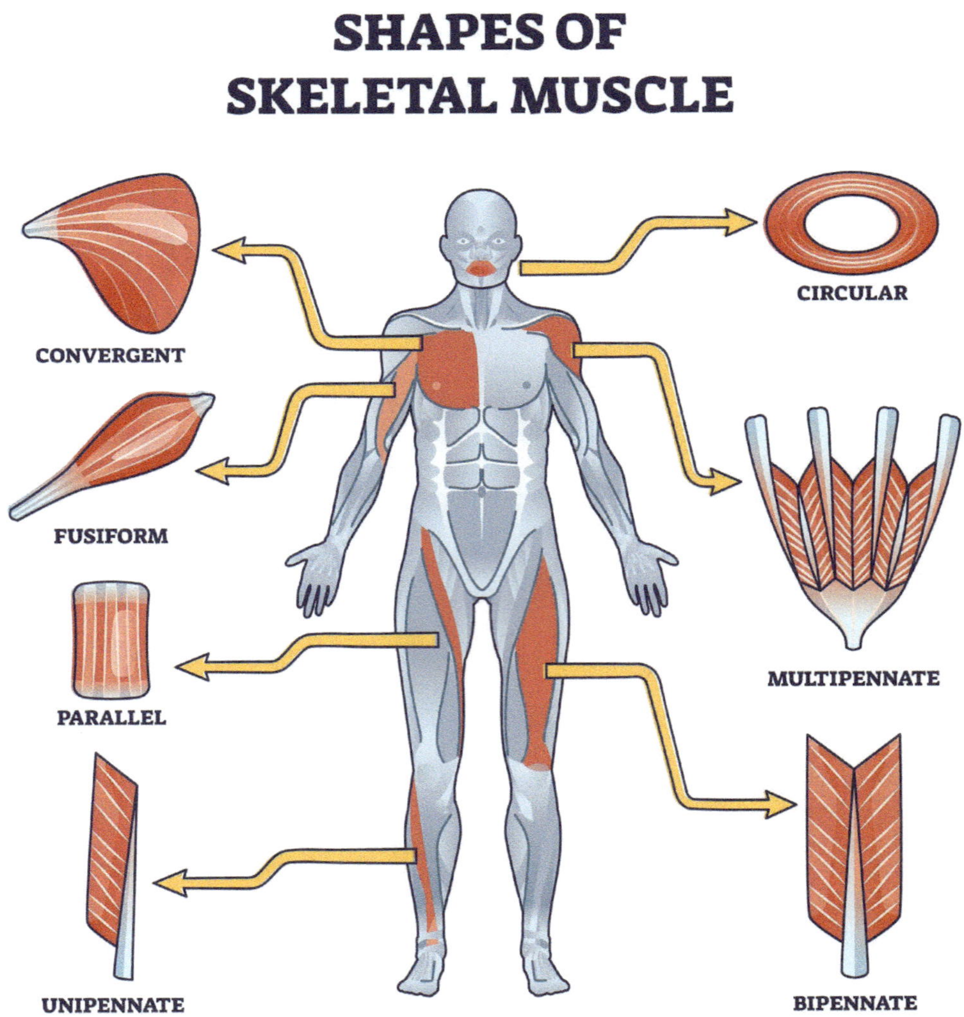

Exhibit 3.8 Skeletal muscle shapes and fiber arrangements

which has an anterior, lateral, and posterior head that come together to form one insertion on the humerus is an example of a multipennate muscle.

Convergent muscles have a broad origin extending over a wide area and the fibers come together at a small insertion site on a bone, which allows for greater force production in one direction. For example, the pectoralis major has a broad origin along the clavicle and sternum, and the fibers come together to insert onto a much smaller area on the humerus, making it a powerful arm flexor.

Circular muscles, also called sphincters, have a concentric muscle fiber arrangement that opens and closes passageways in the body to regulate the flow of substances (e.g., cardiac sphincter of the stomach or external anal sphincter) or can contract to close an opening. For example, the orbicularis oris and orbicularis oculi are circular muscles that close the mouth and eyelids, respectively (McKinley, O'Loughlin, and Pennefather-O'Brien, 2020).

Functional Roles of Muscles, Types of Contraction, and Fiber Types

Muscle contractions can be categorized into several types based on how the muscle changes length during activity. **Concentric contractions** occur when a muscle shortens as it contracts, generating force to produce movement. For example, when performing a biceps curl, the brachialis contracts concentrically to lift the weight upward. In contrast, **eccentric contractions** happen when a muscle lengthens under tension, often to control or decelerate movement. During the lowering phase of a biceps curl, the same brachialis muscle contracts eccentrically to resist gravity and control the descent of the weight. These two types of contractions fall under the broader category of **isotonic contractions**, which involve movement and a change in muscle length, while maintaining a constant tension.

Isokinetic contractions are a unique type of muscle contraction in which the muscle shortens or lengthens at a constant speed throughout the entire range of motion. This requires specialized equipment called **isokinetic dynamometers**, which maintain the selected speed of contraction. These machines are commonly used in rehabilitation and performance testing because they provide precise control over speed, range of motion, and resistance.

Muscles also play specific roles during movement. The **agonist**, or prime mover, is the muscle(s) primarily responsible for producing a specific action. For example, during knee extension, the **quadriceps femoris** functions as the agonist. Muscles that work in opposition to the agonist are called **antagonists**. These muscles help regulate movement by controlling its speed and protect the joint by preventing the agonist from acting too forcefully or overextending the joint. In this case, the **hamstrings** act as the antagonist during knee extension.

Assisting the agonist are **synergists**, which help perform the movement by stabilizing joints or contributing additional force. In a biceps curl, the brachioradialis functions as a synergist, supporting the primary actions of the brachialis and the biceps brachii. These roles ensure smooth, coordinated, and controlled movements throughout the body.

Human skeletal muscles can be classified into two fiber types based on their inherent characteristics. Most muscles are made up of a mixture of fiber types. Slow-twitch (type I) muscle fibers contract slowly, generate small forces, and are fatigue-resistant. Importantly, they rely on oxygen to make ATP for contraction. An example of a muscle with a majority of slow-twitch fibers is the soleus of the calf. The soleus helps generate force to allow us to stand and walk for long periods of time. Fast-twitch (type II) muscle fibers have fast contraction speeds, generate large amounts of force, and fatigue rapidly. These fibers use anaerobic (i.e., without oxygen) pathways to make ATP for contraction. Muscles with a high proportion of fast-twitch fibers are typically those involved with powerful, explosive movements. The tibialis anterior on the anterior leg is primarily composed of fast-twitch fibers. Muscles like the quadriceps femoris in the thigh are considered mixed fiber type, with a distribution of about 40% slow-twitch and 60% fast-twitch fibers but can vary among individuals depending on genetics and training adaptations.

Articulations

An **articulation**, or joint, is defined as a junction between two or more bones and may be classified by structure (i.e., the type of connective tissue that binds it together) or by function (how much movement is permitted). There are six types of freely movable joints, known as

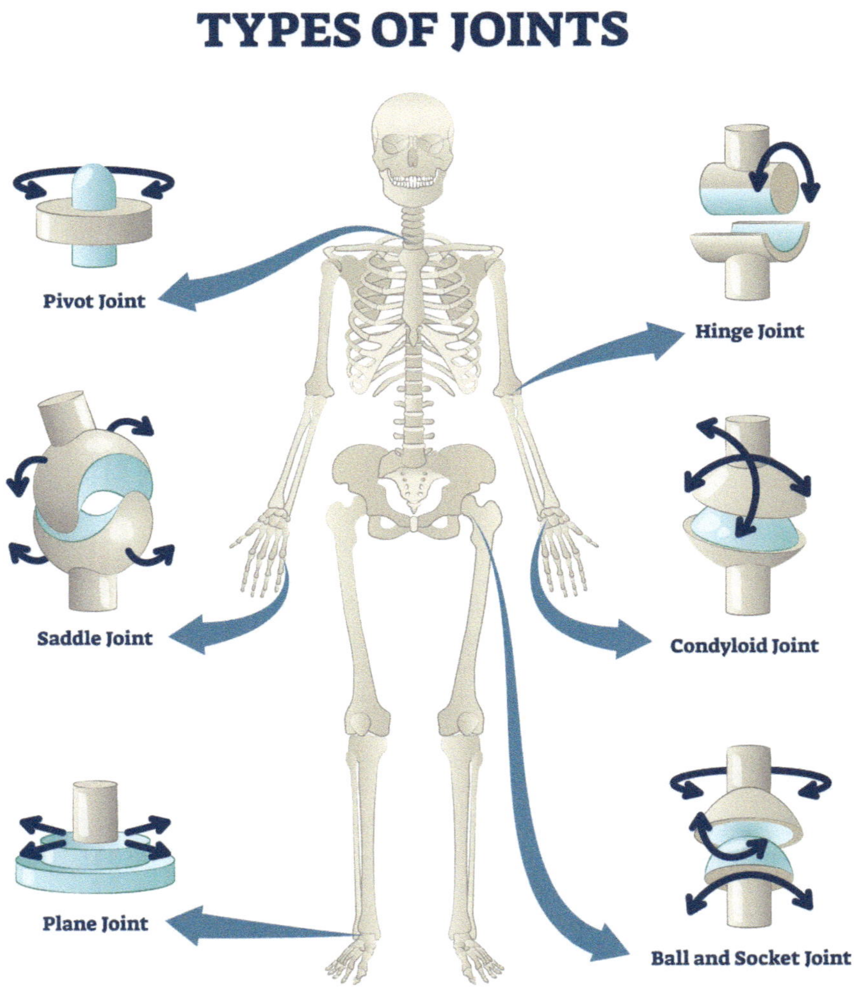

Exhibit 3.9 Muscles involved in movements at synovial joints

Joint	*Movements*	*Primary muscles involved*
Shoulder (ball-and-socket)	Flexion	Deltoid (anterior fibers), pectoralis major (clavicular head), biceps brachii
	Extension	Deltoid (posterior fibers), latissimus dorsi, teres major, triceps brachii (long head)

(*Continued*)

Exhibit 3.9 (Continued)

Joint	*Movements*	*Primary muscles involved*
	Abduction	Deltoid (middle fibers), supraspinatus
	Adduction	Pectoralis major, latissimus dorsi, teres major
	Circumduction	Combination of the above movements, involving all the muscles listed above
	Rotation	Subscapularis (internal rotation), supraspinatus, infraspinatus and teres minor (external rotation)
Elbow (hinge)	Flexion	Biceps brachii, brachialis, brachioradialis
	Extension	Triceps brachii
Knee (hinge)	Flexion	Hamstrings (biceps femoris, semitendinosus, semimembranosus)
	Extension	Quadriceps (rectus femoris, vastus lateralis, vastus medialis, vastus intermedius)
Hip (ball-and-socket)	Flexion	Iliopsoas, rectus femoris, sartorius, pectineus
	Extension	Gluteus maximus, hamstrings
	Abduction	Gluteus medius, gluteus minimus, tensor fasciae latae
	Adduction	Adductor longus, adductor brevis, adductor magnus, gracilis
	Circumduction	Combination of the above movements, involving all the muscles listed above
	Rotation	Gluteus medius and minimus (internal rotation), piriformis and deep rotators (external rotation)
Wrist (condyloid)	Flexion	Flexor carpi radialis, flexor carpi ulnaris, palmaris longus
	Extension	Extensor carpi radialis longus, extensor carpi radialis brevis, extensor carpi ulnaris
	Abduction (Radial deviation)	Flexor carpi radialis, extensor carpi radialis longus and brevis
	Adduction (Ulnar deviation)	Flexor carpi ulnaris, extensor carpi ulnaris
Thumb (saddle)	Flexion	Flexor pollicis brevis, flexor pollicis longus
	Extension	Extensor pollicis brevis, extensor pollicis longus
	Abduction	Abductor pollicis brevis, abductor pollicis longus
	Adduction	Adductor pollicis
	Opposition	Opponens pollicis
Forearm (pivot)	Pronation	Pronator teres, pronator quadratus
	Supination	Biceps brachii, supinator

synovial joints (Marieb and Hoehn, 2022). Exhibit 3.9 provides an overview of each type, the movements they allow, and the major muscles responsible for producing those movements.

Muscle and Joint Actions

As indicated above, muscles cross joints by attaching to the bones that form the joint to produce movement. Recall that when a muscle contracts, it shortens and pulls the moveable bone (insertion) and, thus, its associated body part toward the more stationary bone (origin). The following sections provide a brief overview of the bones, joints, muscles, and their movements at different body regions. It should be noted that the muscles discussed in this section are not exhaustive. Instead, the muscles included will provide the reader with the foundational understanding of major muscle groups and movements created by those muscles.

Axial Muscles that Move the Trunk, Head, and Neck

The muscles associated with the **axial skeleton** provide postural stability and enable movements of the **head, neck, and trunk** (refer to Exhibits 3.3 and 3.4). Muscles of the head and neck include the sternocleidomastoid, the scalenes, and splenius capitis and splenius cervicis. Flexion and extension of the neck and lateral flexion and rotation of the head are movements produced by these muscles. The muscles of the trunk include rectus abdominus, internal and external obliques, and transversus abdominus on the anterior of the body and the erector spinae group (iliocostalis, longissimus, and spinalis) and quadratus lumborum on the posterior. Overall, these muscles are the primary movers of the axial skeleton for flexion, extension, rotation, and stabilization of the torso and the spine. These muscles also assist in breathing related movements.

Muscles that Move the Shoulder (Pectoral) Girdle

Muscles that move the shoulder girdle (see Exhibit 3.5) have an origin on the axial skeleton and insert on the clavicle and/or scapula (i.e., the pectoral girdle) and include the serratus anterior, trapezius, levator scapulae, and rhomboids. Movements produced by these muscles include protraction, retraction, elevation, depression and upward and downward rotation of the shoulder girdle.

Muscles that Move the Shoulder (Glenohumeral) Joint

The major muscles that produce movements of the arm at the shoulder joint include the deltoid, rotator cuff group, pectoralis major, and latissimus dorsi. These muscles have an origin on the axial skeleton or pectoral girdle and insert on the humerus (Exhibit 3.5) and act to flex, extend, abduct, adduct, and rotate the arm.

Muscles that Move the Elbow Joint

The humerus, ulna, and radius bones make up the elbow joint. Although the radius is part of the elbow region, it is not a major contributor to the joint's hinging action, which allows the forearm to flex and extend. The major muscles that produce movements at the elbow joint include the biceps brachii, brachialis, brachioradialis, and triceps brachii (Exhibit 3.5).

Muscles that Move the Hand and Fingers

The muscles of the forearm are responsible for flexion and extension of the hand at the wrist joint. Muscles on the anterior aspect of the forearm generally have a common origin on the medial epicondyle of the humerus or along the ulna and cross the wrist joint on the anterior side, attaching to bones in the hand and fingers. The anterior compartment of the forearm is responsible for flexion of the hand and fingers. The major muscles on the posterior aspect of the forearm generally originate on the lateral epicondyle of the humerus or along the ulna and attach to the bones of the hand and digits resulting in extension of the hand and fingers (Exhibit 3.5).

Muscles that Move the Thigh at the Hip Joint

The major muscles supporting the hip joint are found on the anterior, posterior, medial, and lateral sides of the hip and thigh (Exhibit 3.6). The muscles located on the anterior side of the hip joint include the iliopsoas and rectus femoris, which work together to produce hip flexion, also called thigh flexion, as the movement involves bringing the thigh forward. The muscles that extend the thigh are located on the posterior side of the joint and include the gluteus maximus and the hamstrings (biceps femoris, semitendinosus, and semimembranosus). These muscles produce hip extension, or thigh extension, by moving the thigh backward. In addition to extending the thigh, the hamstrings also flex the leg at the knee joint, since they originate on the hip and insert on the tibia and fibula, crossing both joints. Muscles on the medial side of the thigh, including the adductor longus, adductor brevis, adductor magnus, and gracilis, primarily function to adduct the thigh at the hip joint. In contrast, muscles on the lateral side, such as the gluteus medius and gluteus minimus, are responsible for thigh abduction.

Muscles that Move the Leg at the Knee Joint

The knee is a hinge joint formed by the femur and the tibia. The primary muscle groups that act on the leg at the knee joint are the quadriceps femoris on the anterior thigh and hamstrings on the posterior thigh (Exhibit 3.6). The quadriceps femoris includes the rectus femoris, vastus lateralis, vastus medialis, and vastus intermedius, all of which extend the leg at the knee. The rectus femoris originates on the anterior side of the hip and inserts on a large bump on the anterior side of the tibia (tibial tuberosity) via the patellar tendon. It is the only muscle of the quadriceps group that crosses both the hip and the knee joint and is sometimes referred to as the "kicker's muscle," since it flexes the thigh and extends the leg. The vastus lateralis, vastus medialis, and vastus intermedius all have an origin on the femur and insert on the tibial tuberosity with the rectus femoris via the patellar tendon.

As mentioned above, the hamstrings are located on the posterior thigh and function to extend the thigh at the hip joint and flex the leg at the knee joint. All three muscles in the group originate from the ischial tuberosity, a prominent bump on the ischium that can be felt when sitting; it is sometimes referred to as the "sit bones" in yoga and Pilates. As the name suggests, the biceps femoris has two heads; the long head attaches to the fibula, while the short head attaches to the femur. The semitendinosus and semimembranosus both insert on the medial side of the tibia.

Muscles that Move the Foot at the Ankle Joint

The ankle is a hinge joint that connects the leg (i.e., tibia and fibula) to the foot and allows for plantar flexion (ankle extension) and dorsiflexion (ankle flexion) (Exhibit 3.6).

Talus, however, the tibia and talus are largely responsible for the hinging action at the joint. The tibia (or shin bone) is the largest bone of the leg and is on the medial side. Muscles of the anterior compartment of the leg produce dorsiflexion and extension of the digits (toes) and include the tibialis anterior, extensor hallucis (big toe) longus, and extensor digitorum longus. The two primary muscles that plantarflex the foot, the gastrocnemius and soleus, make up most of the mass of the posterior compartment of the leg.

CARDIORESPIRATORY SYSTEM

The **cardiorespiratory system** consists of the cardiovascular system, which includes the heart, blood vessels, and blood, and the pulmonary system, which includes the airway passages and the lungs. The cardiorespiratory system helps maintain **homeostasis** by delivering oxygen (O_2) and nutrients to the tissues throughout the body and removing carbon dioxide (CO_2) and waste products from the tissues. Homeostasis is the body's ability to maintain a stable environment despite changes in external conditions. This section will serve as an overview of the cardiorespiratory system, anatomy of the major organs, and how the organs work together to maintain homeostasis (McKinley, O'Loughlin, and Pennefather-O'Brien, 2020).

Structure and Function of the Heart

The heart, or **myocardium**, is located in a compartment in the middle of the thoracic cavity called the **mediastinum**. The heart functions as a dual pump system facilitating the

The pathway of blood flow through the heart

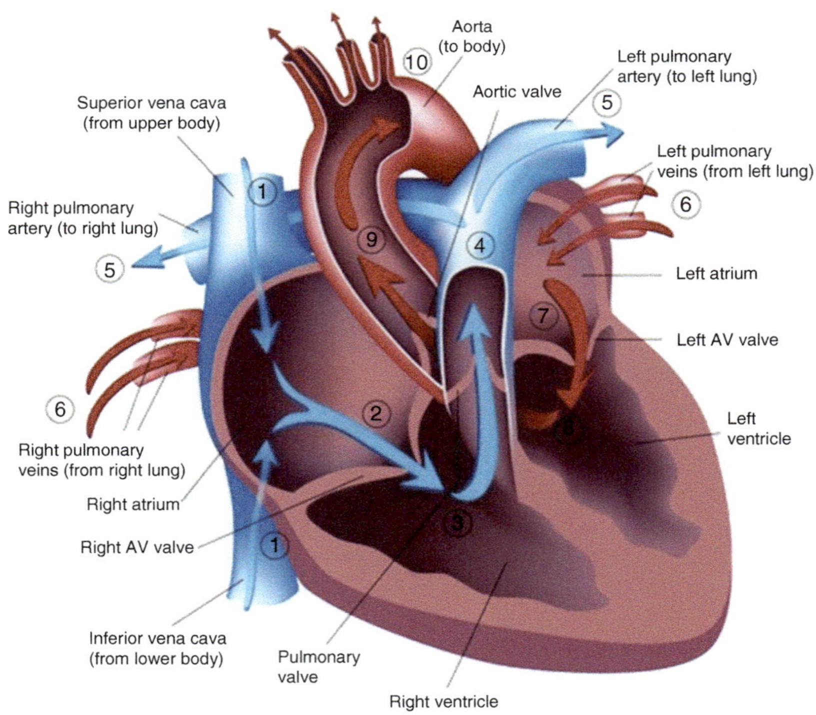

Exhibit 3.10 Anatomy of the heart

Chamber	*Description*
Right Atrium	Receives deoxygenated blood from the superior and inferior vena cava (from body tissues) and the coronary sinus (large vein that drains the heart).
Right Ventricle	Pumps deoxygenated blood into the pulmonary arteries to the lungs (for diffusion of oxygen into and CO_2 out of blood).
Left Atrium	Receives oxygenated blood via the pulmonary veins from the lungs.
Left Ventricle	Pumps oxygenated blood into the aorta and through the systemic circulation (to body tissues).
Valve	***Description***
Right Atrioventricular or Tricuspid Valve	Located between the right atrium and right ventricle, prevents backflow of blood into the right atrium.
Pulmonary Semilunar Valve	Located between the right ventricle and pulmonary artery, prevents backflow of blood into the right ventricle.
Left Atrioventricular or Bicuspid (Mitral) Valve	Located between the left atrium and left ventricle, prevents backflow of blood into the left atrium.
Aortic Semilunar Valve	Located between the left ventricle and aorta, prevents backflow of blood into the left ventricle.

circulation of blood through the pulmonary circuit (blood going to and from the lungs) and the systemic circuit (blood going to and from the body tissues). The heart has four chambers: the right atrium, right ventricle, left atrium, and left ventricle (Exhibit 3.10). Blood flow through these chambers is regulated by four specialized valves which help prevent backflow (Marieb and Hoehn, 2022).

The heart beats on its own due to an intrinsic electrical conduction system which coordinates the contraction of the myocardium (Exhibit 3.11). This intrinsic conduction system is made up of clusters of specialized heart cells, called **cardiomyocytes**, which not only set the heart rate, but also initiate an electrical impulse that is throughout the heart tissue to cause the atria to contract simultaneously, followed by simultaneous contraction of the ventricles. The first specialized cluster of cells make up the **sinoatrial (SA) node**, which is in the right atrium and is known as the pacemaker of the heart because it regulates heart rate. The electrical impulse gets passed from the SA node to the **atrioventricular node**, where there is a brief pause before the impulse travels down the interventricular septum via the **bundle of His**, and out to the walls of the ventricles through the **Purkinje fibers** (Wingerd, 2014).

The complex process of pumping blood involves a coordinated timing of events known as the cardiac cycle. The cycle includes contraction (systole) and relaxation (diastole) of the myocardium. During **systole**, the ventricles contract, increasing the pressure within the chambers, leading to the ejection of blood through the **pulmonary semilunar valve** (right ventricle) to pulmonary circulation or the **aortic semilunar valve** (left ventricle) to systemic circulation. During ventricular contraction, the right and left **atrioventricular valves** close, preventing backflow into the atria. During **diastole**, the ventricles relax, allowing the chambers to fill with blood flowing from the atria (Marieb and Hoehn, 2022).

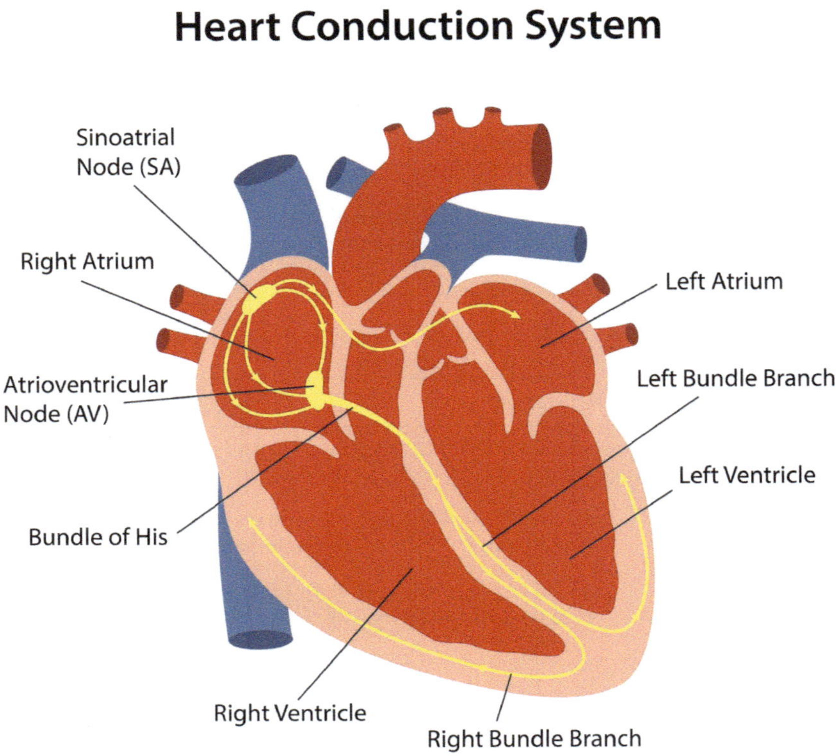

Exhibit 3.11 Conduction system of the heart

Structure and Function of the Lungs

The lungs are located on each side of the heart in the right and left thoracic cavity (Exhibit 3.12). Each lung is divided into regions called **lobes.** The right lung has three lobes (superior, middle, and inferior), while the left lung has only two (superior and inferior) to accommodate space for the heart. The lungs allow for **respiration** (the process of absorbing O_2 and releasing CO_2). During inhalation, air moves into the lungs via the following pathway: nasal/oral cavities → pharynx → larynx → trachea → right/left primary bronchi → secondary bronchi → tertiary bronchi → terminal bronchi → respiratory bronchi → alveoli (Exhibit 3.12).

The airway consists of a **conducting zone** and the **respiratory zone.** The conducting zone begins with the oral and nasal cavities and ends at the terminal bronchioles. The respiratory zone begins with the respiratory bronchioles and ends with the alveoli. Each lung is enclosed by a membrane called the **pleura,** which consists of two layers: the visceral pleura (inner layer covering the lung) and the parietal pleura (outer layer lining the thoracic cavity). Pleural fluid between the two layers helps reduce friction during breathing (Exhibit 3.12).

The primary role of the lungs is to facilitate gas exchange, which takes place in the **alveoli,** tiny air sacs located deep within the lungs. Here, O_2 from inhaled air diffuses across the thin alveolar membrane into the surrounding capillaries, while CO_2 from the blood diffuses in the opposite direction to be exhaled. Air from the surrounding environment is brought into the lungs by a process called **inhalation,** in which the diaphragm

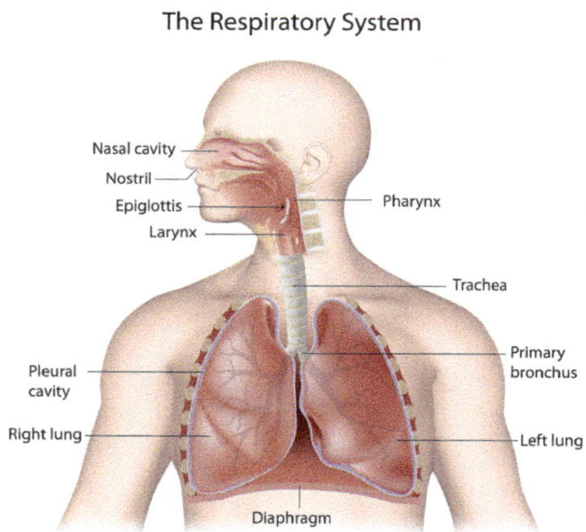

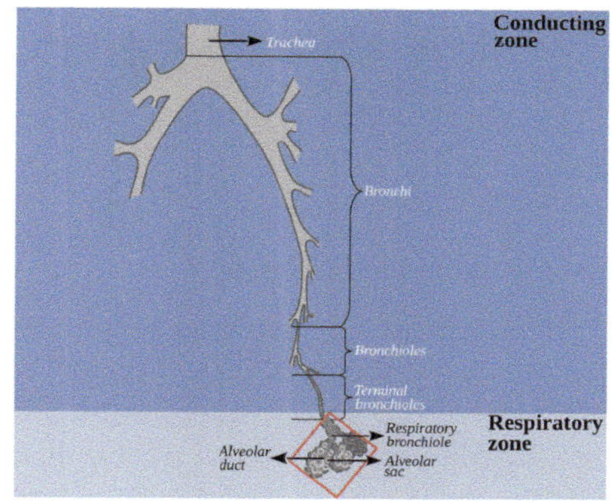

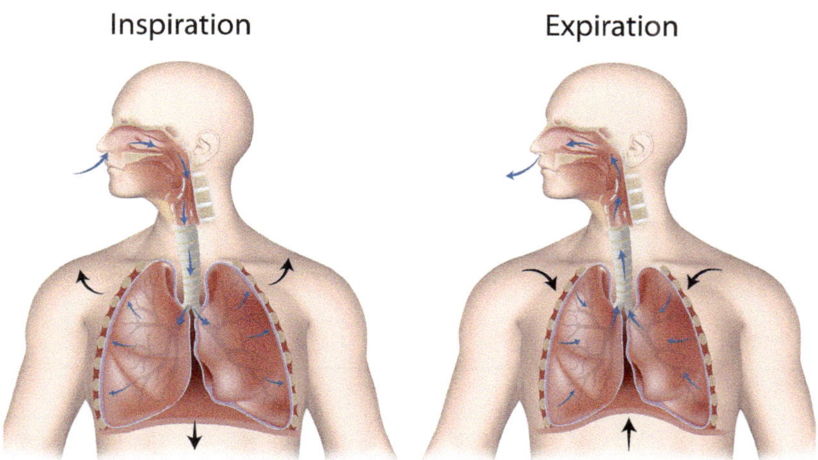

Exhibit 3.12 Anatomy of the respiratory system

Phase	*Process*	*Description*
Inhalation	Air intake	Diaphragm contracts, external intercostal muscles expand chest cavity, air enters alveoli.
Gas Exchange	Diffusion of oxygen and carbon dioxide	Oxygen moves into blood; carbon dioxide moves into alveoli.
Exhalation	Air expulsion	Diaphragm relaxes, internal intercostal muscles contract, air with carbon dioxide is expelled from the lungs.

contracts and flattens, and the external intercostal muscles contract lifting the ribcage to expand the thoracic cavity. As a result, the pressure in the lungs becomes less than the atmospheric pressure, which causes air to rush into the lungs. **Exhalation** occurs upon relaxation of the respiratory muscles which leads to the release of CO_2 from the lungs into the atmosphere (Exhibit 3.12) (McKinley, O'Loughlin, and Pennefather-O'Brien, 2020).

Anatomy of the Blood Vessels

Blood vessels include arteries, veins, and capillaries and each plays an important role in circulation and gas exchange. **Arteries** carry blood away from the heart to the lungs and body tissues and **veins** return blood from the lungs and peripheral tissues back to the heart. **Capillaries** are tiny vessels that connect the arterial and venous networks. They have thin walls and are the site for gas and nutrient exchange between the tissues and the blood. Exhibit 3.13 describes the three tunics (layers) of the walls of arteries and veins.

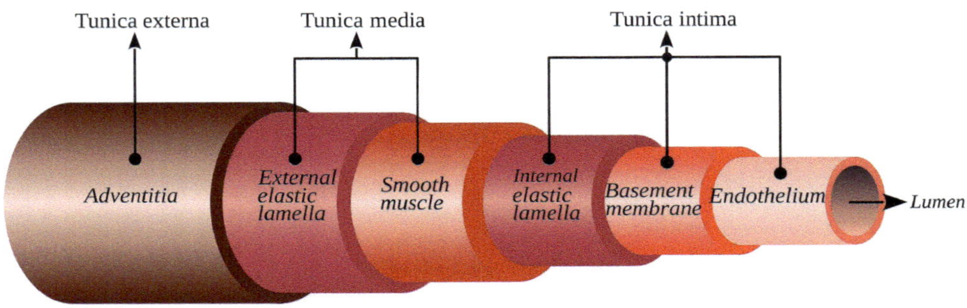

Exhibit 3.13 Anatomy of blood vessels

Layer	*Arteries*	*Veins*
Tunica Intima	Deepest layer of endothelium	Deepest layer of endothelium but thinner than arteries
Tunica Media	Thickest layer. Composed of smooth muscle and elastic fibers essential to withstand high pressure and vasoconstriction or vasodilation	Thinner than in arteries. Less smooth muscle and elastic fibers due to reduced pressure in the veins
Tunica Externa	Connective tissue covering to provide support to prevent overstretching	Thickest layer in veins. Supports the vessel under lower pressure to prevent collapse

The Nervous System

The nervous system is a complex network that coordinates and regulates all body functions and consists of two divisions: the **central nervous system** (CNS) and the **peripheral nervous system** (PNS) (Exhibit 3.14) (Marieb and Hoehn, 2022). The CNS is made up of the brain and spinal cord and is the primary control center for the human body. The PNS is comprised of all nervous tissue outside of the CNS (e.g., cranial nerves, spinal nerves, peripheral nerves) and communicates information between the CNS and the body tissues. The CNS and PNS work together to facilitate sensory perception, motor function, and other complex functions. Within the nervous system, gray matter enables information processing, while white matter provides pathways for communication. **Gray matter** is primarily located in the outer layers of the brain (cerebral cortex), cerebellum, deep within the brain, and the central region of the spinal cord. Gray matter is composed of neuronal cell bodies, dendrites, and ends of axons. It is responsible for processing and integrating information (sensory input and motor control) and is where decision making occurs. On the other hand, **white matter** is found between the cortex and the deep gray matter in the brain and the outer portion of the spinal cord. White matter consists of myelinated axons and functions as a communication route transmitting signals between different regions of the brain and body (McKinley, O'Loughlin, and Pennefather-O'Brien, 2020).

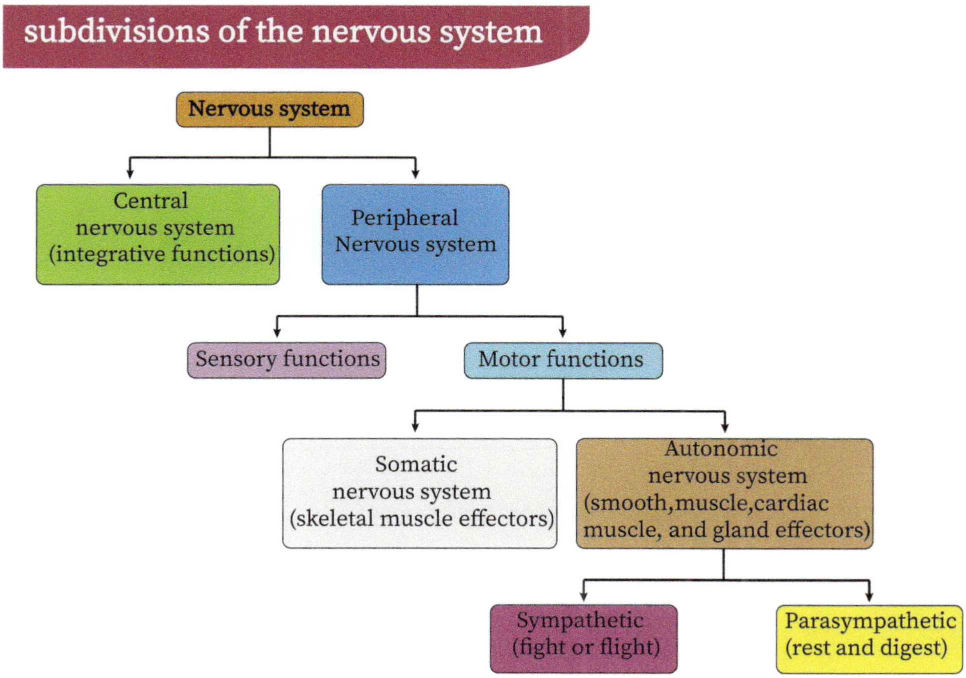

Exhibit 3.14 Organization of the nervous system

Neurons and Neuroglial Cells

A **neuron** is responsible for the transmission of an electrical signal (i.e., action potential) and has several common structural characteristics (Exhibit 3.15). Neuroglial cells, or **glial cells,** are support cells within the nervous system that play an essential role in maintaining the health, structure, and function of neurons. Glial cells do not transmit electrical signals; instead, they provide physical and metabolic support and protection and assist in maintaining homeostasis (Exhibit 3.16).

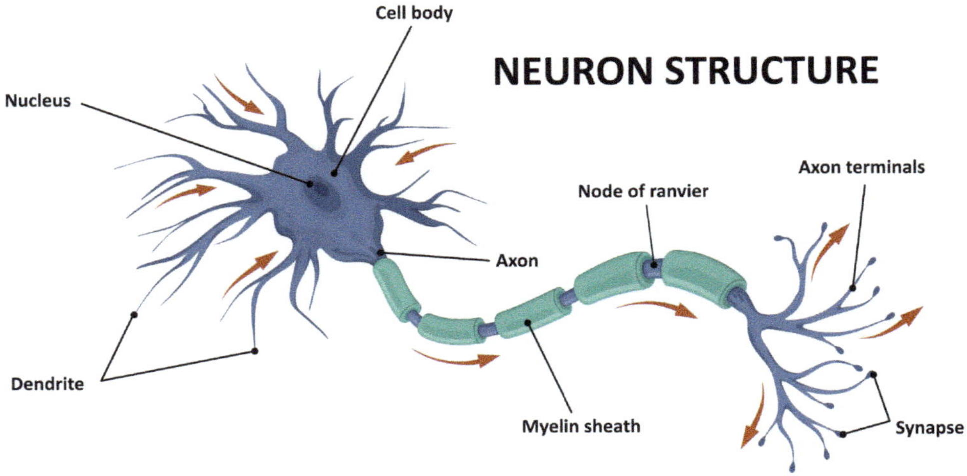

Exhibit 3.15 Anatomy of a neuron

Part of neuron	*Description*
Cell Body (soma)	Contains the nucleus and organelles. Responsible cell metabolic functions and integrating incoming signals
Dendrites	Branch-like extensions that receive signals from other neurons.
Axon	A single, long extension that transmits signals away from the cell body to other neurons, muscles, glands
Axon Terminal	The terminal ends of the axon that release neurotransmitters to communicate with other cells
Myelin Sheath	Insulated covering of the axon by Schwann cells (in the PNS) or oligodendrocytes (in the CNS) that increases signal speed and reduces signal loss

The Structure and Function of the Central Nervous System

As previously mentioned, the CNS consists of the brain and spinal cord and is responsible for receiving and processing information from all over the body and directing an appropriate response to target tissues. The brain is divided into three major regions: the cerebrum (i.e., cerebral cortex), cerebellum, and the brain stem (Exhibit 3.17a). The **cerebrum** has two hemispheres (right and left), and each hemisphere has four lobes: frontal, parietal, occipital, and temporal (Exhibit 3.17b). The **frontal lobe** is located deep to the frontal bone of the skull and is responsible for executive function (i.e., reasoning, judgement, problem solving, emotional responses), language and speech, voluntary movement (motor cortex), and short-term memory. The **parietal lobes** are bilateral (present on left and right sides of the cerebrum), located deep to the parietal bones. The parietal lobe processes sensory information, including touch, temperature, pain, and spatial awareness, enabling perception of the body's position in space. It also plays a role in integrating sensory input with visual information to coordinate movement and navigation. The **occipital lobe** makes up the posterior portion of the cerebrum located deep to the occipital bone. The occipital lobe is primarily responsible for processing visual information, including color, shape, and motion. It interprets signals from the eyes to construct visual

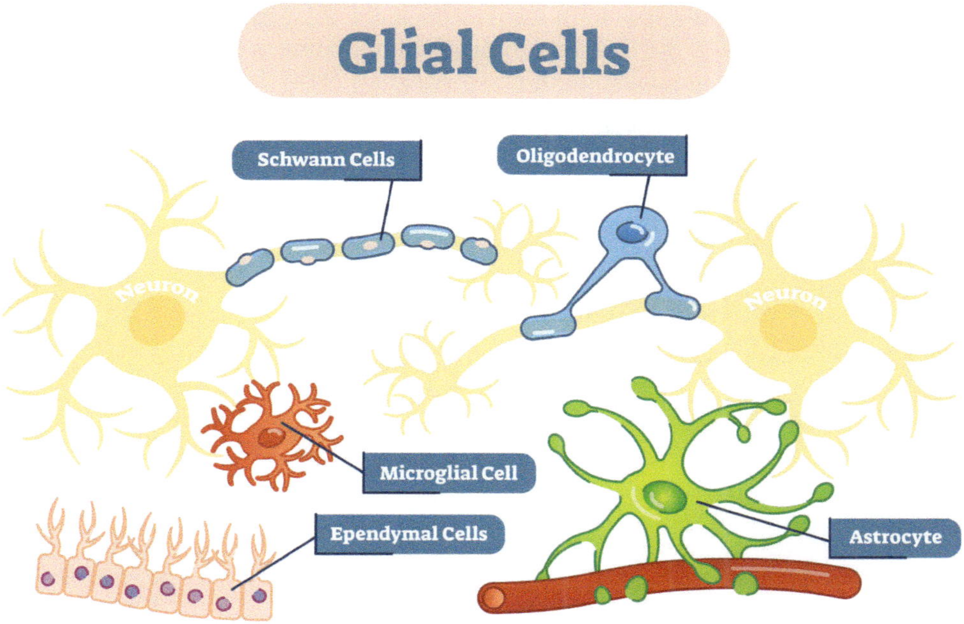

Exhibit 3.16 Support cells of the nervous system

Neuroglial Cell	*Location*	*Function*
Astrocytes	CNS	Support neurons. Help maintain the blood-brain barrier, regulate ion balance and repair nervous tissue
Microglia	CNS	Act as immune cells in CNS
Oligodendrocytes	CNS	Produce myelin to insulate neurons in CNS
Ependymal Cells	CNS	Line the ventricles of the brain and central canal of the spinal cord. They produce and circulate cerebrospinal fluid (CSF)
Schwann Cells	PNS	Produces myelin for axon insulation in PNS
Satellite Cells	PNS	Surround neuron cell bodies in ganglia; regulate the chemical environment around neurons in PNS

perception and support functions like object recognition. The **temporal lobes** are located deep to the temporal bones and are involved in processing auditory information, language comprehension, and memory formation. They also play a role in recognizing faces and interpreting emotions. The **cerebellum** is in the posterior region of the brain inferior to the occipital lobe and is important for coordination and balance of movement and motor learning. Finally, the **brain stem** is located at the base of the brain and is continuous with the spinal cord. The brain stem controls many autonomic functions such as heart rate, breathing, and blood pressure and consists of three regions: the midbrain, pons, and medulla oblongata (Paterno et al., 2025).

The **spinal cord** is continuous to the inferior medulla oblongata and extends inferiorly within the vertebrae (i.e., the vertebral foramen) terminating at the lumbar region. The spinal cord provides communication of nervous signals between the brain and the body, as well as producing reflexes, through 31 pairs of spinal nerves that exit from the cord (Harrow-Mortelliti, Reddy, and Jimsheleishvili, 2023).

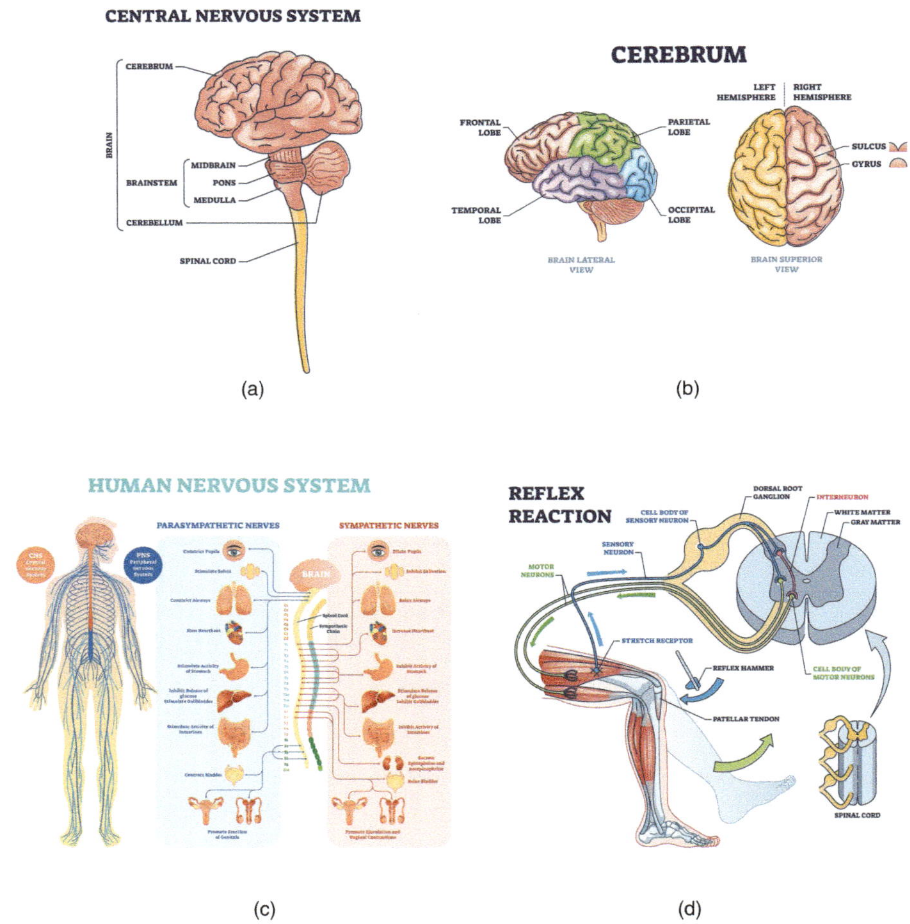

Exhibit 3.17 Anatomy of the nervous system and spinal reflexes

Spinal Reflex	*What it Does*	*How it Works*	*Example*
Stretch Reflex	Helps muscle stay at a constant length	A muscle is stretched → muscle spindle senses it → spinal cord sends signal back to contract the muscle	Doctor taps knee causing leg to kick out
Flexor Withdraw Reflex	Pulls the body away from something painful	Pain receptors activate → signal goes to spinal cord → muscles contract to pull away	Touching a hot stove and pulling the hand away quickly

(*Continued*)

Exhibit 3.17 (Continued)

Spinal Reflex	*What it Does*	*How it Works*	*Example*
Crossed Extensor Reflex	Supports balance when the withdrawal reflex happens	One leg withdraws → spinal cord signals the opposite leg to extend	Step on a tack with your right foot, your left leg stiffens to support your weight
Golgi Tendon Reflex	Prevents muscles from over-contracting and getting damaged	Too much tension in a tendon → Golgi tendon organ senses → spinal cord sends a signal to relax the muscle	When lifting something too heavy, muscles may suddenly relax

The Structure and Function of the Peripheral Nervous System

The PNS is composed of all the nerves outside of the CNS (i.e., cranial, spinal, and peripheral nerves) and it is divided into two parts: the somatic and autonomic systems. The **somatic nervous system** is responsible for voluntary control of skeletal muscles. It transmits sensory information from the skin, muscles, and joints via sensory (or afferent) neurons to the CNS and carries motor commands from the CNS to the skeletal muscles via motor (or efferent) neurons to initiate movement. The **autonomic nervous system** regulates involuntary physiological processes such as heart rate, digestion, respiratory rate, and blood pressure. The motor component of the autonomic nervous system has two divisions: the sympathetic and parasympathetic systems (see Exhibit 3.17 c). The **sympathetic nervous system** is the excitatory division of the autonomic nervous system, and its function is often described as the fight or flight response to stressors. This system responds to stress (e.g., exercise) by increasing heart rate, respiratory rate, and blood pressure to deliver more O_2 to the muscles. The sympathetic division also responds by slowing digestion to allow for more blood to be sent to the working muscles. The **parasympathetic nervous system** works in opposition to the sympathetic division and acts to conserve energy and maximize efficiency of body functions. The parasympathetic division is often given the tag line, rest and digest, which highlights the primary utility of the system to keep heart rate and respiratory rate low and increase digestion. Overall, the autonomic division of the PNS helps the body maintain homeostasis under all conditions, whether calm or stressful (Jänig, 2022).

Neural Control of Movement

Neural control of movement and sensory feedback during movement are intricately linked processes that work together to enable precise and coordinated motor actions (Fox and Rompolski, 2022). Particularly, the **motor cortex** of the brain located in the frontal lobe plays a crucial role in planning and executing movements. When a movement is initiated, populations of neurons in the motor cortex exhibit coordinated activity patterns. This neural activity translates into motor commands that are sent to the muscles via **motor neurons** to produce the desired movement. As movement occurs, various sensory systems provide continuous feedback to the brain, including **proprioception**, visual, and tactile (touch) feedback. Proprioception informs the brain about the position and movement of body parts. The visual feedback provides information about the body's position in relation to the environment, and the tactile feedback comes from touch receptors in the skin, which offer information about contact with objects (Sherwood, 2016).

Spinal Reflexes

Spinal reflexes are rapid, involuntary responses to stimuli that are mediated by neural circuits within the spinal cord, without direct involvement from the brain (Fox and Rompolski, 2022). The four types of spinal reflexes are the stretch reflex, flexor withdrawal reflex, crossed extensor reflex, and Golgi tendon reflex (Exhibit 3.17d). These reflexes are important for protecting the body from harm, helping to maintain posture and balance, and serving as diagnostic tools for neurological examinations. Spinal reflexes demonstrate the remarkable ability of the nervous system to respond quickly and automatically to environmental stimuli, playing a crucial role in our daily functioning and survival.

APPLICATIONS TO EXERCISE SCIENCE

Anatomy and physiology are foundational to exercise science because they provide knowledge of how the human body is structured and how it functions. Understanding anatomy helps exercise scientists identify the roles and relationships of muscles, bones, joints, and other structures involved in movement. Physiology explains how body systems, such as the musculoskeletal, cardiovascular, respiratory, and nervous systems, work together to support physical activity and adapt to exercise. This knowledge is critical for designing effective training programs, preventing injuries, and optimizing performance across diverse populations and activities.

HEALTH/CLINICAL ASPECTS

Anatomy and physiology are fundamental to understanding the clinical and health-related aspects of exercise science, providing essential knowledge for both the prevention and treatment of injuries and chronic conditions. For example, a clear understanding of joint anatomy and muscle function enables physical therapists, athletic trainers, and other rehabilitation professionals to develop effective recovery protocols for patients rehabilitating injuries. In addition, understanding the integrated functions of the cardiovascular and respiratory systems allows practitioners to safely prescribe exercise programs for individuals recovering from cardiorespiratory events, helping to restore functional capacity, and improve overall fitness.

SPORTS/PERFORMANCE ASPECTS

A strong understanding of anatomy and physiology is essential for improving athletic performance, enhancing training outcomes, and minimizing injury risk. For example, strength and conditioning professionals need a solid understanding of muscle anatomy, including attachment sites, primary actions, and the joints they cross, to design effective sport-specific training programs, such as building explosive power in the quadriceps and hamstrings for sprinters. Similarly, understanding joint mechanics, including joint types, ranges of motion, and the muscles responsible for those movements, helps athletic trainers enhance flexibility and reduce the risk of injury.

From a physiological standpoint, knowing how muscles generate force and how that force translates into movement is critical for modifying training to meet an athlete's specific needs. Using the sprinter example above, anaerobic training helps build explosive power, while targeted exercises strengthen the primary muscles involved in sprinting, including the quadriceps, hamstrings, calves, and glutes.

TECHNOLOGY AND RESEARCH TOOLS

Developing technology and research tools allow for improving our understanding of the human body and are presented in more detail in other chapters within this textbook. For example, imaging technologies (e.g., MRI, CT, ultrasound), physiological monitoring systems (e.g., wireless physiological monitors, electromyography (EMG), metabolic carts), digital platforms and software for data analysis, molecular and genetic tools (e.g., polymerase chain reaction (PCR) and gene sequencing, proteomics, metabolomics), wearable technology (e.g., activity trackers, smart fabrics), and virtual and augmented reality (e.g., 3D anatomical models, virtual reality (VR) exercise simulations) enable anatomists, physiologists, and exercise scientists to collect more detailed and accurate data, analyze complex physiological processes, and gain deeper insights into how the human body responds and adapts to exercise.

CAREERS AND EMPLOYMENT OPPORTUNITIES

Training in anatomy and physiology leads to opportunities in a wide range of careers across healthcare, research, education, sports, government, and industry. Professionals in these fields use their knowledge of the human body to promote health, enhance performance, and contribute to scientific innovation.

In **healthcare and clinical settings,** a strong foundation in anatomy and physiology is essential for diagnosing and treating illnesses. Physicians, physical therapists, and occupational therapists rely on this knowledge to assess patients and develop treatment plans, including rehabilitation strategies post-surgery and for injuries and disabilities. Clinical exercise physiologists use their expertise to design safe and effective exercise programs for individuals with chronic conditions. Chiropractors apply detailed knowledge of the musculoskeletal system to treat spine and joint disorders, while respiratory therapists and cardiopulmonary specialists use physiological principles to manage breathing and cardiovascular conditions. The following abstract (Exhibit 3.18) underscores the value of interdisciplinary collaboration between orthopedic surgeons and physical therapists, emphasizing their shared expertise in hip musculature for effective post-surgical recovery.

Exhibit 3.18 Pre-operative gluteus medius tendon degeneration and its impact on strength and functional ability one year after total hip replacement

Juhlin, J., Sernert, N., & Åhlund, K. (2024). Pre-operative gluteus medius tendon degeneration and its impact on strength and functional ability one year after total hip replacement. *Annals of Medicine*, *56*(1), 2388701. https://doi.org/10.1080/07853890.2024.2388701

Abstract

Objective: Hip osteoarthritis is a common cause of disability and surgery is often unavoidable. Patient satisfaction is high, and functional ability improves after surgery. However, residual impairment and pain are common. Degenerative changes in tendons and muscles are probable causes. The aim of this study is to investigate gluteus medius (GMED) tendon degeneration in relation to muscle strength, physical function and walking distance before and one year after total hip replacement.

Material and methods: In total, 18 patients were examined pre- and post-operatively, of whom 15 were available in the final analysis. Muscle strength, physical function and walking distance were assessed. Tendon biopsies were assessed microscopically, and the total degeneration score (TDS) was calculated.

Results: A correlation between the TDS and muscle strength was found for the hamstrings, GMED and quadriceps pre- or post-operatively. No correlations were found between the TDS and functional ability. Functional ability and muscle strength improved significantly after surgery.

Conclusion: Our results indicate a correlation between tendon degeneration and the muscle strength of the hip and knee in patients with hip OA and one year after THR. To minimize post-operative residual discomfort, rehabilitation programs should probably be modified over time to match the pre- and post-operative needs. Further studies are needed.

Key Messages

- There are negative correlations, which suggest patterns between degeneration in the GMED tendon and muscle strength in the muscles acting around the hip in patients with hip OA, before and after THR.
- The strength training of muscles acting around the hip joint may need to be adjusted before and after THR.

Several **support roles in healthcare** also require anatomical and physiological expertise. For example, medical illustrators create accurate visual representations of the human body for use in educational and clinical settings. Pharmaceutical representatives also draw on their understanding of body systems to explain how medications interact with biological processes when working with healthcare providers.

In **research and academic environments**, biomedical scientists study disease mechanisms and contribute to medical innovation. University professors teach anatomy and physiology across disciplines such as medicine, nursing, and exercise science, and often engage in scholarly research. Anatomical technicians support education and research by preparing specimens for laboratory instruction or scientific study. Clinical anatomists offer advanced anatomical insights for medical training, surgical planning, and procedural simulations.

Sports and performance professions rely heavily on a strong foundation in anatomy and physiology. As previously discussed, strength and conditioning specialists use this knowledge to create targeted training programs that enhance performance and minimize injury risk. Sports scientists analyze physical demands and design evidence-based recovery strategies, while athletic trainers apply anatomical and physiological principles to prevent, diagnose, and treat injuries sustained during physical activity.

In **government and industry**, professionals use anatomical and physiological knowledge in a range of specialized roles. Forensic scientists use their expertise to determine causes of injury or death in criminal investigations. Ergonomists draw on principles of anatomy, biomechanics, and physiology to design tools, equipment, and workspaces to reduce physical strain, prevent injury, and improve overall efficiency and safety in the workplace.

EDUCATION REQUIREMENTS

Education requirements for anatomists and physiologists vary depending on their specific career goals. For entry-level positions (e.g., laboratory assistants or anatomical technicians) a bachelor's degree in anatomy, physiology, biology, or a related life science field is typically required. Undergraduate programs often include foundational coursework in anatomy, physiology, biochemistry, and the biological sciences.

For careers in research, academia, or advanced clinical roles, a master's degree (MS) or doctorate (PhD) in anatomy, physiology, or a related discipline is typically necessary. Graduate programs emphasize both advanced knowledge and research skills, requiring students to complete specialized coursework, conduct original research, and formally defend a thesis or dissertation. Individuals with a PhD can pursue careers as biomedical researchers or university professors, where they teach and conduct research.

Healthcare-focused careers, such as physical therapy, clinical exercise physiology, or chiropractic care, typically require a professional degree such as a Doctor of Physical Therapy (DPT), a Master's in Clinical Exercise Physiology, or a Doctor of Chiropractic (DC). These programs integrate anatomy and physiology within clinical practice and require licensure for professional practice.

For those pursuing medical careers, such as becoming a physician or surgeon, completing a medical degree (MD or DO) is necessary. Medical school expands students' knowledge of anatomy, physiology, and pathophysiology, while also requiring hands-on clinical training through internships and residencies.

In summary, education requirements for anatomists and physiologists range from bachelor's degrees for entry-level roles to advanced degrees for specialized careers in research, academia, or clinical practice. The level of education required depends on the complexity and scope of the desired profession.

CERTIFICATIONS AND LICENSURE

While there is no universally recognized certification specifically for clinical anatomists, individuals can demonstrate expertise through advanced education and professional experience. Common pathways include earning a specialized graduate degree (such as a master's or PhD in anatomy), completing university-based certificate programs, and gaining experience in teaching, research, or clinical anatomy-related roles. These qualifications can support careers in academic instruction, surgical education, and anatomical research.

Additionally, Histotechnician (HT) and Histotechnologist (HTL) certifications, offered by the American Society for Clinical Pathology (ASCP) Board of Certification, are closely tied to anatomy and physiology, since they involve the preparation and analysis of tissue samples for microscopic examination, which is essential in diagnosing diseases and conducting medical research. A brief description of the degree requirements for eligibility for the HT and HTL certifications is provided below. Students interested in learning more are encouraged to visit the ASCP website (ASCP, n.d.).

- A histotechnician typically holds an associate degree or a certificate from a program accredited by the National Accrediting Agency for Clinical Laboratory Sciences (NAACLS), which ensures high educational standards in clinical laboratory education. Certification is earned by passing the HT exam through the ASCP.
- A histotechnologist requires a bachelor's degree and more advanced training. They are eligible to take the HTL certification exam (also through ASCP) and are qualified to perform more complex procedures, troubleshoot technical issues, and often take on supervisory or instructional roles in clinical or research settings.

PROFESSIONAL ORGANIZATIONS

American Association for Anatomy (AAA)
American Physiological Society (APS)
Human Anatomy and Physiology Society (HAPS)
American Association of Clinical Anatomists (AACA)
International Federation of Associations of Anatomists (IFAA)
American Society for Clinical Pathology (ASCP)

JOURNALS

Anatomy & Cell Biology
The Anatomical Record
American Journal of Physiology
Journal of Anatomy
Clinical Anatomy
Journal of Applied Physiology
European Journal of Applied Physiology

FUTURE DIRECTIONS

Advances in science and technology are rapidly transforming the fields of anatomy and physiology. These innovations are not only enhancing medical diagnosis and treatment but also expanding opportunities across exercise science, sports performance, and rehabilitation. Emerging tools and research are deepening our understanding of movement, fitness, and health, while shaping how professionals approach injury prevention, recovery, and performance optimization. The following section highlights key trends and their impact on careers in health, fitness, sports, and related fields.

Personalized Medicine and Tailored Exercise Programs

Advances in personalized medicine use genetic, physiological, and lifestyle data to create tailored treatments for individuals. In exercise science, similar approaches are being applied to develop customized exercise and nutrition plans based on a person's unique biology (Nasb et al., 2024). These individualized strategies can be designed to improve fitness, enhance athletic performance, and reduce the risk of chronic conditions such as type 2 diabetes, heart disease, and obesity.

Three Dimensional (3D) Imaging and Virtual Reality (VR)

New technology like 3D imaging and VR is changing the way we learn about the human body (Salimi et al. 2024; Abundez Toledo et al., 2024). In exercise science, these tools help students "see" muscles, joints, and movements in action through interactive visuals. They are also used in clinical and sports settings to improve movement analysis, study biomechanics, and plan effective rehabilitation programs.

Regenerative Medicine and Injury Recovery

Regenerative medicine focuses on helping the body repair or replace damaged tissues and organs. For those working in athletic training, physical therapy, or orthopedics, this type of research has the potential to change how injuries are treated and how recovery is managed. Understanding how the body heals at the cellular level can help guide effective post-injury exercise programs and reduce long-term complications (Zhang et al., 2024).

Artificial Intelligence (AI) in Exercise and Health Monitoring

Artificial intelligence is becoming a valuable tool in both healthcare and fitness (Sujith et al., 2022). In exercise science, AI can support real-time monitoring of exercise performance, analyze physical activity data, identify injury risks, and help customize training programs. It is also becoming an essential tool for developing digital health solutions and virtual coaching platforms (Baca, 2025).

Human Performance in Extreme Environments

Research in space physiology and other extreme environments helps scientists understand how the body adapts to physical stressors like microgravity, high altitude, and extreme temperatures. This knowledge applies to exercise science by informing training and safety strategies for elite athletes, military personnel, firefighters, and others working in demanding conditions (Schmidt, Jones, and Mason 2023).

SUMMARY

An understanding of anatomy and physiology is fundamental to the study of exercise science. These disciplines explain how the body is structured, how it functions, and how it adapts to physical activity, injury, and disease. Whether applying this knowledge in clinical, athletic, research, or educational settings, a strong foundation in anatomy and physiology supports informed decision-making and evidence-based practice. As the field continues to evolve with advances in technology and personalized approaches to health, a systems-level perspective of the human body remains essential for improving performance, promoting wellness, and enhancing quality of life.

STUDY QUESTIONS

1. How are joints classified based on structure and function? List the major synovial joints in the body and describe the types of movements each allows (e.g., flexion, extension, rotation).
2. Choose a sport or exercise movement (e.g., throwing a ball, performing a squat, doing a jumping jack). Identify the major joints involved, the muscles that cross the joints, and describe the types of movement occurring at each joint during the activity.
3. Describe the pathway of blood flow through the heart and body. Why is this circulation important during physical activity or exercise?
4. What is the role of the lungs in gas exchange, and how do the respiratory and cardiovascular systems work together to deliver oxygen to working muscles during exercise?
5. What is the difference between the central and peripheral nervous systems? How does the nervous system contribute to voluntary muscle movement?

LEARNING ACTIVITIES

1. Body Systems Concept Map
    a. Create a list of the four body systems discussed in the chapter (musculoskeletal, cardiovascular, respiratory, and nervous) and their major organs and functions.
    b. Create a concept map or diagram showing how the systems interact. For example, how the cardiovascular and respiratory systems work together to deliver oxygen to the body.

2. Homeostasis Tracker
    a. Practice measuring heart rate by placing your index and middle fingers over the carotid artery in your neck (Figure 3.15) and measure by counting heart beats for 15 seconds and multiplying by 4 (to get how many beats per minute [BPM]).
    b. Monitor your heart rate and breathing rate after performing the following activities for 1 minute:
        i. Sitting, walking, and jumping jacks.
        ii. A partner could simultaneously count breathing rate (breaths per minute).
    c. Reflect on how your body maintained homeostasis, and what signals might have caused the changes (e.g., increased oxygen demand).

SUGGESTED READING AND RELATED WEBSITES

Neumann, D.A. (2016). *Kinesiology of the musculoskeletal system: Foundations for rehabilitation* (3rd ed.). Amsterdam: Elsevier.

Saladin, K.S. (2021). *Anatomy & physiology: The unity of form and function* (9th ed.). New York: McGraw-Hill Education.

Tortora, G.J., and Derrickson, B. (2021). *Principles of anatomy and physiology* (16th ed.). New York: Wiley.

Supplementary Books

Delavier, F., and Gundill, M. (2018). *The strength training anatomy workout III: Advanced programming for serious strength and power*. Champaign, IL: Human Kinetics.

Kapit, W., and Elson, L.M. (2013). *The anatomy coloring book* (4th ed.). London: Pearson.

Drake, R.L., Vogl, W., and Mitchell, A.W.M. (2024). *Gray's anatomy for students* (5th ed.). Amsterdam: Elsevier.

Fremgen, B. F. and Frucht, S.S. (2019). *Medical terminology: A living language* (7th ed.). London: Pearson Education.

Interactive Learning Tools

BioDigital Human

- https://www.biodigital.com
- a free, interactive anatomy platform with 3D visualizations and quizzes

GetBodySmart

- https://www.getbodysmart.com
- animated tutorials and quizzes to reinforce anatomy and physiology concepts

TeachMeAnatomy

- https://teachmeanatomy.info
- clear explanations and diagrams geared toward learners of all levels

Visible Body

- https://www.visiblebody.com
- interactive 3D models of the human body with explanations of systems and functions

REFERENCES

Abundez Toledo, M., Ghanem, G., Fine, S., Weisman, D., Huang, Y.M., and Rouhani, A.A. (2024). Exploring the promise of virtual reality in enhancing anatomy education: A focus group study with medical students. *Frontiers in Virtual Reality*, 5.1369794. https://doi.org/10.3389/frvir.2024.1369794

ASCP. (n.d.) American Society for Clinical Pathology website. Available at: https://www.ascp.org (Accessed September 9, 2025).

Baca, A. (2025). Perspectives of artificial intelligence in training and exercise. In M.J. Blondin, I. Fister Jr., and Pardalos, P.M. (Eds.), *Artificial intelligence, optimization, and data sciences in sports* (pp. 265–274). Cham: Springer Nature Switzerland. DOI: 10.1007/978-3-031-76047-1_9

Chien, S., and Gargus, J.J. (1987). Molecular biology in physiology. *FASEB Journal*, 1(2), 97–102. https://doi.org/10.1096/fasebj.1.2.2886391

Conti, A.A., and Paternostro, F. (2019). Anatomical study in the Western world before the Middle Ages: Historical evidence. *Acta Bio-Medica: Atenei Parmensis*, 90(4), 523–525. https://doi.org/10.23750/abm.v90i4.8738

Davies, K.J. (2016). Adaptive homeostasis. *Molecular Aspects of Medicine*, 49, 1–7. https://doi.org/10.1016/j.mam.2016.04.007

Denkler, K., and Norman, M.A. (2012). Nerve and arterial supply to the hand in *Vesalius's De Humani Corporis Fabrica. Hand* (New York, N.Y.), 7(2), 224–228. https://doi.org/10.1007/s11552-012-9394-4

Ford, B.J. (1991). *The Leeuwenhoek legacy*. Bristol: Biopress & Farrand Press. Available at: https://www.brianjford.com/wlegacya.htm (Accessed September 9, 2025).

Fox, S.I., and Rompolski, K.L. (2022). Muscle: Mechanisms of contraction and neural control. In *Human physiology* (16th ed., pp. 359–376). New York: McGraw-Hill.

Franzini-Armstrong, C. (2018). The relationship between form and function throughout the history of excitation–contraction coupling. *Journal of General Physiology*, 150(2), 189–210. https://doi.org/10.1085/jgp.201711889

Friedland, G. (2009). Discovery of the function of the heart and circulation of blood. *Cardiovascular Journal of Africa*, 20(3), 160. https://pmc.ncbi.nlm.nih.gov/articles/PMC3721262/

Harrow-Mortelliti, M., Reddy, V., and Jimsheleishvili, G. (2023). Physiology, spinal cord. *StatPearls* [Internet]. StatPearls Publishing. https://www.ncbi.nlm.nih.gov/books/NBK544267/

Jänig, W. (2022). *The integrative action of the autonomic nervous system: Neurobiology of homeostasis*. Cambridge: Cambridge University Press.

Lakhtakia, R. (2014). A trio of exemplars of medieval Islamic medicine: Al-Razi, Avicenna and Ibn Al-Nafis. *Sultan Qaboos University Medical Journal*, 14, e455–e459. https://doi.org/10.18295/2075-0528.1618

Li, K.H.C., Kui, C., Lee, E.K.M., Ho, C.S., Wong, S.H., Wu, W., Wong, W.T., Voll, J., Li, G., Liu, T., Yan, B., Chan, J., Tse, G., and Keenan, I.D. (2017). The role of 3D printing in anatomy education and surgical training: A narrative review. *MedEdPublish*, 6, 92. https://doi.org/10.15694/mep.2017.000092

Marieb, E.N., and Hoehn, K. (2022). *Human anatomy & physiology* (12th ed.). London: Pearson.

McKinley, M., O'Loughlin, V., and Pennefather-O'Brien, E. (2020). *Human anatomy* (6th ed.). New York: McGraw-Hill.

Nasb, M., Wei, M., Lin, B., and Chen, N. (2024). Unraveling precision exercise: A journey from efficacy to molecular insights. *Advanced Exercise and Health Science*, 1(1), 3–15. https://doi.org/10.1016/j.aehs.2024.01.004

Piccolino, M. (1997). Luigi Galvani and animal electricity: Two centuries after the foundation of electrophysiology. *Trends in Neurosciences*, 20(10), 443–448. https://doi.org/10.1016/s0166-2236(97)01101-6

Paterno, G., Buccilli, B., Iess, G., Montano, S., Vitali, V., Cevik, O., Babur, M., Orhun, O., and Ascenzi, B. (2025). Chapter 5a – Functional anatomy of the brainstem. In B. Ascenzi (Ed.), *From anatomy to function of the central nervous system: Clinical and neurological applications* (pp. 129–161). Amsterdam: Elsevier. https://doi.org/10.1016/B978-0-12-822404-5.00023-1

Rühli, F., van Schaik, K., and Henneberg, M. (2016). Evolutionary medicine: The ongoing evolution of human physiology and metabolism. *Physiology*, 31(6), 392–397. https://doi.org/10.1152/physiol.00013.2016

Sujith, A.V.L.N., Sajja, G.S., Mahalakshmi, V., Nuhmani, S., and Prasanalakshmi, B. (2022). Systematic review of smart health monitoring using deep learning and artificial intelligence. *Neuroscience Informatics*, 2(3), 100028. doi:10.1016/j.neuri.2021.100028

Sherwood, L. (2016). The peripheral nervous system: Afferent division; special senses. In *Human physiology: From cells to systems* (9th ed., p. 186). Boston, MA: Cengage Learning.

Salimi, S., Asgari, Z., Mohammadnejad, A., Teimazi, A., and Bakhtiari, M. (2024). Efficacy of virtual reality and augmented reality in anatomy education: A systematic review and meta-analysis. *Anatomical Sciences Education*, 17, 1668–1685. https://doi.org/10.1002/ase.2501

Schmidt, M.A., Jones, J.A., and Mason, C.E. (2023). Optimizing human performance in extreme environments through precision medicine: From spaceflight to high-performance operations on Earth. *Cambridge Prisms: Precision Medicine*, 1, e27. doi:10.1017/pcm.2023.16

Wingerd, B.D. (2014). *The human body: Concepts of anatomy and physiology*. Alphen aan den Rijn: WoltersKluwer.

Zhang, Z., Yao, P., and Fan, S. (2024). Advances in regenerative rehabilitation in the rehabilitation of musculoskeletal injuries. *Regenerative Medicine*, 19(6), 345–354. https://doi.org/10.1080/17460751.2024.2357956

4 Exercise and Sport Nutrition

Joan M. Eckerson and G. Patrick Lambert

LEARNING OBJECTIVES

After studying this chapter, the student will be able to:

- identify the six classes of nutrients and describe their roles in energy production, exercise performance, and overall health
- compare and contrast the three energy systems and explain how each contributes to physical activity at different intensities and durations
- interpret the concepts of glycemic index and glycemic load and evaluate their application to exercise and sport performance
- assess personal dietary intake using consumer nutrition tools and apply the Acceptable Macronutrient Distribution Ranges (AMDR) to develop a balanced, goal-specific meal plan
- outline the academic and professional steps required to pursue careers such as registered dietitian nutritionist (RDN), sports dietitian, or nutrition specialist
- describe emerging technology such as nutrigenomics and metabolomics and discuss their relevance to personalized nutrition and exercise science

INTRODUCTION

The role of nutrition in health, physical activity, and sports performance has gained increasing attention, particularly with advances in exercise physiology and a growing understanding of how diet influences athletic outcomes and chronic disease risk. **Nutrition** is the science of food and the physiological processes involved in ingestion, digestion, absorption, metabolism, and nutrient utilization. **Dietetics** is a specialized field that applies this knowledge to promote health, manage disease, and improve quality of life. **Dietitians** are experts in nutrition and dietetics who have completed specific education requirements to earn the Registered Dietitian and Nutritionist (RDN) credential and are recognized as medical professionals within the field. **Nutritionists** are individuals who have a strong interest in food and nutrition but have varying levels of education and training and are not typically recognized as health professionals.

Dietitians work in a variety of settings, including hospitals, clinics, schools, universities, public health programs, the military, corporate wellness programs, research institutions, and private practice. While responsibilities vary by setting, most dietitians are involved in meal planning, medical nutrition therapy, food service management, and the promotion of healthy eating habits. They play a central role in preventing and managing

DOI: 10.4324/9781032697185-4

chronic conditions such as coronary heart disease (CHD), obesity, and diabetes through individualized nutrition counseling and evidence-based dietary strategies. Many also pursue advanced credentials to specialize in areas such as clinical nutrition, obesity and weight management, eating disorders, and **sports dietetics**.

Exercise and sport nutrition is a growing field that integrates principles of nutrition with exercise science to support physical performance, optimize training adaptations, and reduce the risk of injury and illness. This chapter introduces the basic principles of exercise and sport nutrition, highlights current research, and outlines career paths for students interested in working in this exciting and growing field.

HISTORICAL PERSPECTIVES

Nutrition science has evolved over centuries, developing from early observational practices to a formal scientific discipline grounded in medicine, biochemistry, and the biological sciences. The importance of diet for maintaining health can be traced back thousands of years to ancient civilizations such as Egypt, Greece, and Rome when early physicians used dietary interventions, including enemas and clysters (injections of fluids such as wine, whey, and milk into tissue spaces, the rectum, or abdominal cavity) to treat illness (Brooks and Kearns, 1996). However, nutrition was not officially recognized as an independent scientific discipline until 1928 with the establishment of the American Institute of Nutrition, now known as the American Society for Nutrition (n.d.).

The early 20th century is often called the "vitamin era," since this is when the discovery of many essential vitamins and minerals occurred, and early nutrition research focused on preventing deficiency diseases such as scurvy from a lack of Vitamin C and rickets, due to inadequate intake of Vitamin D. During World War II, many soldiers failed military physicals because of deficiencies in protein and vitamins and minerals, which led to the development of the first edition of the Recommended Dietary Allowances (RDA) published in 1943 (Hasler, Brown, and Burns, 2009; Leveille, 2016). By the 1960s, research shifted from deficiency diseases to studying the effects of excessive nutrient intake, particularly fat, cholesterol, and sodium, and their relationship to chronic diseases like CHD, hypertension, and cancer. Nutrition research in the late 20th century led to the discovery of **functional foods** (i.e., enriched, fortified, and whole foods that have health benefits beyond basic nutrition) and nutraceuticals (i.e., plant chemicals or "**phytochemicals**") that may have pharmacological effects when consumed in adequate amounts. For example, carotenoids found in carrots, tomatoes, and green leafy vegetables may have antioxidant effects and protect cells from damage. The evolution of functional foods and nutraceuticals contributed to a boom in the dietary supplement industry, as well as changes in food labeling laws and the development of the Dietary Supplement Health and Education Act in 1994 (Hasler, Brown, and Burns, 2009).

In the 21st century, "omics" technologies, including nutrigenomics, proteomics, and metabolomics, have revolutionized nutrition science. These fields examine how nutrients interact with genes, proteins, and metabolism, paving the way for precision nutrition (Ferguson et al., 2016). "Foodomics" is a newer discipline and described as a holistic approach to improving human nutrition, since it integrates these technologies to improve a person's overall well-being by connecting food, food components, and the individual, to health and disease (Capozzi and Bordini, 2013; Bordini and Capozzi, 2014).

The history of nutrition in exercise science dates back to 1904 with the establishment of the Nutrition Laboratory at the Carnegie Institute in Washington, DC. However, major strides in sport nutrition began with the creation of the Harvard Fatigue Laboratory in 1927 under the direction of Dr. David Bruce Dill. Research conducted there laid the groundwork for modern exercise physiology, particularly in areas like metabolism, environmental physiology, physical fitness, and nutrition (McCardle, Katch, and Katch, 2023). Ancel Keys, a renowned biochemist and physiologist associated with the Harvard Fatigue Laboratory, contributed to the field with the development of Key's or K-rations that were used by soldiers during World War II, and were replaced by the MRE (Meal, Ready-to-Eat) in the early 1980s (Buskirk, 1992). His research on starvation and the recovery that followed also resulted in the classic work, *The Biology of Human Starvation* in 1950 (Keys et al., 1950).

Epidemiological studies, which examine the distribution of disease in a large population, have also significantly impacted nutrition guidelines and public health. Two major studies, the Framingham Heart Study and the National Health and Nutrition Examination Survey (NHANES), have shaped our understanding of the role of nutrition in chronic disease prevention. The Framingham Heart Study (n.d.), which began in 1948, provided critical insights into the health behaviors and genetic factors associated with cardiovascular disease and the information obtained from this long-term study has been instrumental in identifying the lifestyle behaviors (risk factors) and genetic patterns associated with the development of CHD.

The NHANES is a large cross-sectional epidemiological program of studies, interviews, and physical examinations designed to assess the health and nutrition status of adults and children in the United States and is considered the cornerstone for national nutrition monitoring and the development of public health policies related to nutrition and the prevention of chronic disease (Ahluwalia et al., 2016). The NHANES is conducted as part of the Center for Disease Control and Prevention (CDC) and has been collecting data since the 1970s. Data from the NHANES surveys is also used in other epidemiological studies and clinical research to develop health policies, as well as health programs and services such as the National Cholesterol Education Program and the National High Blood Pressure Education Program.

The relationship between diet and sports performance also dates back thousands of years, but it is only within the past 60 to 70 years that sports nutrition has emerged as a distinct science. Although studies examining the role of carbohydrate in muscle glycogen storage began in the early 1900s, significant advancements came in the 1960s with the introduction of muscle biopsy techniques when Swedish researchers used the procedure to study **glycogen** depletion, which led to the development of classic carbohydrate loading protocols in endurance sports to supersaturate the muscles with glycogen (McCardle, Katch, and Katch, 2023). Further research in the 1970s refined these methods, emphasizing the importance of eating a high-carbohydrate diet and tapering exercise before competition to delay fatigue (Sherman et al., 1981).

Fluid balance during exercise has been another focal point of sports nutrition research thanks to the commercial producers of sports drinks. Probably one of the most widely known sports drinks is Gatorade®, which was developed by a University of Florida research team to help prevent dehydration and improve performance. The drink was first tested on University of Florida Gator football players in 1965 and was shown to delay fatigue and prevent heat-related illness. The creation of the Gatorade Sports Science Institute (GSSI) in 1985 significantly advanced research surrounding hydration, electrolyte balance, and the effects of carbohydrate intake during prolonged exercise, and has been instrumental in developing guidelines for fluid replacement to prevent dehydration and enhance performance.

As exercise physiology and nutrition science have advanced, so has the development of ergogenic aids, substances or techniques that enhance athletic performance. Some of the most researched supplements include creatine, caffeine, beta-alanine, beetroot juice, and whey protein. While many supplements have been studied, ongoing research is needed to clarify their effectiveness and potential applications in sports and exercise performance.

In summary, nutrition science has evolved from early observational practices to a multidisciplinary field shaped by advances in biochemistry, epidemiology, and genomics. Key developments include the discovery of vitamins, the emergence of functional foods and nutrigenomics, and the establishment of evidence-based dietary guidelines. In sport nutrition, research on carbohydrate loading, hydration, and ergogenic aids has enhanced our current understanding of how diet influences exercise performance and recovery.

FUNDAMENTAL CONCEPTS

Bioenergetics and Metabolism

A strong foundation in bioenergetics and metabolism is essential for understanding how the body utilizes nutrients to fuel activity, promote recovery, and support overall health. **Bioenergetics** refers to the transfer (or conversion) of **energy** from one form to another within biological (living) systems, while **metabolism** encompasses the chemical processes that break down nutrients to produce energy (catabolism) and build complex molecules for growth and repair (anabolism) (Fink and Mikesky, 2025).

Energy is essential for the body to perform **work**, which occurs in three main forms: **mechanical work**, such as muscular contractions; **chemical work**, like the synthesis of biomolecules; and **transport work**, which involves moving substances across cell membranes (McArdle et al., 2023). The primary types of energy used by the body to accomplish these tasks are **mechanical energy** (including kinetic and potential energy) and **chemical energy** (stored in chemical bonds) (Powers, Howley, and Quindry, 2024). Kinetic energy drives movements, such as those generated by muscle contractions, enabling the performance of physical work. Potential energy, stored within the body in the form of fats, carbohydrates, and proteins, can be converted into both chemical energy and kinetic energy to meet the body's energy demands.

Fat provides most of the energy for the body's daily processes and is stored as **triglycerides** in fat cells called adipocytes. **Carbohydrates** are also a primary energy source for the body and are stored in the liver and skeletal muscles as glycogen (long branches and chains of **glucose** molecules) or in the blood as blood glucose. **Protein** is found in the tissues of the body and in the blood but is not a major energy source under normal conditions; however, it can provide energy when necessary (Powers, Howley, and Quindry, 2024).

When energy is released from the above "fuels" it becomes stored as chemical energy in high energy bonds in a molecule called adenosine triphosphate (ATP). When ATP bonds are split by an enzyme called **ATPase**, released energy can be used for work, like exercise (Exhibit 4.1). Most of the reactions that produce ATP are organized into chains of reactions called **metabolic pathways**.

ATP can be produced under **anaerobic** (without adequate oxygen in the cells) and **aerobic** (with adequate oxygen in the cells) conditions. Anaerobic ATP production occurs when there is insufficient time for oxygen to be consumed by the body to allow for sufficient ATP to be produced to perform the work aerobically. There are two pathways

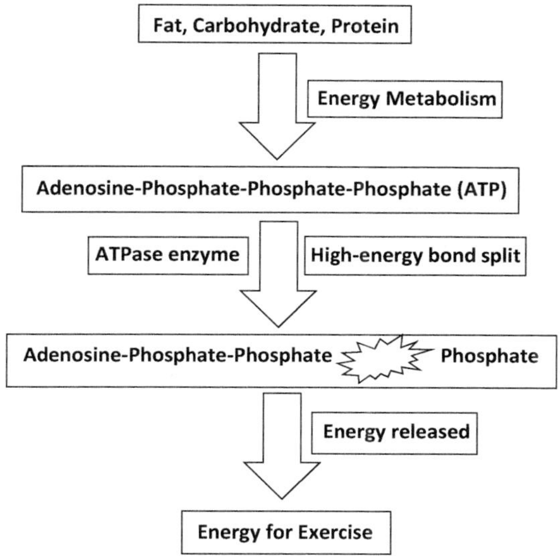

Exhibit 4.1 ATP production and energy release for exercise

that supply ATP anaerobically: 1) the **ATP-creatine phosphate (CP) system** (also called the "**phosphagen system**") which is used at the onset of exercise, and during short bursts of high-intensity exercise (e.g., 5–15 seconds) and, 2) the **anaerobic system** (also called the "**glycolytic system**") that is the predominant system for ATP production during high-intensity exercise lasting up to approximately 1–3 minutes (Fink and Mikesky, 2025).

With the ATP-CP system, a small, limited amount of stored ATP is split by ATPase to adenosine diphosphate (ADP) and phosphate (P), and the energy released is used for immediate muscular contractions. CP is subsequently split by the enzyme **creatine kinase** and provides both additional energy and a phosphate to produce a "new" ATP allowing for a few additional seconds of muscle contraction (Exhibit 4.2) (Fink and Mikesky, 2025).

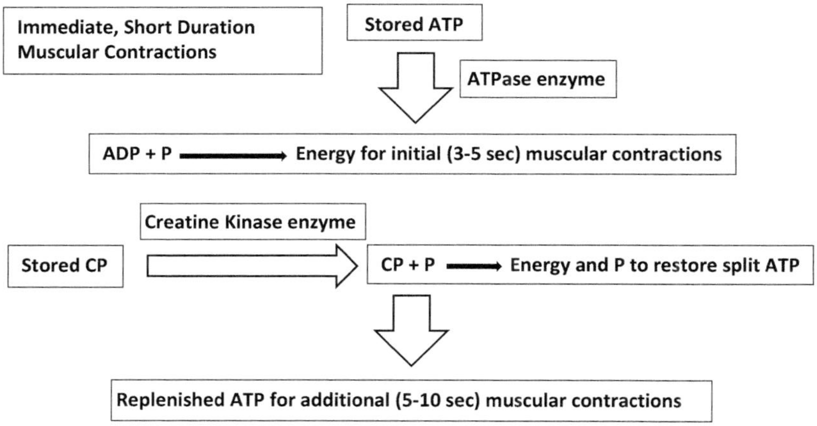

Exhibit 4.2 ATP-CP system (phosphagen system) for ATP

In the anaerobic system, the metabolic pathway **glycolysis** (i.e., **anaerobic glycolysis**) is utilized to produce ATP rapidly to allow for continued muscular contractions under low oxygen conditions (Powers, Howley, and Quindry, 2024). This process utilizes either muscle glycogen or blood glucose as the fuel source. Initially, 1–2 ATP must be utilized to get the reactions started (depending on whether it starts with glycogen or glucose) but, ultimately, 4 ATP are produced for a net gain of 2–3 ATP by the muscle cells. However, a byproduct of this process is lactic acid, which creates an acidic environment in the muscle cells ultimately inhibiting muscular contractions and leading to fatigue (Smith et al., 2022) (Exhibit 4.3).

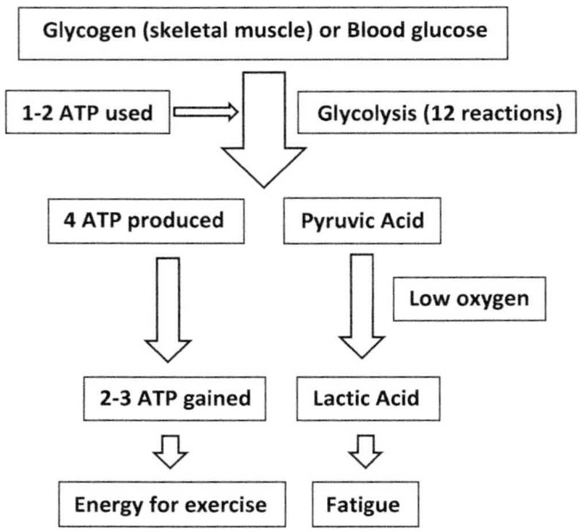

Exhibit 4.3 Anaerobic system (glycolytic system) for ATP

For sustained exercise, ATP production relies progressively more on the **aerobic system**, in which oxygen consumption by the cells is sufficient to produce ATP "oxidatively." Carbohydrate, fat, and protein are all energy sources for the aerobic system (Smith et al., 2022). Carbohydrate in the form of glucose (from glycogen and/or blood glucose) can be "oxidized" through the process of **aerobic glycolysis** in the cytoplasm of the muscle cell to **pyruvate** molecules. Pyruvate then enters the mitochondria and are converted to **acetyl coA** molecules. Acetyl coA enters a metabolic pathway called the **Kreb's cycle** where reactions produce ATP and **reduced coenzyme molecules** ("electron carriers"). Reduced coenzymes carry electrons (and hydrogen ions) to a chain of reactions referred to as the **electron transport system**. The movement of hydrogens and electrons through this chain results in the production of many ATP with oxygen ultimately being used to accept the hydrogens and electrons to form water (H_2O) (Smith et al., 2022) (Exhibit 4.4).

During fat utilization, triglycerides are split into a glycerol molecule and three fatty acid molecules. The fatty acids are broken down through a process called **beta oxidation** which results in the production of numerous acetyl coA molecules allowing for production of many ATP molecules (via the Kreb's Cycle and electron transport system, as described above) (Smith, Plowman, and Ormsbee, 2022).

Protein is made up of amino acid molecules. It is only used sparingly for ATP production during exercise. For it to be utilized, protein is broken down into individual amino acids which produce ATP in similar manner to carbohydrate and fat (i.e., via glycolysis, the Kreb's Cycle, and the electron transport system) (Smith, Plowman, and Ormsbee, 2022) (Exhibit 4.4).

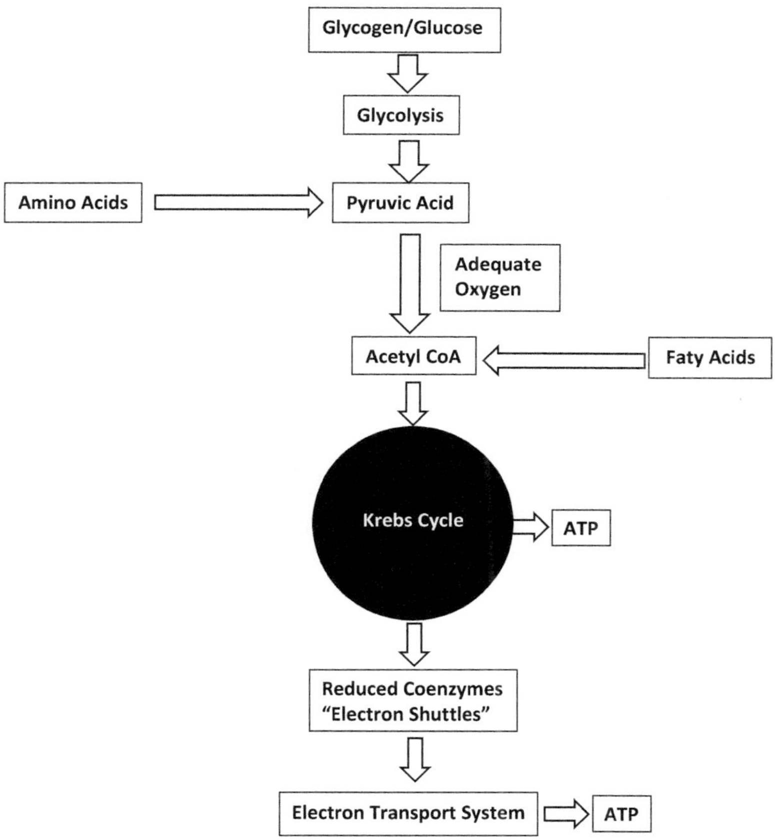

Exhibit 4.4 Aerobic system for ATP

As mentioned above, energy metabolism is comprised of many chemical reactions and metabolic pathways. The reactions are catalyzed by proteins called enzymes. These "catalysts" must be controlled precisely to allow for the right amount of ATP to be available under all conditions. Thus, the control of bioenergetics is achieved by influencing the ability of certain enzymes to catalyze specific reactions. In energy metabolism, this is primarily achieved by control of a rate-limiting enzyme in a pathway and are commonly influenced by the level of ATP (and ADP+P) in the cell and can adjust their catalytic pace based on those levels (e.g., low ATP and high ADP + P increase the rate) (Powers, Howley, and Quindry, 2024).

In summary, it is important that students interested in exercise science develop a strong understanding of bioenergetics and metabolism, since it is essential for evaluating energy needs and allows professionals to tailor dietary recommendations based upon an individual's energy requirements, activity level, and personal goals. It also aids in optimizing nutrient timing by providing insights into how and when carbohydrates, proteins, and fats are utilized for energy, recovery, and performance. This knowledge is also important for promoting health by identifying how imbalances in energy intake and expenditure can lead to conditions such as obesity, diabetes, and metabolic disorders.

Energy Needs, Energy Balance, and Energy Availability

The term used in nutrition and physiology to measure the energy content of food and energy expenditure is the Calorie (with a capital C) or kilocalorie (kcal) and is defined as the amount of heat necessary to raise the temperature of 1 liter of water by 1° Celsius. In an everyday nutritional context, kcals are typically expressed as Calories. For example, if a food label states that a serving contains 140 Calories, it really means that it contains 140 *kcals* (1 Calorie (big C) = 1 kcal = 1000 calories (small c)).

Getting enough energy through food, known as **energy intake (EI)**, is the foundation of good nutrition. Adequate EI is essential not only for peak performance but also for supporting the body's normal physiological and metabolic functions. How much energy a person needs depends on several factors, such as age, sex, body composition, environmental conditions (like altitude or temperature), and their level of physical activity. If someone does not consume enough energy, it can lead to poor performance, slower recovery, loss of muscle mass and bone strength, as well as increase the risk of injury, illness, or result in menstrual problems in females (Thomas et al., 2016).

Energy balance occurs when EI through food matches the energy used by the body, referred to as **total daily energy expenditure (TDEE)**. Tools like food diaries, 24-hour diet recalls, and interviews are often used to estimate EI, although it is not uncommon for athletes and other highly active people to underreport how much they eat (Thomas et al., 2016).

TDEE consists of three main components:

1. **Basal Metabolic Rate (BMR)**: this is the energy (i.e., Calories) the body needs to perform basic functions, like breathing and maintaining heart rate, while at complete rest. BMR is difficult to measure directly because strict conditions are required (i.e., measured after overnight fasting and no recent exercise). Instead, **Resting Metabolic Rate (RMR)**, which is about 10% higher than BMR, is often measured since testing only requires about 10–20 minutes. For sedentary people, RMR makes up about 60–80% of their TDEE, but for very active individuals, it may represent only 38–47% (Thomas et al., 2016).
2. **Thermic Effect of Food (TEF)**: this refers to the energy used to digest, absorb, and store food and accounts for about 10% of TDEE.
3. **Thermic Effect of Activity (TEA)**: this encompasses all energy used during physical activity and includes:

    a. **exercise energy expenditure (EEX)**: energy used during structured exercise
    b. **excess post-exercise oxygen consumption (EPOC)**: the extra energy used to recover after exercise, which can contribute up to 15% of TDEE in active individuals (Thomas et al., 2016)
    c. **non-exercise activity thermogenesis (NEAT)**: energy used for everyday activities like walking, standing, housekeeping, yardwork, and spontaneous movements like fidgeting

Together, these components determine TDEE, showing that energy expenditure involves much more than just structured exercise.

Measuring Energy Needs

In laboratory settings, TDEE can be measured using methods like **direct and indirect calorimetry** or **doubly labeled water,** which tracks how quickly certain isotopes leave the body (Heydenreich et al., 2017). These methods are accurate but expensive and impractical for everyday use. Instead, simple equations like the revised Harris-Benedict equation (Mifflin et al., 1990), Cunningham equation (Cunningham, 1980), or Mifflin-St Jeor equation (Mifflin et al., 1990) are commonly used to estimate RMR, which is then multiplied by an activity factor to estimate TDEE.

Exhibit 4.5 Calculating energy requirements

Revised Harris-Benedict Equation

Adult Males	Adult Females
RMR = 13.397 (weight in kg) + 4.799 (height in cm) – 5.677 (age) + 88.362	RMR = 9.247 (weight in kg) + 3.098 (height in cm) – 4.33 (age) + 447.593

Mifflin-St Jeor Equation

Adult Males	Adult Females
RMR = 10 (weight in kg) + 6.25 (height in cm) – 5 (age) + 5	RMR = 10 (weight in kg) + 6.25 (height in cm) – 5 (age) -161

Cunningham Equation

Males and Females
RMR = 500 + 22 FFM (kg)

Dietary Reference Intakes (DRI) Method: Estimated Energy Requirements for Adults

Males	Females
662–9.53 (age) + PA x (15.91 x (weight in kg) + 539.6 x (height in meters))	354–6.91 (age) + PA x (9.36 x (weight in kg) +726 x (height in meters))
PA (physical activity)	PA (physical activity)
Sedentary: 1.0	Sedentary: 1.0
Low active: 1.11	Low Active: 1.12
Active: 1.25	Active: 1.27
Very Active: 1.48	Very Active: 1.45

Source: Institute of Medicine (2005).

Resting Energy Expenditure (REE) Calculations and Activity Factors

Gender and Age (years)	*Equation (BW in kilograms)*	*Activity Factor*
Males, 10 to 18 years old	REE = (17.5 x BW) + 651	1.6 – 2.4
Males, 19 to 30 years old	REE = (15.3 x BW) + 679	1.6 – 2.4
Males, 31 to 60 years old	REE = (11.6 x BW) + 879	1.6 – 2.4
Females, 10 to 18 years old	REE = (12.2 x BW) + 749	1.6 – 2.4
Females, 19 to 30 years old	REE = (14.7 x BW) + 496	1.6 – 2.4
Females, 31 to 60 years old	REE = (8.7 x BW) + 829	1.6 – 2.4

Source: World Health Organization (1985).

Energy Availability (EA)

Another important concept in understanding energy needs is **energy availability (EA)**. EA refers to the energy left over for normal body functions after subtracting the energy used during exercise (EEX), standardized to kilograms of fat-free mass (FFM, i.e., muscle, bone, connective tissue). It is calculated using the formula: *EA = (EI – EEX) / fat-free mass (FFM)*.

The concept of EA emerged from studies on the **Female Athlete Triad.** Scientists found that an EA of 45 kcal/kg FFM per day supports health and energy balance. On the other hand, long-term low EA (≤30 kcal/kg FFM per day) can lead to serious health problems, including slower metabolism, weaker bones, and issues with the endocrine, cardiovascular, and reproductive systems (Loucks, Kiens, and Wright, 2011).

Dietary Guidelines

Nutrients are the nourishing substances found in food that the body uses for vital body processes. Therefore, for optimal health, it is important to consume a balanced diet that includes fruits, vegetables, whole grains, healthy fats, and protein. Carbohydrates, fats, and protein are referred to as **macronutrients,** because the body needs them in large amounts to function and provide fuel (i.e., Calories). **Micronutrients** include vitamins and minerals such as iron, zinc, and vitamins A, D, E, and K, that the body needs in very small amounts. Although they have no caloric value, they are essential for health and metabolism since they primarily serve as regulators in metabolic reactions. The Dietary Guidelines for Americans (DGA) and MyPlate® (Exhibit 4.6) and The New Pyramid (released in January 2026), are all useful tools developed by the US government to help Americans develop eating habits that stress balance, variety, and moderation to promote health and prevent disease. Interested readers are encouraged to visit the DGA (n.d.) and MyPlate® (n.d.) websites to learn more.

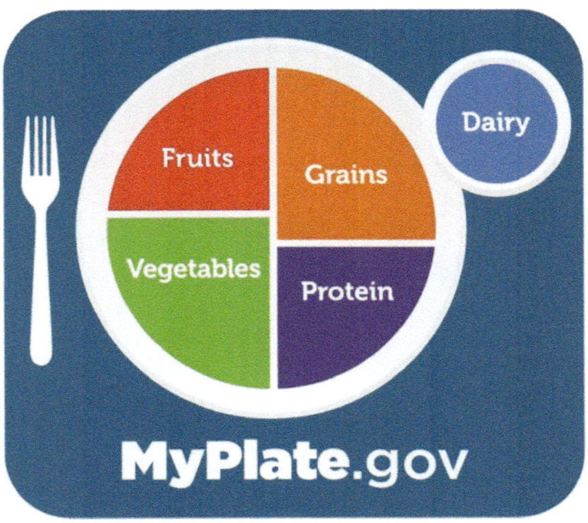

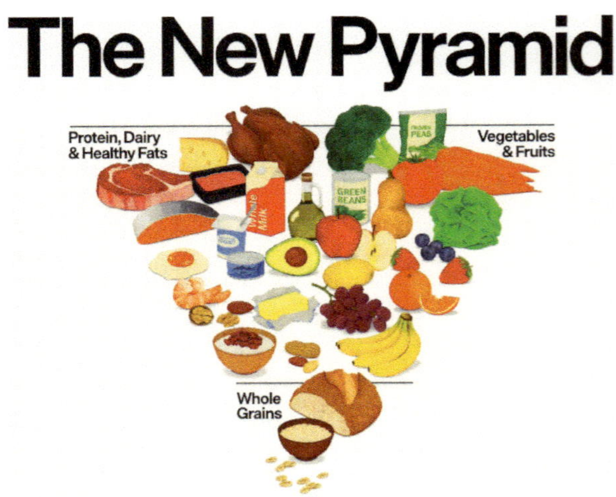

Exhibit 4.6 MyPlate® and The New Pyramid

Carbohydrates

Carbohydrates are composed of carbon, hydrogen, and oxygen (CHO) and are often referred to as the master fuel because they serve as the primary source for energy. Carbohydrates are classified into two main types: **simple** and **complex**, both of which play important roles in nutrition.

Simple carbohydrates are smaller, basic forms of carbohydrates and include **monosaccharides**, or single sugar units, such as glucose (the body's primary energy source), fructose (found in fruits), and galactose (found in dairy products), and the **disaccharides**, which are formed when two monosaccharides bond together. Common disaccharides include sucrose (table sugar, glucose + fructose), lactose (milk sugar, glucose + galactose), and maltose (found in malted foods and beverages, glucose + glucose).

Complex carbohydrates are larger molecules made up of long chains of simple sugars. These include **starches** (found in foods like bread, rice, and potatoes) and **glycogen**, which is the storage form of glucose in the body. Glycogen is a glucose polymer, meaning it consists of many glucose molecules linked together in a repeating chain. Due to their larger size and heavier molecular weight, complex carbohydrates take longer to break down, providing a more sustained release of energy compared to simple carbohydrates (Fink and Mikesky, 2025).

Another key category of complex carbohydrates includes **fibrous carbohydrates**, which are primarily found in plant-based foods like vegetables, fruits, legumes, and whole grains. Fibrous carbohydrates contain dietary fiber that cannot be fully broken down by digestive enzymes. Fiber types include **soluble fiber**, which dissolves in water and helps regulate blood sugar and cholesterol levels, and **insoluble fiber**, which adds bulk to stool and supports healthy digestion. Unlike other carbohydrates, fiber does not provide energy directly, but it plays an important role in maintaining gut health and preventing diseases like heart disease and diabetes (Fink and Mikesky, 2025).

The **glycemic response** refers to the change in blood glucose levels following the consumption of carbohydrate-containing foods. Simple carbohydrates, including glucose, table sugar, and foods made with refined flour, are digested and absorbed quickly, leading to a rapid rise in blood sugar. In contrast, complex carbohydrates, such as those found in whole grains, legumes, and vegetables, are broken down more slowly, resulting in a more gradual increase in blood glucose. To classify these differences, nutrition scientists developed the concepts of **glycemic index (GI)** and **glycemic load (GL)**. These tools help evaluate both the quality and quantity of carbohydrates in foods and are useful for managing blood sugar, appetite, and the risk of chronic disease.

The GI ranks carbohydrate containing foods based on how quickly they raise blood glucose levels compared to glucose or white bread, which are given a standardized GI of 100, and are classified as high GI (>70), medium GI (56–69), or low GI (<55) (Beavers and Leutholtz, 2008). In addition to the type of carbohydrate consumed, several other factors influence GI including the amount of fiber, cooking method, food processing, and whether it is eaten with fat, protein, or other foods. For example, the GI of a potato can vary depending on how it is cooked (mashed vs. baked vs. fried) and what types of toppings may be added (butter vs. sour cream vs. ketchup). Foods that are **nutrient dense** (i.e., low in Calories and high in nutrients) like fruit, whole grains, and legumes have a low GI because they are digested slowly resulting in a lower, more controlled rise in blood glucose. In contrast, foods with a high GI such as white bread, jellybeans, and sports drinks are rapidly digested and absorbed leading to a quick spike in blood glucose.

Glycemic load considers both the quality (i.e., the GI) and the *quantity* of carbohydrates in a food. It is calculated by multiplying the GI by the number of grams of carbohydrate in a serving and dividing by 100 and is also classified as high (>20), medium (11–19), or low (≤10) (Beavers and Leutholtz, 2008). Foods with a low GI also have a low GL. However, foods with an intermediate or high GI may have a GL that ranges from low to high. For example, as shown in Exhibit 4.7, one slice of Wonder™ white bread contains 14.5 g of carbohydrate and has a high GI (77) and a medium GL (12) (The University of Sydney, n.d.).

Exhibit 4.7 Glycemic index and glycemic load of selected foods

Food Item	*Carbohydrate Content (g)*	*Glycemic Index (GI)*	*Glycemic Load (GL)*
Wonder White Bread (1 slice)	14.5	77	12
Mashed potato	24.0	73	17
Garbanzo beans	30.0	31	9
Jellybeans	28.0	80	22

Source: University of Sydney (n.d.).

Understanding both GI and GL is important for long-term health and also has implications for enhancing sports performance and recovery. For example, diets that are lower in GI and GL have been shown to improve insulin sensitivity, reduce hunger, and maintain blood glucose levels, which is important for weight control and preventing chronic diseases. In contrast, diets that are higher in GI and GL may increase the risk of heart disease and type 2 diabetes by promoting oxidative stress, inflammation, and excess insulin demand (Marsh et al., 2011). For athletes, consuming high GI foods and beverages may be beneficial during or after intense exercise to quickly replenish glycogen stores.

According to the DGA, the **Acceptable Macronutrient Distribution Range (AMDR)** for carbohydrates is **45–65% of total daily Calorie intake** to ensure that the body has enough energy for physical activity, brain function, and other essential processes. Within that range, it is recommended that the majority of daily Calories come from complex carbohydrates and that no more than 10–15% come from added sugars. Therefore, a person consuming 2,000 Calories per day should aim for about 900–1,300 Calories from carbohydrates, which is equivalent to 225–325 g since the energy value of digestible carbohydrates is 4 Calories per gram.

Because carbohydrate needs vary widely between individuals, recommendations can also be made based on body weight (BW). A general recommendation for athletes is 5–10 g per kilogram (kg) of BW; however, elite athletes who train several hours a day may need as much as 12 g/kg to meet daily Calorie needs. In general, recreational athletes who exercise 3–5 days per week can usually meet their carbohydrate requirements at the lower end of the range, while competitive athletes who may train up to 6 days per week or participate in multiple workouts throughout the day would require amounts at the higher end (Fink and Mikesky, 2025). For example, if a recommendation of 5–7 g/kg was made for a 70 kg individual who is performing moderate-to-high intensity exercise 4–5 times per week, they would need to consume between 350–490 g per day, which is equivalent to 1400–1960 Calories. Keep in mind that value does not account for Calories needed from protein and fat and demonstrates that active individuals need to consume more Calories compared to sedentary individuals who may need ≤ 4 g/kg to meet daily Calorie needs.

Protein

Protein is a major component of the body structure and has a role in virtually every body process including immune and endocrine function, and in tissue growth, maintenance, and repair. It can also serve as an energy source during prolonged exercise (when glycogen stores become depleted) or during periods of starvation.

Proteins are composed of carbon, hydrogen, oxygen, and nitrogen, with nitrogen being the distinguishing feature compared to CHO and fats. These elements combine to form **amino acids**, the building blocks of protein. Proteins are created when amino acids link together, forming dipeptides (two amino acids) or polypeptides (many amino acids).

There are 20 amino acids needed for protein synthesis, including **nine essential amino acids** that must be obtained through the diet and **11 non-essential amino acids** that the body can create (Exhibit 4.8). During periods of severe illness, physiological stress, or rapid growth, the body may be unable to produce certain non-essential amino acids quickly enough to meet its needs. In these situations, they become **conditionally essential,** meaning they must be obtained through the diet. Examples include arginine, cysteine, glutamine, tyrosine, glycine, proline, and serine. **Complete proteins**, such as those found in animal products, contain all nine essential amino acids in the right amounts to support life and growth. **Incomplete proteins**, often found in plant sources, lack one or more essential amino acids but can be combined with other plant foods to provide all the necessary amino acids for optimal nutrition. Soy protein, for example, is a plant protein that is nearly equivalent to animal protein in quality, although it has small amounts of methionine (Fink and Mikesky, 2025).

Exhibit 4.8 Essential and non-essential amino acids

Essential Amino Acids	*Non-essential Amino Acids*
Isoleucine	Alanine
Leucine	Arginine
Valine	Asparagine
Histidine	Aspartic Acid
Tryptophan	Cysteine
Threonine	Glutamine
Phenylalanine	Glutamic Acid
Methionine	Glycine
Lysine	Proline
	Serine
	Tyrosine

High-quality protein sources include animal-based foods such as meat, fish, poultry, eggs, and dairy products. Plant-based sources like legumes (beans, lentils, soybeans), nuts, and seeds are good sources, although they often contain less protein per serving compared to animal products. Grains, fruits, and vegetables, while nutritious, have relatively low protein content. In practice, consuming a variety of animal and plant proteins ensures adequate intake of essential amino acids while also providing additional nutrients like fiber, vitamins, iron, and calcium.

Protein needs vary based on age, activity level, and physiological demands. The RDA for the average adult is 0.8 g/kg/BW (0.36 g/lb.), however, athletes and elderly adults require higher amounts typically ranging from 1.2–2.0 g/kg or higher (Baum, Kim, and Wolfe, 2016; Thomas et al., 2016). For children, the requirements range from

0.85–0.95 g/kg depending on their stage of growth (Trumbo et al., 2002). The AMDR for protein is **10–35% of daily Calorie intake**, with an average intake of about **12–15%** for most individuals. Similar to carbohydrates, the energy value of protein is 4 Calories per gram.

Fats

Although the terms are often used interchangeably, "fat" is actually a specific type of lipid, a broader category that also includes oils, sterols, and related compounds. Lipids are primarily composed of carbon and hydrogen atoms and are characterized by their inability to dissolve in water, making them hydrophobic in nature. Lipids are an essential macronutrient that provide a concentrated source of energy and serve many critical functions in the body.

Triglycerides are the predominant type of lipid, making up the majority of dietary fats as well as the fat stored in the body. Triglycerides are found in small amounts in the muscles and liver where they serve as a readily available source of energy; however most are stored in the adipose tissue surrounding the organs and under the skin (i.e., subcutaneous fat). As described earlier, a triglyceride molecule consists of one glycerol backbone attached to three fatty acids, which can vary in length and saturation. These fatty acids are the main fuel source during periods of rest and prolonged, low-intensity physical activity (Fink and Mikesky, 2025).

In addition to serving as a major energy reserve, lipids are essential for physiological processes, including the absorption of fat-soluble vitamins (A, D, E, and K), insulation to regulate body temperature, and protection of vital organs. Dietary fat provides more than twice the energy per gram (9 Calories per gram) than carbohydrate or protein, which explains why it is the major storage form of energy for the body.

The AMDR for fats is **20–35% of total daily Calorie intake**. For a person consuming 2,000 Calories per day, this equates to 400–700 Calories from fats, or about 44–78 g per day. A balanced fat intake should include sources of healthy fats, such as unsaturated fats from nuts, seeds, avocados, and fatty fish, while limiting saturated fats from animal products and trans fats found in butter and margarine, to reduce the risk of chronic disease.

Water

Water is often overlooked as a nutrient, yet it is the most vital for life, since even mild dehydration can significantly hinder physical performance and daily activities, while severe dehydration can be life-threatening. Water comprises 55–60% body weight and, therefore, is a key component of body composition, particularly in muscle tissue where it accounts for about 75% of muscle mass (McCardle, Katch, and Katch, 2023).

Water has several major functions in the body, including stabilizing body temperature. For example, water dissipates heat through mechanisms like conduction, convection, radiation, and evaporation during sweating. Water also acts as a solvent, facilitating the transport of nutrients and the removal of waste products. As a structural component of cells, water supports tissue integrity and contributes to proper cellular function. Additionally, it lubricates and cushions joints, reducing friction and enabling smooth movement.

The body gets water through the consumption of beverages and foods high in water content, such as fruits and vegetables. However, water is continuously lost through various processes, including urine excretion, sweating, and smaller amounts through feces and water vapor during respiration. The kidneys play a central role in maintaining body water balance by regulating urine production based on hydration status. Two practical ways to help ensure proper hydration are to monitor BW, since daily weight fluctuations are typically caused by changes in water status, and to subjectively evaluate urine color. When adequately hydrated, urine color is either clear or pale yellow, whereas dark, concentrated urine indicates dehydration. Other methods of assessing hydration related to urine include measuring specific gravity and volume. While rare, it is possible to become overhydrated (i.e., water intoxication) and the symptoms are similar to those associated with dehydration including mental confusion, nausea and vomiting, seizures, and unconsciousness (Fink and Mikesky, 2025).

Daily water needs vary from person to person depending upon several factors including activity level, climate, age, medications, altitude, metabolism, and overall health. Because of these interindividual differences, an **Adequate Intake (AI)** (discussed later in this section) has been established instead of an RDA, with general guidelines of 11.5 cups (2.7 L) per day for women and 15.5 cups (3.7 L) for men (Fink and Mikesky, 2025).

Vitamins and Minerals

Vitamins and minerals are essential micronutrients required by the body in small amounts for optimal health and functioning. Vitamins are organic compounds, meaning they contain carbon and hydrogen, and are categorized as either water-soluble (e.g., B-complex vitamins and vitamin C) or fat-soluble (e.g., vitamins A, D, E, and K). Minerals are inorganic elements like calcium, potassium, and iron, classified as either macrominerals (required in larger amounts such as potassium, magnesium, and calcium) or trace minerals (required in smaller quantities such as iron, copper, and zinc) (Fink and Mikesky, 2025).

Both vitamins and minerals play critical roles in metabolism, acting as coenzymes or cofactors that facilitate biochemical reactions involved in energy production, protein synthesis, and the breakdown of macronutrients. For example, B vitamins are essential for converting carbohydrates into usable energy, while minerals like magnesium and zinc regulate enzymatic activity.

In addition to their important role in metabolism, vitamins and minerals support many physiological functions. Vitamins contribute to immune function, vision, blood clotting, and cellular repair, while minerals are vital for bone health, oxygen transport (via hemoglobin), fluid balance, and nerve signaling (Fink and Mikesky, 2025). A balanced intake of vitamins and minerals through diet or supplementation (i.e., multivitamin/multimineral) is crucial to maintaining health and performance, and preventing deficiencies that can lead to various diseases.

Key Dietary Reference Terms

When evaluating an individual's nutrient intake, the RDA is typically used as the primary reference standard. The RDA is not a minimum requirement but, rather, an intake level that exceeds the needs of most (97–98%) healthy individuals. While it is not necessary to meet the RDA each day, an individual's average intake should meet the RDA over a

5–8-day period. Registered dietitians generally become concerned if someone consistently consumes less than two-thirds of the RDA for a particular nutrient. Other dietary reference values, such as the **Estimated Average Requirement (EAR)**, **Tolerable Upper Intake Level (UL)**, and **AI**, are used primarily in clinical or population-based assessments and are defined below:

- **Estimated Average Requirement (EAR):** the daily intake value estimated to meet the nutrient requirement of 50% of healthy individuals within a specific group and must be known to establish the RDA
- **Adequate Intake (AI):** established when there is not enough evidence to develop an EAR/RDA and represents the average daily intake based on current data to be sufficient to meet the nutritional needs of most healthy individuals in a specific group
- **Tolerable Upper Intake Level (UL):** the maximum daily level of nutrient intake that is unlikely to cause harmful health effects in most individuals

The **Dietary Reference Intake (DRI)** is an umbrella term used to describe guidelines for nutrient intake that includes the RDA, EAR, AI, and UL.

To help consumers make informed dietary choices, food labels use **Daily Values (DVs)**, which are based on two components: **Reference Daily Intakes (RDIs)** and **Daily Reference Values (DRVs)**. RDIs are derived from the RDAs and apply to vitamins and minerals. In contrast, DRVs are used for nutrients that do not have RDAs, such as total fat, saturated fat, cholesterol, carbohydrate, fiber, sodium, potassium, and protein. These values are shown as percentages on food labels and are typically based on a 2,000-Calorie diet. For example, the DRI for carbohydrate is 130 g per day (based on the minimum amount needed by the brain), however, the DV listed on food labels is 300 g, reflecting the higher intake recommended for a general healthy diet (The Food and Nutrition Board of the National Academies of Sciences, Engineering, and Medicine, n.d.).

The Nutrition Facts Label

Food labeling in the United States is regulated by the Food and Drug Administration (FDA). The Nutrition Labeling and Education Act of 1990 mandated standardized labeling on most packaged foods, leading to the introduction of the Nutrition Facts label in 1994. Prior to this, food labels lacked consistency and comprehensive nutritional information. The FDA updated the label in 2016 to reflect advances in nutrition science and changes in consumer eating habits. Currently, the Nutrition Facts label must include the following components to comply with FDA guidelines:

- **statement of identity**: the common or descriptive name of the food product (e.g., "whole grain cereal")
- **net contents**: the quantity of food in the package, shown by weight, volume, or count (e.g., "16 oz" or "12 cookies"), usually located on the front bottom edge
- **manufacturer information**: the name and address of the manufacturer, packer, or distributor, usually listed near the ingredient list
- **ingredient list**: lists all ingredients in descending order by weight. This is especially helpful for identifying potential allergens (e.g., nuts, gluten) or additives, and assessing the overall nutritional quality of the food

The **Nutrition Facts Panel** is usually on the back or the side of the packaging and provides the following dietary information:

- **serving size and servings per container:** standardized to reflect what people typically eat vs. the recommended intake, so that nutrition comparisons across similar products are easier to make
- **Calories:** the total number of Calories per serving is prominently displayed
- **nutrients listed:** includes total fat, saturated fat, trans fat, cholesterol, sodium, total carbohydrates, dietary fiber, total sugars, added sugars, and protein
- **micronutrients:** required micronutrients include vitamin D, calcium, iron, and potassium (vitamin A and C were previously required but are now optional unless added to the product)
- **% daily values (%DV):** based on a 2,000-kcal daily diet to help consumers gauge how much a nutrient in a serving of food contributes to their total daily intake. As previously discussed, the %DV is based on either RDIs for vitamins and minerals or DRVs for nutrients without established RDAs (FDA, n.d.c).

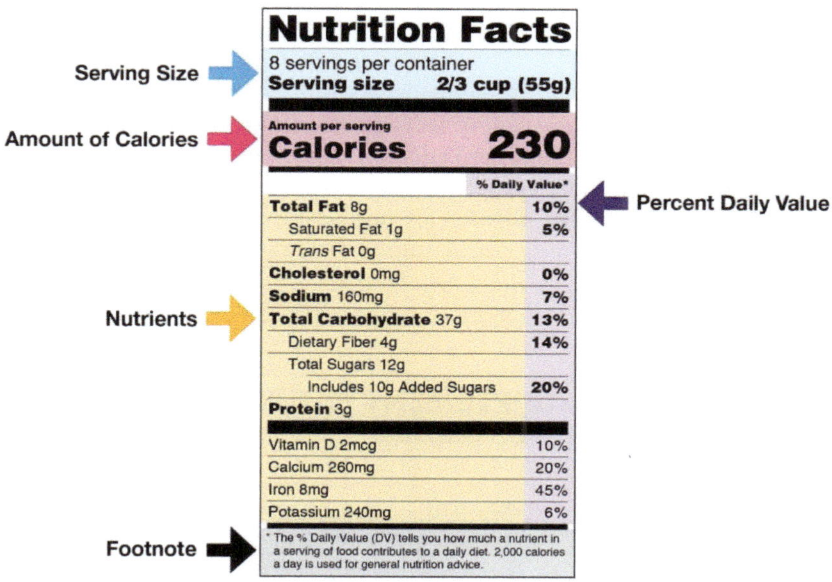

(For educational purposes only. These labels do not meet the labeling requirements described in 21 CFR 101.9.)

Exhibit 4.9 Nutrition facts panel

The new regulations also allow food manufacturers to make nutrient content and health claims on packaging, but only if they meet specific criteria established by the FDA. Nutrient content claims such as low fat, high fiber, or reduced sodium must adhere to clearly defined thresholds for the amount of the nutrient per serving. Health claims, which link a food or nutrient to a reduced risk of a disease or health-related condition (e.g., calcium may reduce the risk of osteoporosis), are permitted only when supported by significant scientific agreement and reviewed by the FDA. These standards help prevent misleading information and ensure that any claims made on packaging are truthful and based on scientific evidence (FDA, n.d.b).

Dietary Supplements

Dietary supplements have become increasingly popular among individuals who want to improve their health and/or physical performance. While many supplements are marketed as natural and beneficial, their safety and effectiveness are not always well understood or well-studied. Unlike prescription drugs, dietary supplements do not require FDA approval before reaching the market, which makes it especially important for consumers to be informed. To provide a legal framework for the production and sale of these products, Congress passed the Dietary Supplement Health and Education Act (DSHEA) in 1994, which defines a dietary supplement as a product that contains one or more dietary ingredients, such as a vitamin, mineral, herb or botanical, amino acid, or other substances that supplement the diet. Unlike traditional foods, supplements cannot be marketed as a conventional food or as the sole item of a meal or diet. Examples include multivitamin/multimineral supplements, herbal remedies (e.g., ginseng, echinacea), protein powders, ready-to-drink (RTD) shakes, energy bars, and beverages like Gatorade® and Red Bull®.

As mentioned above, dietary supplements are not regulated like drugs and are not required to undergo the rigorous safety testing and clinical trials that are standard for medications. Instead, the FDA and the **Federal Trade Commission (FTC)** share responsibility for oversight. The FDA enforces labeling standards and requires manufacturers to notify the agency within 30 days of marketing a new supplement that makes statements describing how a nutrient or ingredient may affect normal body structure

SUPPLEMENT FACTS
Serving Size: 1 Capsule
Servings Per Container: 60

Amount Per Serving	% Daily Value
Vitamin C (as Ascorbic Acid) – 100 mg	111%
Vitamin D3 (Cholecalciferol) – 25 mcg (1000 IU)	125%
Zinc (as Zinc Gluconate) – 11 mg	100%
Magnesium (as Magnesium Oxide) – 100 mg	24%
Ashwagandha Root Extract – 300 mg	*
Turmeric Root Powder – 200 mg	*
Black Pepper Extract – 5 mg	*

*Daily Value not established.

Exhibit 4.10 Dietary supplement facts panel

or function (i.e., **structure/function claims**). Products can claim to help with general conditions associated with life stages, such as pregnancy, menopause, or aging, but they may not claim to diagnose, treat, cure, or prevent disease. For example, the claim that "glucosamine helps support joint health" is acceptable, whereas a claim stating that "glucosamine *cures* arthritis" is not. To clarify this, all supplement labels must include a disclaimer, such as: "This statement has not been evaluated by the Food and Drug Administration. This product is not intended to diagnose, treat, cure, or prevent any disease."

The FTC is responsible for regulating the advertising of dietary supplements and ensures that marketing claims made on product packaging, in print, online, or in commercials are truthful and not misleading. If a company makes exaggerated or unsubstantiated claims, it may face fines, lawsuits, or forced product recalls. Weight-loss supplements are among the most frequently targeted by the FTC for making deceptive claims or promoting results that are not supported by scientific evidence.

Because dietary supplements are not required to demonstrate safety or effectiveness before being sold, their quality and content can vary widely. For example, the ingredients listed on the label may not accurately reflect what is in the product. Supplements may also be contaminated or contain illegal substances, and there can be inconsistencies between different batches of the same product (Exhibit 4.10). Therefore, consumers should be cautious and seek guidance from healthcare professionals when considering supplement use, especially if taking prescription medications or managing a chronic condition (FDA, n.d.a).

APPLICATIONS TO EXERCISE SCIENCE

Nutrition plays a vital role in health, physical activity, and athletic performance, making it a foundational area of study in exercise science. Whether the goal is to improve general fitness, enhance athletic performance, or prevent and manage chronic disease, understanding how dietary strategies support movement, recovery, and overall well-being is essential. The following sections explore the health and clinical applications of nutrition, followed by its application in sports and performance.

HEALTH/CLINICAL ASPECTS

Epidemiological, animal, clinical, and metabolic studies consistently demonstrate that both diet and physical activity play vital roles in promoting health and preventing disease. Clinical research, in particular, shows that diet and exercise work synergistically to prevent and manage conditions such as high cholesterol (hyperlipidemia), high blood pressure (hypertension), type 2 diabetes, osteoporosis, and certain types of cancer. Chronic low-grade inflammation has been associated with the development of many of these diseases. Diets, including the Mediterranean diet (Exhibit 4.11), DASH (Dietary Approaches to Stop Hypertension) diet, and vegetarian diets, that are rich in fruits, vegetables, whole grains, omega-3 fatty acids, and antioxidants may help reduce systemic inflammation, whereas diets high in refined carbohydrates, trans fats, and added sugars are pro-inflammatory (van Zonneveld et al., 2024). In short, current evidence suggests that individuals who are physically active and consume diets lower in saturated fat and refined carbohydrates, and higher in whole foods tend to have lower mortality rates and a reduced risk of chronic disease compared to their sedentary peers (O'Sullivan et al., 2013; Shivappa et al., 2016; Fishman et al., 2016).

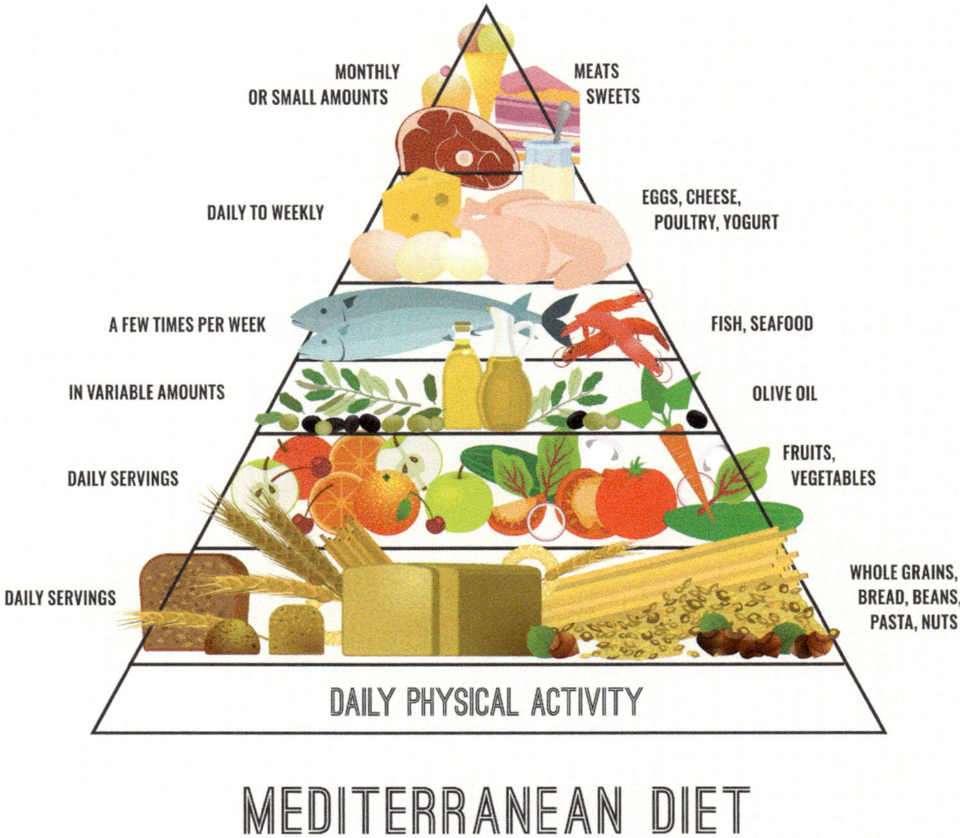

Exhibit 4.11 Mediterranean diet food pyramid

Nutrigenomics

Chronic diseases such as CHD and type 2 diabetes develop through complex interactions between genes and the environment, including diet (Ferguson et al., 2016; Neeha and Kinth, 2013; Capozzi and Bordoni, 2013; Roberts and Barnard, 2005). Recent advances in molecular biology, including completion of the Human Genome Project and the International HapMap Project, have improved our understanding of how nutrients affect gene expression. This emerging field, known as nutritional genomics or **nutrigenomics**, investigates how an individual's genetic makeup influences their response to nutrients and how those nutrients may, in turn, regulate gene expression. This research has paved the way for **personalized nutrition**, where dietary recommendations are tailored to a person's unique genetic profile to help prevent disease and improve health outcomes (Isaak and Siow, 2013).

Obesity

Obesity continues to be one of the most pressing public health concerns in the United States and other industrialized countries. According to NHANES data from 2021–2023, the prevalence of obesity (BMI ≥ 30) among adults aged 20 and older was 40.3%, which is relatively unchanged from the 2013–2014 report. However, the prevalence of severe obesity (BMI ≥ 40) increased from 7.7% to 9.7% during that period (Emmerich et al., 2024). In response to these trends, there is increasing interest in the development of fat substitutes, weight-loss medications, and dietary interventions aimed at reducing body weight and fat mass. Research in this area often examines the roles of nutrition and metabolism, including how specific nutrients influence energy balance, fat storage, hormonal regulation, and inflammation.

Gut Microbiota and Digestive Health

The gut microbiome is the diverse community of microorganisms including bacteria, yeast, and viruses that live in the digestive tract. These microbes play essential roles in breaking down food, regulating metabolism, and supporting immune function. Probiotics and prebiotics are parts of food that work symbiotically to maintain a healthy microbiome and are often referred to as gut flora or gut microbiota. **Probiotics** are live beneficial bacteria found in fermented foods like yogurt, kefir, kimchi, sauerkraut, and pickles. **Prebiotics**, on the other hand, are types of dietary fiber that serve as fuel for probiotics and help them thrive. Research suggests that exercise and a diet rich in prebiotics, probiotics, fiber, fermented foods, and plant-based nutrients can positively influence the composition and diversity of gut bacteria, which is associated with improved immune function, reduced inflammation, and better overall metabolic health (van Zonneveld et al., 2024). The following abstract suggests that long-term sauerkraut supplementation may have positive effects on gut microbiota in athletes (Exhibit 4.12).

Exhibit 4.12 The short- and long-term effects of a short course of sauerkraut supplementation on the gut microbiota of active athletes: a pilot follow-up study

Zonjić, J., Karačić, A., Brodić, I., Starčević, A., Renko, I., Krznarić, Ž., Ivančić, M., Liberati Pršo, A. M., and Šatalić, Z. (2025). The short- and long-term effects of a short course of sauerkraut supplementation on the gut microbiota of active athletes: a pilot follow-up study. *Nutrients*, *17*(5), 929. https://doi.org/10.3390/nu17050929

Abstract

Objectives: The application of whole fermented foods in sports nutrition for gut microbiota personalization is a promising area of investigation. Sauerkraut, a traditional fermented food, has not been extensively studied in this context. This study aimed to replicate earlier findings of a proof-of-concept study on the potential of sauerkraut for gut microbiota personalization in active athletes.

Methods: A pilot follow-up study was conducted on active recreational athletes who consumed 250 g of organic pasteurized sauerkraut daily for 10 days. Changes in gut microbiota composition and functionality were assessed using 16S rRNA sequencing and metabolic pathway analysis across three time points: pre-intervention, postintervention, and one-month postintervention. Laboratory parameters, bowel function, and side effects were monitored throughout the study.

Results: In total, 11 male participants with an average age of 30 years completed the study. The pilot follow-up study did not replicate the original study's findings on sauerkraut's short-term effects on β-diversity and taxonomic and functional groups. However, long-term effects of sauerkraut supplementation were demonstrated, including a significant reduction in β-diversity variance and increased gut microbiota composition similarity (β-diversity) as well as several significant changes in bacterial taxa and metabolic pathways after a washout period. The intervention also induced a transient decrease in B12 vitamin levels and a short- and long-term increase in leukocyte concentrations. The probability for physiological types of stools increased after one week of sauerkraut supplementation as well as the incidence of gastrointestinal side effects, such as bloating, diarrhea, pain, nausea, and constipation.

Conclusions: This study suggests that the short-term effects on the gut microbiota of sauerkraut supplementation depend on its baseline status, but it can induce long-term effects. Sauerkraut supplementation requires a seven-day adaptation period. Further research is needed to explore the mechanisms behind the short-and long-term effects of sauerkraut supplementation.

Keywords: athletes; fermented food; microbiota; personalization; sauerkraut; sports nutrition; whole food.

Sarcopenia and Aging

Sarcopenia (also discussed in Chapter 5) is the age-related loss of skeletal muscle mass, strength, and function, which can contribute to decreased mobility, frailty, and an increased risk of falls, fractures, and loss of independence in older adults. This gradual decline typically begins in the fourth decade of life and accelerates with advancing age, particularly in individuals who are physically inactive or have poor nutritional habits. One of the primary nutritional strategies for delaying sarcopenia is ensuring adequate protein intake, which supports muscle protein synthesis and helps preserve lean body mass. Research suggests that older adults may require more protein than younger individuals to achieve the same anabolic effect, and that distributing protein intake evenly throughout the day may be particularly beneficial. When combined with resistance training, protein intake in the range of 1.2 to 1.6 g/kg BW per day has been shown to support muscle maintenance and growth (Bauer et al., 2013; Tieland et al., 2012). In addition to protein, nutrients such as vitamin D and omega-3 fatty acids have also been associated with improved muscle health. Vitamin D plays a role in muscle function and balance, while omega-3 fatty acids may reduce inflammation and enhance the muscle-building response to protein and exercise (Smith et al., 2011). Collectively, these nutrition and exercise strategies can help reduce the risk of sarcopenia and promote functional independence in aging populations.

Bone Health

In addition to preventing osteoporosis, adequate intakes of calcium and vitamin D, as well as magnesium, phosphorus, and vitamin K, are essential for maintaining bone health across the lifespan. Calcium plays a central role in bone mineralization, while vitamin D enhances calcium absorption and supports bone remodeling. Deficiencies in either nutrient are associated with reduced bone mass and an increased risk of fractures, particularly among older adults and postmenopausal women who are at greater risk of bone loss due to hormonal changes (Cashman, 2007; Weaver et al., 2016); whereas, supplementing with both calcium and vitamin D has been shown to reduce bone turnover and lower the incidence of osteoporotic fractures in older adults (Exhibit 4.13) (Tang et al., 2007).

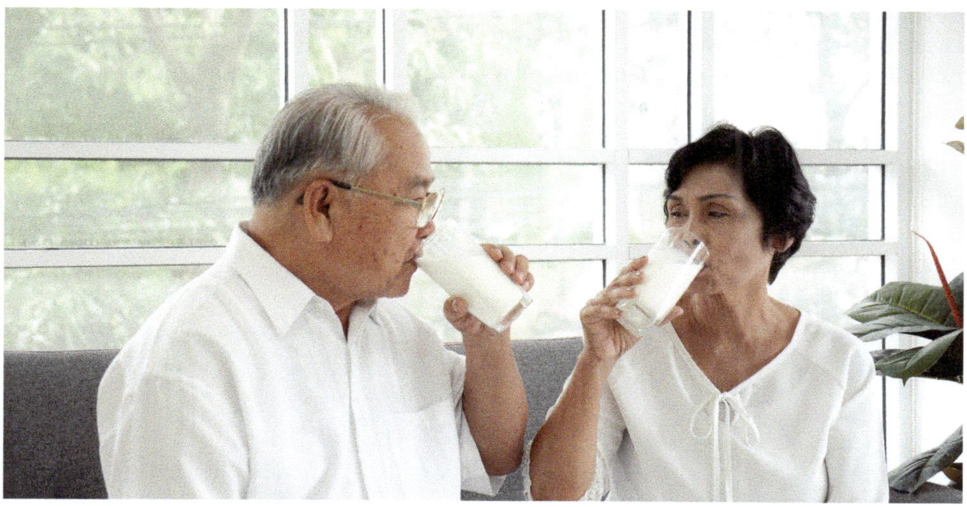

Exhibit 4.13 Elderly couple drinking milk

Nutrition in Recovery and Clinical Rehabilitation

Nutritional support plays a key role in recovery from illness, surgery, and injury. Clinical nutrition interventions, particularly those involving protein, amino acids, vitamins (such as C and A), and minerals (such as zinc), can improve wound healing, reduce recovery time, and preserve muscle mass in hospitalized or injured patients (Seth et al., 2024). This aspect of nutrition is particularly relevant to students pursuing careers in medicine, physical therapy, occupational therapy, or physician assistant studies, where integrating evidence-based nutritional strategies into treatment plans can enhance recovery and patient outcomes.

SPORTS/PERFORMANCE ASPECTS

Although genetic endowment plays an important role in determining athletic potential, nutritional status also has a significant impact on performance. True athletic potential may not be fully realized if an athlete lacks sufficient fuel stores or essential nutrients. Inadequate intake of nutrients, electrolytes, and water can impair performance, while excessive intake of certain nutrients can also be detrimental, potentially disrupting physiological function or contributing to undesirable changes in body composition (Rawson, Branch, and Stephenson, 2023).

Carbohydrate Intake and Performance

All biological functions require energy; therefore, the use of dietary manipulation to determine how the body uses and stores energy for biological work continues to be a main focus in human performance research. In approximately 1939, Christensen and Hansen were among the first to study the effects of dietary manipulation on exercise performance (Costill, 1994) and, today, it is well established that carbohydrate availability is a limiting factor during prolonged, moderate-intensity exercise.

From a practical standpoint, research in this area has led to carbohydrate guidelines for athletes. For example, endurance athletes are advised to consume 5–10 g/kg of carbohydrate per day to maintain glycogen stores. During events lasting more than 60–90 minutes, consuming 30–60 g of carbohydrate per hour has been shown to help maintain performance. Additionally, post-exercise glycogen resynthesis is optimized when carbohydrates are consumed within 30 minutes after exercise, especially when paired with a small amount of protein (Fink and Mikesky, 2025). These strategies are commonly used by athletes to improve training outcomes, support recovery, and delay the onset of fatigue (Exhibit 4.14).

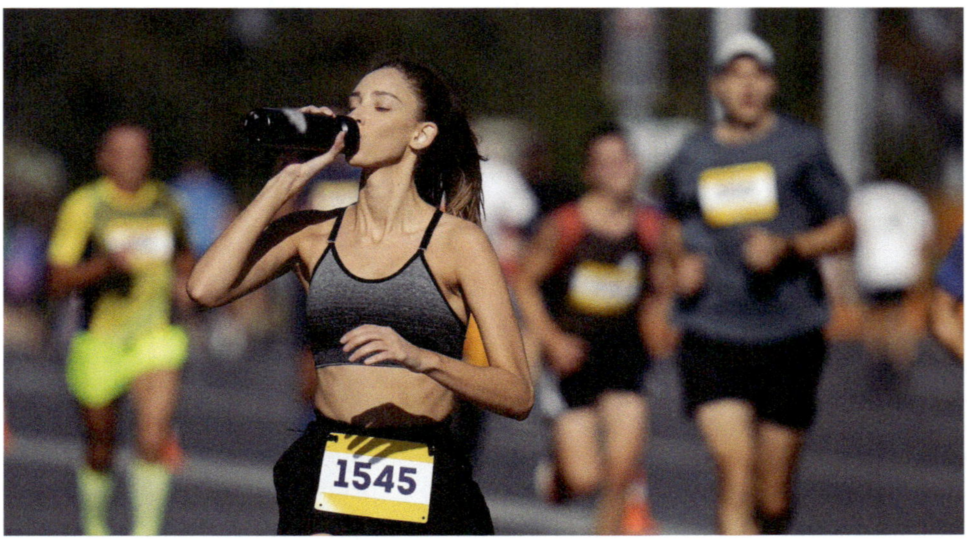

Exhibit 4.14 Endurance athlete consuming a carbohydrate beverage during competition

Protein Intake and Performance

Research on protein intake continues to generate interest among athletes, coaches, and trainers. Strength athletes, such as bodybuilders and weightlifters, often consume large quantities of protein because they believe it enhances muscle growth and performance. Many protein supplements also claim to stimulate muscle protein synthesis through improved absorption or reduced protein breakdown. Although athletes and active individuals require more protein than the general population, their needs are not dramatically higher. While the RDA is 0.8g/kg/body weight (BW), a joint position stand by the American College of Sports Medicine (ACSM), Academy of Nutrition and Dietetics (AND), and Dietitians of Canada recommends 1.2–2.0 g/kg/BW per day for athletes (Thomas et al., 2016) (Exhibit 4.15).

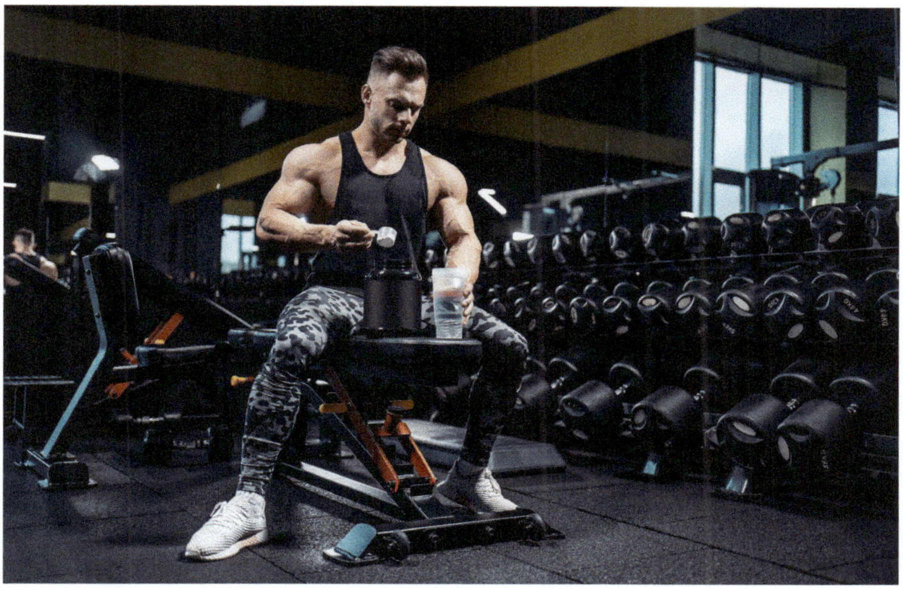

Exhibit 4.15 Strength athlete supplementing with whey protein

Many studies also suggest that the *timing* of protein intake following exercise is more important than the *quantity* ingested for increasing protein synthesis and does not require the purchase of expensive over the counter (OTC) supplements (Borsheim et al., 2002; Tipton et al., 2004; Escobar, McLain, and Kerksick, 2015). For example, Prichett et al. (2009) found that low-fat chocolate milk was just as effective as an OTC carbohydrate replacement drink on post-exercise recovery and endurance cycling performance in trained cyclists and triathletes. Upshaw et al. (2016) also reported that chocolate milk, low-fat milk, and a chocolate soy and chocolate hemp beverage were equally effective for improving cycling performance following an exhaustive bout of exercise compared to a placebo drink.

Fat Intake and Performance

Fat is a major source of energy for muscles, particularly at low intensities, and training improves the muscle's ability to utilize FFA as an energy source during exercise. Research examining the use of high-fat diets to improve athletic performance has yielded mixed results. For example, Jacobs et al. (2004) reported that a short-term (about 10 days) high-fat diet resulted in significant increases in fat oxidation and reduced carbohydrate oxidation without negatively impacting high-intensity time trial performance, and Lambert et al. (2001) found that a 10-day high-fat diet followed by 3 days of carbohydrate loading significantly improved cycling time trial performance by more than 1 minute. Other studies also suggest that highly trained endurance athletes tolerate short-term high-fat diets better than untrained individuals (Erlenbusch et al., 2005; Yeo et al., 2011) and that endurance training blunts the potential deleterious effects of high-fat diets on mitochondrial efficiency (Edwards et al., 2011). However, the metabolic adaptations that can occur following a high-fat diet, including ketosis and enhanced FFA oxidation, do not always translate to enhanced performance, since studies also show that both acute (Okano et al., 1996; Okano, Sato, and Yoshihisa, 1998) and chronic high-fat diets (Burke et al., 2000; Fleming et al., 2003; Havemann et al., 2006) have negative effects on exercise performance. Although there has been renewed interest in the theory that fat adaptation can enhance exercise performance (Burke, 2015), the majority of evidence suggests that high carbohydrate diets are superior to high fat diets for optimal training and performance outcomes.

Vitamin and Mineral Intake and Performance

As discussed earlier in this chapter, vitamins and minerals do not provide energy, but they do play crucial roles in metabolic processes that release energy from carbohydrates, fats, and proteins. With the possible exception of vitamin D, athletes who eat a well-balanced diet generally do not need vitamin supplementation, even though many believe that it is essential for improving general overall health and performance. While the general consensus is that vitamin supplementation does not significantly enhance either anaerobic or aerobic exercise performance, research is inconclusive, especially with regard to the dosages that would be necessary to elicit an ergogenic effect, the effects of mega-doses, time of administration, and use of different forms of vitamins (Rawson, Branch, and Stephenson, 2023).

Antioxidant vitamins, such as E, C, and beta-carotene, have been widely studied because of their ability to protect the body from free radicals, which are highly reactive molecules produced during metabolism that have been linked to aging, cancer, CHD, and other chronic diseases. Fortunately, the body has natural defenses in the form of antioxidants (e.g., vitamins E and C) and protective enzymes that neutralize free radicals and help minimize cellular damage (Dolara et al., 2012). As with the general population, athletes are encouraged to consume a diet rich in antioxidant-containing foods such as fruits, nuts, dark leafy greens (e.g., spinach, kale, collard greens), and cruciferous vegetables (e.g., broccoli, cauliflower, Brussels sprouts) to support overall health and recovery.

Vitamin D is an important fat-soluble vitamin involved in several physiological functions, including calcium absorption, but it is difficult to get in adequate amounts unless the diet is high in fatty fish such as trout and salmon. In fact, vitamin D deficiency is very common in athletes as well as the general population, particularly during the winter months (Cannell et al., 2009; Holick, 2007). The RDA for vitamin D for men and women between the ages of 19 and 70 years is 600 IU per day. However, because vitamin D deficiency can impair athletic performance and most athletes are vitamin D deficient, many sports nutrition and health professionals recommend at least 1,000–2,000 IU per day.

Minerals are also vital for body structure and function, including metabolism. However, female athletes, in particular, have an increased risk for iron and calcium deficiencies, which may be due, in part, to an inadequate intake of total Calories. The Female Athlete Triad (Exhibit 4.16) describes the interrelationship between low EA (with or without disordered eating), menstrual dysfunction (irregular or absence of menstrual cycles), and low bone mineral density. Treatment of female athletes with the triad requires a multidisciplinary approach involving medical providers, dietitians, mental health professionals, coaches, and family members. The primary goals are the return of regular menstrual cycles and improved bone mineral density. Increasing EA is the first step, typically by reducing training and increasing caloric intake, and a threshold of at least 30 kcal/kg FFM per day may be needed to resume menstruation. Although no specific drug

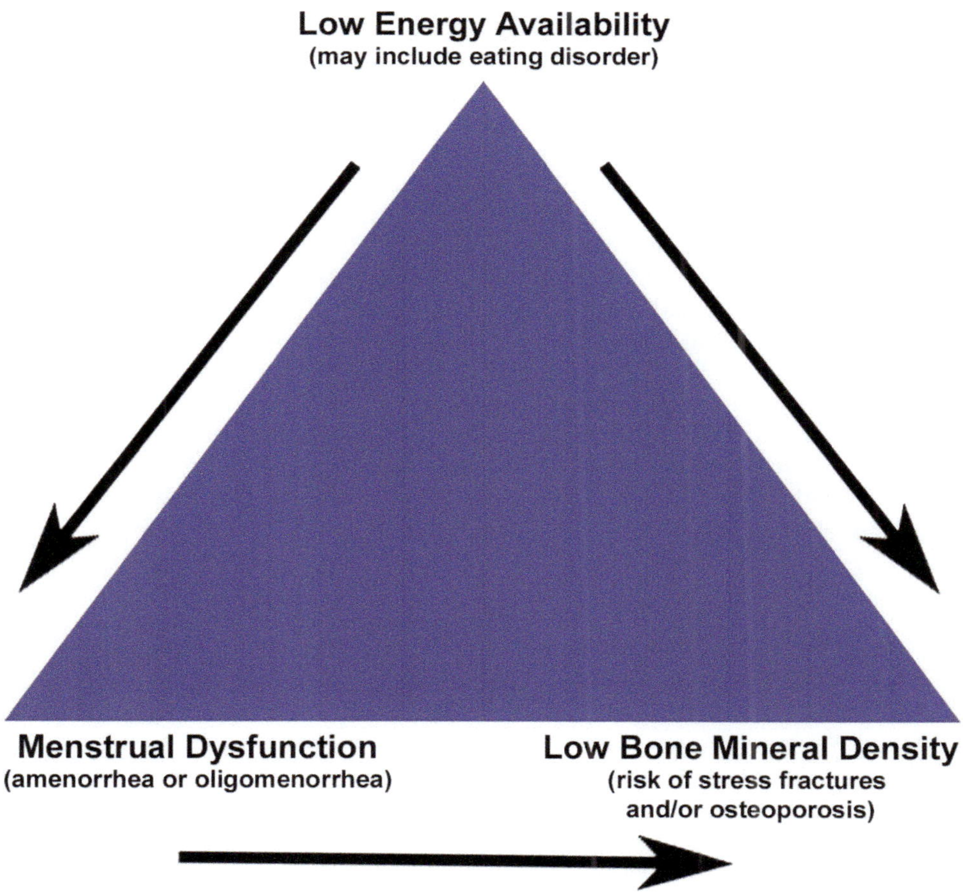

Exhibit 4.16 The Female Athlete Triad

intervention has been found to consistently improve bone density in this population, maximizing EA and optimizing vitamin D and calcium intake are key components of the treatment plan (Nazem and Ackerman, 2012).

Iron supports many important functions in the body, including oxygen transport, energy production in cells, muscle performance, immune health, and mental focus. It is a key component of both hemoglobin and myoglobin, which carry oxygen in blood and muscles, respectively. Without enough iron, athletes may experience fatigue, slower recovery, poor training response, and a greater risk of illness. Iron deficiency is the most common nutrient deficiency worldwide, and endurance athletes are at higher risk. It is estimated that 15–35% of female athletes and 3–11% of male athletes may be iron deficient, compared to about 5% of the general population (Nolte et al., 2024).

Because long-term iron deficiency can lead to anemia, athletes should take steps to maintain healthy iron levels through their regular diet. At a minimum, athletes should be meeting the current RDA, which is 8 mg per day for adult males and 18 mg per day for premenopausal females. Choosing iron-rich foods is especially important. Heme iron, found in animal sources such as red meat, poultry, and seafood, is more easily absorbed by the body than non-heme iron found in plant-based foods. To further enhance iron absorption, athletes can also pair iron-rich foods with food high in vitamin C, such as citrus fruits, bell peppers, and tomatoes at mealtimes, while limiting foods and beverages known to reduce absorption including dairy products, whole grains, legumes, tea, and coffee (Nolte et al., 2024; Solberg and Reikvam, 2023).

Building on the discussion above, it is also important to recognize that athletes may be affected by **Relative Energy Deficiency in Sport (RED-S)**. RED-S evolved from the Female Athlete Triad but is different in that it is recognized as a broader syndrome that results from inadequate caloric intake and/or excessive energy expenditure, leading to impaired physiological functioning and decreased athletic performance that affects both men and women. RED-S also shares several of the same symptoms as overtraining, including a common hypothalamic–pituitary axis origin and an association with low carbohydrate intake and overall EA. Therefore, identifying and addressing RED-S requires a multidisciplinary approach that emphasizes proper fueling, adequate recovery, and individualized monitoring of both performance and health indicators (Dipla et al., 2021).

Water and Electrolytes

Normal body function depends on maintaining a proper balance between water and electrolytes. Electrolytes are substances that, when dissolved in fluid, conduct an electrical current. Key electrolytes involved in biological processes include sodium, potassium, chloride, and calcium. Among all nutrients, water is especially critical for physically active individuals and is one of the few that can enhance performance when consumed in adequate amounts before and during exercise.

The effects of exercise on fluid balance and the role of water in thermoregulation have been major areas of research. Studies have shown how environmental conditions such as heat, cold, dehydration, and hypohydration can impair physical performance. In response, researchers have developed guidelines for maintaining hydration and electrolyte balance during various forms of exercise and under different environmental conditions (Thomas et al., 2016). Understanding these principles is essential for athletes and active individuals aiming to prevent performance decline and avoid heat-related illnesses.

Ergogenic Aids

Nutritional ergogenic aids refer to any supplement, food, or dietary strategy that improves performance. During the past century, a considerable number of dietary supplements have been studied for their potential ergogenic effect. Aside from carbohydrate feeding, fluid and electrolyte replacement via sports drinks, and creatine supplementation, few have been shown to delay the onset of fatigue and/or to be of practical value for improving performance.

Application to Injury Rehabilitation in Sports Medicine

Nutrients can also support recovery from musculoskeletal injuries. For example, research has shown that certain nutrients can accelerate healing rates and shorten recovery to full function for sports injuries such as bruises, strains, sprains, lacerations, concussions, and fractures. Nutrient combinations for these types of injuries include anti-oxidative vitamins and minerals (i.e., zinc, vitamins C, E, and A), protein and amino acids, and omega-3 FFAs (Brown and Phillips, 2010; Kavalukas and Barbul, 2011; Tipton, 2015). Although nutrients should not be used as replacements for drugs or medical care, they may have the potential to significantly affect healing and return the athlete to competition sooner than traditional rehabilitation programs.

TECHNOLOGY AND RESEARCH TOOLS

Nutrition scientists use a wide variety of tools and techniques to investigate how dietary intake affects metabolism, performance, health, and disease. These methods range from traditional laboratory techniques to advanced molecular approaches that are essential to understanding the complex interactions between diet and human physiology. This section highlights several key tools used in exercise and sport nutrition research.

Muscle Biopsy Technique

One of the foundational tools in exercise nutrition research is the muscle biopsy technique. As discussed earlier, this method was instrumental to researchers in establishing the role of diet and exercise on muscle glycogen depletion and repletion and has led to effective applications of specific dietary techniques to enhance both high-intensity and endurance activities. Furthermore, the muscle biopsy technique has been vital for advancing our understanding of the molecular pathways (i.e., "omics") involved in muscle adaptation to both exercise and nutritional interventions. The procedure involves removing a very small piece of tissue from the belly of the muscle using a hollow needle. After the area is numbed with a local anesthetic, a small incision is made, and the needle is inserted to collect the sample (Exhibit 4.17). Biochemical assays are then performed to determine glycogen content and other indicators of substrate utilization.

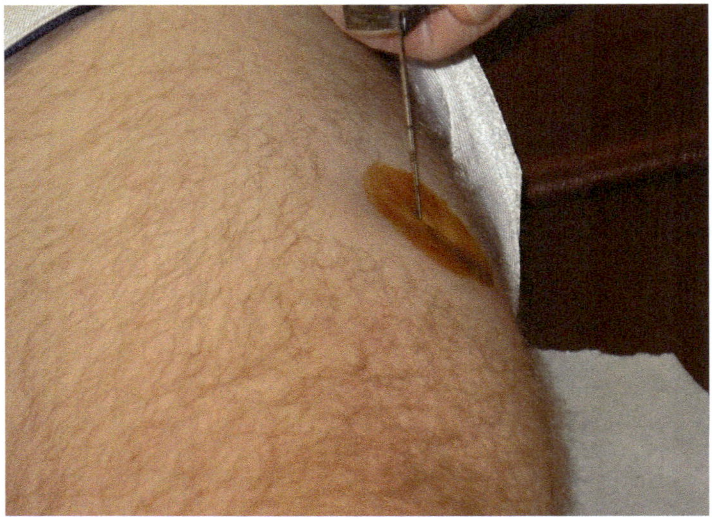

Exhibit 4.17 Muscle biopsy technique

Blood and Urine Analyses

Blood and urine samples are widely used in nutrition research to monitor biochemical responses to diet, supplements, drug therapy, and exercise. For example, researchers can assess markers of muscle damage (e.g., creatine kinase, lactate dehydrogenase), protein degradation (e.g., 3-methylhistidine), or oxidative stress (e.g., malondialdehyde) (Rawson, Branch, and Stephenson, 2023). These analyses can also measure hormone concentrations such as insulin, glucagon, testosterone, cortisol, and growth hormone to understand the body's metabolic adaptations to exercise and diet. Blood and urine testing are also used in clinical studies to evaluate the effectiveness of diet and exercise intervention programs in the development, prevention, and treatment of certain metabolic diseases, such as type 2 diabetes, hyperlipidemia, or CHD.

Metabolic Measurements

To assess energy expenditure at rest and during exercise, researchers often use calorimetry. Direct calorimetry measures heat production inside an insulated chamber, but because of its complexity and cost, it is rarely used and, instead, researchers use indirect calorimetry (McCardle, Katch, and Katch, 2023). When using indirect calorimetry, a technician measures the exchange of respiratory gases, since there is a predictable relationship between the body's use of energy and its use of oxygen or production of carbon dioxide. Instruments used to measure respiratory gases (gas analyzers) are widely available and much less expensive than direct calorimeters. These instruments can be mounted on carts and placed near laboratory equipment including treadmills and cycle ergometers, while portable models may be carried in backpacks or strapped to the body for measurements while a person is engaged in sports activities.

Another approach to indirect calorimetry involves the use of isotopes, such as hydrogen-2 (deuterium, or ^{2}H), as tracers that may be followed in the body. Isotopes are elements with an atypical atomic weight and may be radioactive (radioisotopes) or non-radioactive (stable isotopes). The use of doubly labeled water is a common tracer technique to monitor energy expenditure. In this technique, the subject consumes a known quantity of water labeled with two isotopes ($^2H_2{}^{18}O$), thus the term *doubly labeled water*. The deuterium (^2H) diffuses through the water content of the body, while the oxygen 18 (^{18}O) diffuses through both the water and bicarbonate stores. The rate at which the two isotopes leave the body is then measured by determining their presence in a series of blood, urine, or saliva samples. These turnover rates are then used to calculate how much carbon dioxide is produced, and this value is converted to energy expenditure using calorimetric equations (McCardle, Katch, and Katch, 2023). Because isotope turnover is relatively slow, this technique is not used for measurements of acute exercise metabolism. However, because of its accuracy and the low amount of risk involved to the subject, this technique is well suited for determining energy expenditure over an extended period of time.

Dietary Recall and Analysis

Accurate assessment of dietary intake is essential in both clinical and research settings. Common tools include food records (usually 3- or 7-day records), food frequency questionnaires, and 24-hour recalls. The 24-hour recall requires that individuals remember all the foods and beverages they consumed within the past day, which can be obtained by a face-face interview, phone interview, or guided online programs. Food frequency questionnaires (FFQ) are typically used to examine food intake over a longer period of time (i.e., weekly, monthly, or yearly) and, thus, provide information about long-term dietary patterns.

The development of digital tools such as the Automated Self-Administered 24-hour Dietary Recall (ASA24®) developed by the National Cancer Institute (NCI), has made dietary data collection more efficient. This web-based platform allows participants to log

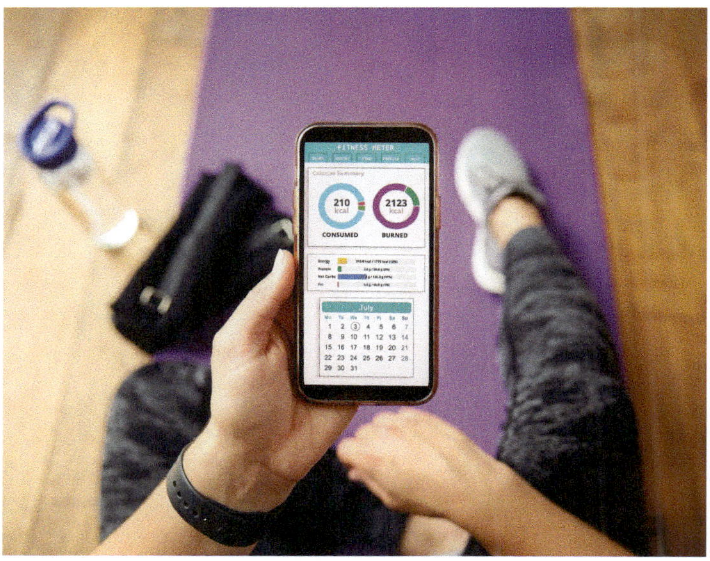

Exhibit 4.18 Using a smartphone application to assess dietary intake

their dietary intake using a computer, tablet, or smartphone, making it especially useful for large-scale research trials. For more information, visit the NCI website (NCI, n.d.).

Apps like MyFitnessPal®, YAZIO™, MyNetDiary™, and Cranometer™ can be useful for increasing dietary awareness and are reasonably accurate for tracking overall Calorie and macronutrient intake (Exhibit 4.18). However, their accuracy for monitoring micronutrients is less reliable due to incomplete databases and user errors and, therefore, they are not typically used for clinical research (Zhang et al., 2021; Gioia et al., 2023).

Body Composition Assessment

Assessing body composition (both percent body fat and lean mass) is important for monitoring the effects of dietary and exercise interventions. Common laboratory techniques include hydrostatic (underwater) weighing, air displacement plethysmography (e.g., BOD POD; Exhibit 4.19), and dual x-ray absorptiometry (DEXA), which also provides measurements of bone mineral density. Other laboratory methods for assessing body composition include radiography, magnetic resonance imaging, hydrometry (for measuring total body water), photon absorptiometry, and total body electrical conductivity (McCardle, Katch, and Katch, 2023).

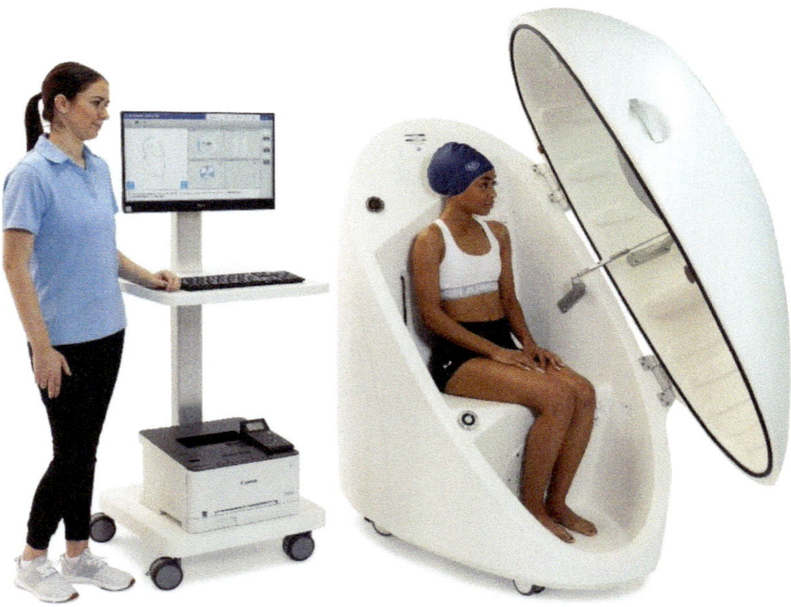

Exhibit 4.19 Air displacement plethysmography (BOD POD) to estimate body composition

Source: Photo courtesy of COSMED USA

Field techniques, such as skinfold measurements, circumferences, and bioelectrical impedance analysis (BIA) are more accessible than laboratory techniques because the equipment is less expensive, more portable, and convenient to use when testing large groups of people. Although they are less precise than laboratory methods, field techniques are commonly used in athletic and clinical settings to monitor body composition and hydration status.

Nutrigenomics and Molecular Tools

As discussed earlier in this chapter, **nutrigenomics** is the study of how nutrients influence genes (genomics), proteins (proteomics), gene expression (transcriptomics), and metabolism (metabolomics) to better understand the links between diet, health, and disease. The HapMap Project and genome-wide association studies (GWAS) have identified common genetic variants, such as single nucleotide polymorphisms (SNPs), that help explain individual differences in responses to bioactive food components and disease risk. These advances have made it possible for individuals to purchase commercially available DNA kits that analyze a small blood sample and offer insights into diet, exercise, medication response, and chronic disease risk (Isaak and Siow, 2013; Neeha and Kinth, 2013).

Common tools in nutrigenomic research include nuclear magnetic resonance spectroscopy, infrared spectroscopy, high-performance liquid chromatography, and bioinformatics for analyzing biochemical data. In the future, these technologies may allow dietitians and nutritionists to replace traditional dietary assessments, such as food records and FFQs, with blood-based micronutrient screening. This could also lead to a shift from general dietary guidelines such as RDAs to precision nutrition, where recommendations are tailored to individual genetic profiles (Isaak and Siow, 2013).

CAREER AND EMPLOYMENT OPPORTUNITIES

Dietetics

According to the US Bureau of Labor Statistics, employment of dietitians is projected to grow 7% from 2023 to 2033, which is higher than the average for all occupations, and may be explained by the increasing emphasis on the role of food and nutrition in preventing and treating disease, an aging population, and growing public interest in health and wellness (Academy of Nutrition and Dietetics, n.d.).

Clinical dietitians have important roles as members of medical teams in hospitals, nursing homes, health maintenance organizations (HMOs), and other healthcare facilities. They work with doctors, nurses, and therapists to speed recovery following illness or injury and set goals for long-term health. Community dietitians are primarily employed in public and home health agencies; daycare centers; health and recreation clubs; and government-funded programs that feed and counsel families, the elderly, pregnant women, children, and disabled or underprivileged individuals (Academy of Nutrition and Dietetics, n.d.).

Dietitians involved in the business world work in food and nutrition-related industries. Their primary responsibilities include product development, sales, marketing, advertising, public relations, and purchasing. Management dietitians play a key role wherever food is served and work mainly in healthcare institutions, schools, cafeterias, and restaurants, where they are responsible for such things as personnel management, menu planning, budgeting, and purchasing (Academy of Nutrition and Dietetics, n.d.).

Consultant dietitians may work full- or part-time in private practice or under contract with a healthcare facility (Exhibit 4.20). Those in private practice typically perform nutrition screenings and provide counseling for clients who seek their services directly or are referred by a physician. They offer guidance on a range of diet-related concerns, such as weight management, cholesterol reduction, and chronic disease prevention (Academy of Nutrition and Dietetics, n.d.). In most cases, dietitians provide individualized recommendations tailored to each client's unique needs and health goals.

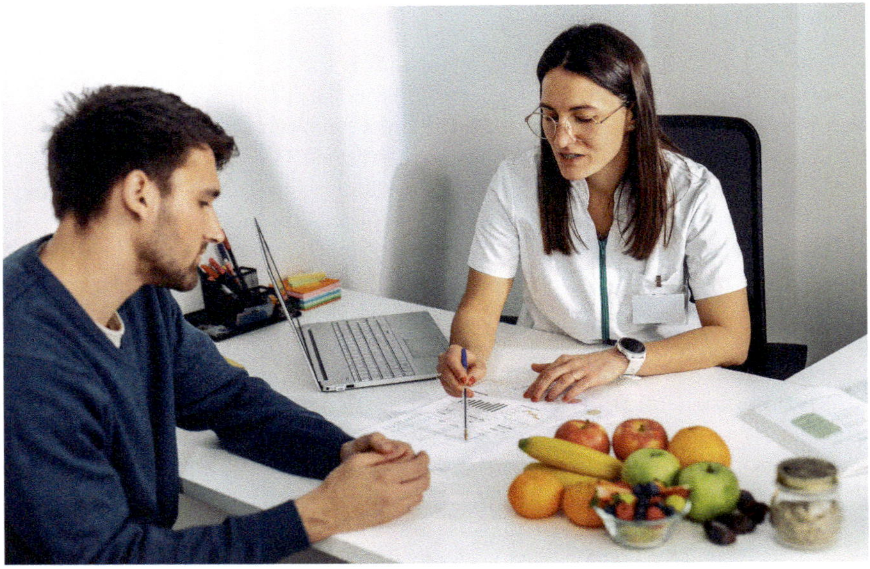

Exhibit 4.20 Dietitians work one-on-one with clients to develop personalized nutrition

Plans

Dietitians who are educators work in colleges, universities, and community or technical schools and teach future doctors, nurses, exercise physiologists, dietitians, and dietetic technicians the complex science of foods and nutrition. Research dietitians work in major universities and medical centers, government agencies, and food and pharmaceutical companies and conduct investigations to answer critical nutrition questions and find alternative foods or dietary recommendations for the public (Academy of Nutrition and Dietetics, n.d.).

A dietetic technician typically works independently or in partnership with a Registered Dietitian Nutritionist (RDN) in many of the same settings described above. In clinical settings, technicians assess the nutritional status of clients and patients and assist in the development, implementation, and review of nutrition care plans. As part of food service management teams, dietetic technicians help to supervise food production and monitor the quality of food service in schools, daycare centers, correctional facilities, restaurants, corporations, nursing homes, and hospitals. Dietetic technicians who are interested in health and wellness teach nutrition classes at health clubs, weight-management clinics, and community wellness centers (Academy of Nutrition and Dietetics, n.d.).

Exercise and Sport Nutrition

Exercise nutrition, as an independent discipline, is practiced in many different settings by individuals with a wide variety of educational backgrounds and sub-specializations in nutrition. Primary employment is usually teaching and/or performing research at a college or university, acting as a sports dietitian for athletic teams, consulting within a private practice, working in cardiac rehabilitation in a hospital, or working in a corporate wellness or fitness center or health club.

Teaching and Research

A teaching position within a college or university typically requires at least a master's degree; however, a doctoral degree is often preferred, especially at large institutions. Certification as an RDN may or may not be a requirement, depending on the department in which one is employed. For example, teaching a nutrition course as a faculty member in a department of exercise science or department of kinesiology does not necessarily require certification. However, it does require a strong background in nutrition principles as they relate to health and human performance. In contrast, the RDN credential may be a requirement for individuals teaching courses in a department of food science or dietetics that prepares their students to take the national registration exam to become an RDN.

Exercise and Sport Nutrition Specialists

Athletic departments in colleges and universities recognize the value of sports dietitians in providing clinical nutrition services and team-based education for athletes, coaches, and trainers. While small colleges often employ part-time consultants, large NCAA Division I programs typically hire at least one full-time sports dietitian to oversee meal planning, performance nutrition, and education.

Full-time sports dietitians frequently work long hours, 6 to 7 days a week, year-round, and their responsibilities change with the athletic calendar. During the off-season, they focus on supporting training goals, optimizing body composition, and providing nutrition education. This may include dietary assessments, body composition testing, and workshops on topics like disordered eating, weight management, and fueling strategies. They may also offer practical guidance, such as grocery store tours and food prep education, especially in the summer when athletes are off campus. In-season, the emphasis shifts to maintaining athletes' performance, eating habits, and body composition. Sports dietitians also coordinate team meals, communicate with hotels and restaurants, and pre-arrange menus to ensure athletes have access to familiar and nutritious foods while traveling.

Many professional teams also employ RDNs either full-time or as part-time consultants. While their core responsibilities are similar across teams, their duties often vary depending on the season and the specific needs of the team. For example, during the off-season, a sports dietitian may work one day per week to deliver educational sessions on topics like ergogenic aids, macronutrients, and meal planning. These sessions typically include Q&A, one-on-one counseling, dietary recall and analysis, guidance on weight management, grocery store tours, and cooking demonstrations. During training camp, dietitians collaborate with food service staff to plan menus rich in carbohydrates and lean protein while keeping fat content low. Because teams invest heavily in nutrition, it is essential that athletes eat at the training table rather than resorting to fast food. To encourage this, menus often include regional favorites that appeal to a diverse roster. In-season, dietitians coordinate with caterers, airlines, and hotels to ensure consistent, performance-focused meals during travel and practice. Many consultants who work with professional athletes also hold advanced credentials in sports dietetics and this is discussed later in the chapter.

Cardiac Rehabilitation

Registered dietitians who work in cardiac rehabilitation facilities typically work as a team with nurses and exercise specialists to educate patients about the synergistic effect of exercise and nutrition as it relates to primary and secondary prevention of cardiovascular disease. The responsibilities of the clinical dietitian include providing one-on-one nutrition counseling, lipid management, cooking demonstrations using low-fat and low-sodium foods and recipe modification, and teaching patient education classes on topics such as risk-factor modification and weight management.

Corporate Fitness and Health Clubs

Employment in a corporate or community fitness or wellness facility or commercial health club typically requires a bachelor's degree in exercise science or related degree with a strong background in nutrition. Job responsibilities include personal training, teaching exercise classes, health promotion, nutrition education, fitness testing, and health screening. In addition to nutrition education, professionals in the corporate fitness setting may assist in the planning and implementation of meals served in the company cafeteria. Certifications through the ACSM (e.g., Certified Exercise Physiologist; Certified Personal Trainer), the NSCA (e.g., Certified Personal Trainer; Certified Strength and Conditioning Specialist), or the American Council on Exercise (ACE) (e.g., Certified Personal Trainer) may also be a requirement for employment.

EDUCATION REQUIREMENTS

Dietetics

Individuals interested in dietetics are typically credentialed as an RDN or a Nutrition and Dietetics Technician, Registered (NDTR). These credentials indicate that an individual has completed an approved educational program in dietetics that meets certification requirements set forth by the Commission on Dietetic Registration (CDR) and are also accredited by the Accreditation Council for Education in Nutrition and Dietetics (ACEND) of the Academy of Nutrition and Dietetics (AND). The AND was founded in 1917 by a group of women committed to improving the health and nutrition of US citizens during World War I when the government was trying to conserve food. Today, the AND is the world's largest organization of dietetics professionals with over 100,000 credentialed practitioners (Academy of Nutrition and Dietetics, n.d.).

Academic Preparation of Registered Dietary Nutritionists

To become an RDN, students must meet the following requirements:

1. **Earn a Graduate Degree**
   Students seeking an RDN must complete a master's degree from an ACEND-accredited dietetics program. Coursework typically includes topics in nutrition and food science, biochemistry, physiology, and other sciences, as well as communication, business, and foodservice systems. Some programs offer an integrated master's, while others require the completion of an undergraduate degree in dietetics followed by a master's in a related field.

2. **Complete Supervised Practice**
   Students must also complete at least 1,000 hours of supervised practice in various settings to apply classroom knowledge to real-world experiences.

3. **Pass the National Registration Exam**
   After completing the master's degree and supervised practice, candidates are eligible to take the CDR's Registration Examination for Dietitians to earn the RDN credential.

4. **Meet State Licensure Requirements**
   Many states require licensure to practice and the RDN credential is accepted in all states with regulatory requirements.

5. **Maintain Continuing Education**
   RDNs must complete ongoing professional development to stay current with research and best practices in nutrition.

To help students understand the different routes to becoming an RDN, the following section briefly describes ACEND-accredited education pathways that meet the eligibility requirements. Students interested in obtaining more detailed information are encouraged to visit the AND website (Academy of Nutrition and Dietetics, n.d.).

Coordinated Program

Coordinated programs integrate both the academic coursework and supervised practice required for RDN eligibility into a single degree program, typically at the graduate level. This streamlined approach allows students to complete all required components within one institution, eliminating the need to apply separately for a dietetic internship (DI). Upon graduation, students are immediately eligible to take the national RDN credentialing exam.

Didactic Program in Dietetics + Dietetic Internship

This two-step pathway involves completing academic coursework through an ACEND-accredited Didactic Program in Dietetics (DPD), followed by acceptance into a separate DI program for supervised practice. A master's degree may be completed before, during, or as part of the DI. Admission into DI programs is competitive and typically involves a national matching process, similar to residency placement in medical fields. This pathway offers flexibility and is a common route for students who complete an undergraduate degree in dietetics and later apply to internship and graduate programs separately.

Future Education Model Graduate Program (GP) in Nutrition and Dietetics

These ACEND-accredited programs are designed to integrate advanced coursework with supervised experiential learning into a single graduate degree. Future Education Model Graduate Programs streamline the educational process by combining both the academic and practical components required for RDN eligibility into one integrated program. Upon graduation, students meet all eligibility requirements to sit for the national RDN exam. This pathway reflects a shift in dietetics education toward competency-based learning and is well-suited for students seeking a direct, graduate-level route into the profession (Academy of Nutrition and Dietetics, n.d.).

Academic Preparation of Nutrition and Dietetics Technicians

There are two primary routes that lead to eligibility to take the national registration exam for the NDTR credential. One option is to complete an accredited dietetic technician program approved by the ACEND and the AND that combines didactic instruction with a minimum of 450 hours of supervised practice experience and earn at least a 2-year associate's degree at a US accredited college or university. The other avenue is to obtain a bachelor's degree in an accredited DPD program and complete an ACEND-accredited Dietetic Technician supervised practice program similar to what is required for the 2-year program (Academy of Nutrition and Dietetics, n.d.).

Exercise and Sport Nutrition

Becoming a well-qualified sports dietitian requires an extensive background in nutrition, particularly as it relates to athletic performance, experience with athletes, and the ability to effectively communicate with both coaches and athletes. The best and, perhaps, most marketable strategy for securing a position as a sports dietitian is to obtain the RDN certification through one of the pathways described above. However, it is possible for individuals without the RDN credential to find jobs in exercise and sports nutrition, depending on their education and experience. For example, an individual with a master's or doctoral degree in exercise science or human nutrition with certifications, licensure, and/or relevant experience would be well-qualified for many positions in the field of sports nutrition.

Undergraduate Programs

Academic preparation for a career in exercise and sport nutrition begins with a strong foundation in the sciences. Courses in biology, physiology, chemistry, and biochemistry form the framework, while additional coursework in math, English, sociology, psychology, and business help build communication, analytical, and interpersonal skills. An undergraduate degree in exercise science is particularly valuable for students interested in sports or exercise nutrition because it emphasizes the physiological and biomechanical principles of human movement and performance. It also complements further graduate study or professional certification in dietetics, sports nutrition, or related fields.

Students are also encouraged to stay current with the latest issues in sport nutrition by reading scientific literature, reputable sport magazines, and sports-related newsletters. Understanding the unique demands of different sports and the stress of competition is essential for working effectively with athletes. Valuable experience may also be gained by volunteering nutrition-related services with high school or university athletic teams, youth sports leagues, or club sports.

Students who do not wish to attend graduate school or obtain the RDN credential but would like to be more marketable following graduation may consider becoming a Licensed Nutrition Therapist or becoming certified through organizations such as the AND, ACSM, or the NSCA. The Medical Commission of the International Olympic Committee (IOC) also offers a distance-learning postgraduate-level program in sport nutrition on a part-time basis that takes 2 years to complete. The program is designed for sports nutrition professionals who work with athletes and coaches to enhance their knowledge and experience in nutrition. Applicants must have an undergraduate degree or equivalent in nutrition or dietetics, the biological sciences (e.g., physiology, exercise science, biology, biochemistry), or medicine and, upon successful completion of the program, graduate with the IOC Committee's Diploma in Sports Nutrition. For more information, visit the IOC website (IOC, n.d.).

Graduate Programs

Many colleges and universities offer graduate programs in exercise science and/or nutrition. Most programs require certain prerequisites for admission; therefore, it is important to establish professional goals before completing an undergraduate degree. Admission requirements for graduate school at most universities require an earned bachelor's degree in a related discipline, a strong overall grade point average, and satisfactory Graduate Record Examination scores. The curriculum for a master's or doctoral degree in nutrition generally has a strong foundation in biological sciences, chemistry, clinical nutrition, nutrition education, and nutrition research. However, if a person is interested in exercise and nutrition or sport nutrition, a program that combines aspects of both disciplines may be more appropriate. Universities offering these types of graduate programs are often offered through a collaborative effort between a department of nutrition or food science and a department of kinesiology, health sciences, or exercise science. This is an example of an interdisciplinary program that also provides a pathway to become an RDN. Other departments combine the two disciplines, such as the Department of Nutrition, Food, and Exercise Sciences at Florida State University, which offers an MS in food and nutrition with a specialization in sports nutrition.

Although a few programs specifically offer a doctoral degree in exercise nutrition, many universities allow a person to tailor their program through elective courses to help meet his or her professional goals. Admission requirements generally require an earned master's degree with the completion of a thesis. A thesis is often required as a prerequisite for programs that confer the Doctor of Philosophy (PhD) degree, since they prepare students to perform independent research, analyze data, and competently evaluate research conducted by their peers. Doctoral programs in both exercise physiology and nutrition typically require 40+ credit hours beyond a master's degree.

CERTIFICATIONS AND LICENSURE

A number of specialty certifications are available through the AND that are accredited by the CDR including the Certified Specialist in Sport Dietetics (CSSD). To become eligible to take the CSSD exam, an individual must be certified as an RDN for a minimum of 2 years and acquire 2,000 hours of documented specialty practice within a 5-year period. Upon successful completion of the exam, the individual may then use the designation "RDN, CSSD" in their title. Currently, RDNs working at the United States Olympic Training Center and those working with military combat units are required to have the CSSD certification. See the CDR website for further details (CDR, n.d.).

The AND also encourages dietitians to pursue licensure in their state of residence. The purpose of licensure is to ensure that only qualified, trained professionals provide nutrition counseling to individuals seeking nutrition care or advice. Non-licensed dietetics professionals who practice nutrition counseling or therapy may be subject to prosecution. States with certification laws restrict the use of titles such as dietitian or nutritionist to persons meeting specific requirements. Eligibility to take a licensing exam varies from state to state. Some require the RDN credential, whereas others allow individuals with a bachelor's, master's, or doctoral degree in human nutrition or a related field to take a licensing exam. Most states confer some form of licensure under titles such as licensed medical nutrition therapist (MNT) and licensed dietitian (LD), depending on the state in which licensure is obtained. Because each state's licensure program is different, interested individuals should contact the licensure division affiliated with their State Department of Health.

The International Society of Sports Nutrition (ISSN) offers two certifications in sports nutrition: the CISSN, or Certified Sports Nutritionist from the ISSN, and the Sports Nutrition Specialist (SNS). The SNS focuses on applied aspects of sports nutrition and is intended for individuals who may not have an undergraduate degree. The primary purpose of the SNS is to provide personal trainers and other fitness professionals with a working knowledge of sports nutrition and supplementation strategies. The CISSN is more advanced and typically requires a 4-year undergraduate degree in any discipline. Individuals who do not have a bachelor's degree may also be eligible if they have been practicing in the field for at least 5 years, are certified by the ACSM, NSCA, or ACE, and meet specific membership requirements of the ISSN. Successful completion of the CISSN exam indicates that an individual possesses a fundamental understanding of the role that nutrition plays in the acute and chronic response to exercise. See the ISSN website for more information (ISSN, n.d.).

PROFESSIONAL ORGANIZATIONS

Academy of Nutrition and Dietetics (AND)

The Academy of Nutrition and Dietetics is the world's largest organization of food and nutrition specialists. The aim of the Academy is to influence the public's food choice and nutritional status. Membership includes sport dietitians, dietetic technicians, and others who hold advanced degrees in nutrition and dietetics (Academy of Nutrition and Dietetics, n.d.).

International Society of Sports Nutrition (ISNN)

The ISSN is an academic society dedicated solely to sport nutrition. Membership includes exercise physiologists, strength and conditioning professionals, personal trainers, and nutritionists interested in sports and exercise (ISNN, n.d.).

American Society for Nutrition (ASN)

The American Society for Nutrition supports nutrition research, education, and collaboration to improve health by promoting scientific discovery, providing accurate nutrition information, and advocating for evidence-based policies and practices (American Society for Nutrition, n.d.).

National Dairy Council (NDC)

The NDC is a non-profit organization supported by dairy farmers that provides science-based education on the health and nutrition benefits of dairy foods. Staffed by RDNs and nutrition scientists, the NDC promotes practical guidance on how dairy supports wellness and sustainable food systems (NDC, n.d.).

International Society of Nutrigenetics/Nutrigenomics (ISNN)

The ISNN promotes research and education about how genetic differences influence dietary responses and how nutrients affect gene expression to advance personalized nutrition for both professionals and the general public (ISSN, n.d.).

JOURNALS

General Nutrition and Dietetics

Journal of Nutrition
Journal of the Academy of Nutrition and Dietetics
Journal of the American College of Nutrition
Nutrition Reviews
Journal of Nutrition Education and Behavior

Clinical and Medical Nutrition

Journal of the American Medical Association (JAMA)
Nutrition and Metabolism
American Journal of Clinical Nutrition
Advances in Nutrition

Sports and Exercise Nutrition

International Journal of Sport Nutrition and Exercise Metabolism
Journal of the International Society of Sports Nutrition
Medicine and Science in Sports and Exercise
Journal of Strength and Conditioning Research
Sports Medicine
British Journal of Sports Medicine

Food Science and Technology

Trends in Food Science & Technology
Food Chemistry
Journal of Food Science & Technology

Obesity and Weight Management

International Journal of Obesity
Diabetes, Obesity, and Metabolism
Obesity

FUTURE DIRECTIONS

Given the prevalence of obesity and obesity-related chronic diseases in the United States, nutrition professionals will continue to play an important role in public health efforts focused on prevention, treatment, and health promotion. This includes contributing to the development and implementation of nutrition education programs, personalized dietary interventions, and long-term behavior change strategies in both clinical and community settings.

To help reduce the prevalence of childhood obesity, future studies will likely emphasize school- and community-based interventions that integrate nutrition education with opportunities for physical activity. The aging population also presents another critical focus for nutrition research. Investigations will continue to explore how nutrition, particularly protein intake and micronutrient support, can help maintain muscle mass, bone health, and functional independence in older adults.

One of the most rapidly evolving areas of nutrition research is *nutrigenomics*, which examines how nutrients interact with genes to influence health outcomes. Advances in genomic technology have laid the foundation for precision nutrition and have the potential to revolutionize dietary assessment and disease prevention. In the future, dietitians may use genetic information to create more targeted and effective nutrition plans. However, ethical, regulatory, and practical challenges must be addressed before precision nutrition becomes a standard part of practice.

In sport nutrition, researchers will continue to investigate how nutrient timing, hydration, dietary manipulation, and ergogenic aids affect performance, recovery, and body composition. In addition, tools such as metabolomics and wearable technologies may allow for more personalized nutrition recommendations and real-time monitoring of an individual's nutritional status and response to training.

Because the field of exercise and sport nutrition is constantly evolving, it is essential for professionals to stay up to date with the latest research and practice guidelines. Students and practitioners are encouraged to become active members in professional organizations, attend scientific conferences, read peer-reviewed journals, and participate in continuing education opportunities to remain current and competitive in their chosen career.

SUMMARY

Exercise and sport nutrition is an interdisciplinary field that combines principles of nutrition and physical activity to support athletic performance, optimize health, and prevent disease. Career opportunities span teaching and research roles in higher education, as well as applied positions in collegiate and professional sports, corporate wellness programs, and community health settings. With increasing public interest in nutrition for both general wellness and performance enhancement, exercise and sport nutrition will continue to grow as a dynamic and influential sub-discipline within exercise science.

STUDY QUESTIONS

1. What is the relationship between nutrition and exercise performance, and how can diet be adjusted to support different types of physical activity?
2. Explain how protein intake and resistance training work together to prevent age-related muscle loss (sarcopenia). What nutrients may also play a role in preserving muscle function?
3. Compare and contrast the Female Athlete Triad and Relative Energy Deficiency in Sport (RED-S). How do these conditions impact performance and long-term health?
4. Describe the role of iron in exercise performance. Why are female and endurance athletes at greater risk for iron deficiency, and how can diet help prevent it?

5. What is nutrigenomics, and how might this emerging field influence personalized nutrition recommendations in the future?
6. Discuss the hydration needs of athletes. What are the potential risks of dehydration, and what strategies can be used to maintain fluid and electrolyte balance during exercise?
7. Why might an undergraduate degree in exercise science be a good foundation for a career in sport or exercise nutrition? What other credentials are commonly required for professional practice?
8. Determine your professional goals for a career in exercise and sport nutrition and develop a course of study designed to meet those goals: desired degree(s) and courses needed, certifications, etc. If you are interested in an area other than nutrition, write about how nutrition will impact your field.

LEARNING ACTIVITIES

3-Day Dietary Record and Self-Analysis

Objective: increase awareness of personal eating patterns and nutritional adequacy.

- track everything you eat and drink for two typical weekdays and one weekend day
- use an app like MyFitnessPal™ or Cronometer™ to analyze your intake
- record total calories, macronutrient breakdown (grams and % of energy), and micronutrients of concern (e.g., iron, calcium, vitamin D)
- write a brief reflection on whether your intake meets the AMDR and RDAs and identify at least two areas for improvement

Label Comparison Activity

Objective: practice reading and interpreting Nutrition Facts labels.

- choose two products from the same food category (e.g., granola bars, yogurt, protein shakes, or sports drinks)
- compare their serving sizes, calories, macronutrients, vitamins/minerals, and added sugar
- identify which product would be a better choice for a pre-workout snack and why
- summarize your findings in a one-page comparison chart or brief report

Calculate Your Protein Needs

Objective: estimate protein needs based on body weight and activity level.

- using your current body weight, calculate your recommended protein intake based on different goals (e.g., general health = 0.8 g/kg, active individual = 1.2–2.0 g/kg)
- review your 3-day food log or current eating habits to estimate whether you are meeting your protein needs
- identify one way to increase or optimize your protein intake through food (not supplements)

Sports Supplement Evaluation

Objective: explore evidence-based recommendations on supplements.

- choose a supplement you have heard about or seen marketed to athletes (e.g., creatine, collagen, caffeine, whey protein)
- research the supplement using a credible source like Examine.com, NIH Office of Dietary Supplements (NIH, n.d.), or a peer-reviewed article
- write a short summary that includes what it claims to do, what the evidence shows, and your recommendation for or against use

Build a 1-Day Performance Meal Plan

Objective: apply nutrition strategies for fueling training and recovery.

- create a 1-day meal plan that includes pre-exercise, during-exercise, and post-exercise meals/snacks
- assume moderate to high-intensity training (~60–90 minutes)
- use the recommendations relative to BW for carbohydrate (5–10 g/kg) and protein (1.2–2.0 g/kg) intake and compare them to AMDR guidelines
- include hydration and timing strategies

SUGGESTED READING

Benardot, D. (2024). *ACSM's nutrition for exercise science*. New York: Wolters Kluwer Health.

Campbell, B. (Ed.) (2020). *NSCA's guide to sport and exercise nutrition* (2nd ed.). Champaign, IL: Human Kinetics.

Clark, N. (2020). *Nancy Clark's sports nutrition guidebook* (6th ed.). Champaign, IL: Human Kinetics.

Dwyer, J. T. and Betz, J. M. (2023). *Health professional's guide to dietary supplements*. United States: Academy of Nutrition and Dietetics.

Lagoumintzis, G., and Patrinos, G. P. (2023). Triangulating nutrigenomics, metabolomics and microbiomics toward personalized nutrition and healthy living. *Human Genomics*, *17*(1), 109. https://doi.org/10.1186/s40246-023-00561-w

Stout, J. R., Kreider, R. B., Candow, D. G., Forbes, S. C., Rawson, E. S., Antonio, B., and Antonio, J. (2025). The birth of modern sports nutrition: tracing the path from muscle biopsies to creatine supplementation—A narrative review. *Journal of the International Society of Sports Nutrition*, *22*(sup1), 2463373. https://doi.org/10.1080/15502783.2025.2463373

REFERENCES

Academy of Nutrition and Dietetics. (n.d.). Academy of Nutrition and Dietetics website. Available at: www.eatright.org (Accessed September 9, 2025).

Ahluwalia, N., Dwyer, J., Terry, A., and Johnson, C. (2016). Update on NHANES dietary data: Focus on collection, release, analytical considerations, and uses to inform public policy. *Advances in Nutrition*, *7*, 121–134.

American Society for Nutrition. (n.d.). American Society for Nutrition website. Available at: www.nutrition.org (Accessed September 9, 2025).

Bauer, J., Biolo, G., Cederholm, T., Cesari, M., Cruz-Jentoft, A. J., Morley, J. E., Phillips, S., Sieber, C., Stehle, P., Teta, D., Visvanathan, R., Volpi, E., and Boirie, Y. (2013). Evidence-based recommendations for optimal dietary protein intake in older people: A position paper from the PROT-AGE Study Group. *Journal of the American Medical Directors Association*, *14*(8), 542–559. https://doi.org/10.1016/j.jamda.2013.05.021

Baum, J. I., Kim, I. Y., and Wolfe, R. R. (2016). Protein consumption and the elderly: What is the optimal level of intake? *Nutrients*, *8*(6), 359. https://doi.org/10.3390/nu8060359

Beavers, K. M. and Leutholtz, B. (2008). Glycemic load food guide pyramid for athletic performance. *Strength and Conditioning Journal*, *30*(3), 10–14.

Bordini, A. and Capozzi, F. (2014). Foodomics for healthy nutrition. *Current Opinion in Clinical Nutrition and Metabolic Care*, *17*, 418–424.

Borsheim, E., Tipton, K. D., Wolf, S. E., and Wolfe, R. R. (2002). Essential amino acids and muscle protein recovery from resistance exercise. *American Journal of Physiology, Endocrinology and Metabolism*, *283*(4), E648–E657.

Brooks, S., and Kearns, P. (1996). Enteral and parental nutrition. In E. E. Ziegler and L. J. Filer, Jr. (Eds.), *Present knowledge in nutrition* (7th ed., p. 530). Washington, DC: ILSI Press.

Brown, K. and Phillips, T. (2010). Nutrition and wound healing. *Clinics in Dermatology*, *28*, 432–439.

Burke, L. M. (2015). Re-examining high-fat diets for sports performance: Did we call the "nail in the coffin" too soon? *Sports Medicine*, *45*(Suppl), S33–S49.

Burke, L., Angus, D., Cox, G., Cummings, N., Febbraio, M., et al. (2000). Effect of fat adaptation and carbohydrate restoration on metabolism and performance during prolonged cycling. *Journal of Applied Physiology*, *89*, 2413–2421.

Buskirk, E. R. (1992). From Harvard to Minnesota: Keys to our history. *Exercise and Sports Science Reviews*, *20*, 1–26.

Cannell, J., Hollis, B., Sorenson, M., Taft, T., and Anderson, J. (2009). Athletic performance and vitamin D. *Medicine and Science in Sports and Exercise*, *41*(5), 1102–1110.

Capozzi, F. and Bordoni, A. (2013). Foodomics: A new comprehensive approach to food and nutrition. *Genes and Nutrition*, *8*,1–4.

Cashman K. D. (2007). Diet, nutrition, and bone health. *The Journal of Nutrition*, *137*(11 Suppl), 2507S–2512S. https://doi.org/10.1093/jn/137.11.2507S

CDR. (n.d.). Commission on Dietetic Registration website. Available at: https://www.cdrnet.org/ (Accessed September 9, 2025).

Costill, D. L. (1994). Applied exercise physiology. In *American College of Sports Medicine—40th anniversary lectures*, pp. 69–79. Indianapolis, IN: American College of Sports Medicine.

Cunningham J. J. (1980). A reanalysis of the factors influencing basal metabolic rate in normal adults. *The American Journal of Clinical Nutrition*, *33*(11), 2372–2374. https://doi.org/10.1093/ajcn/33.11.2372

DGA. (n.d.). Dietary Guidelines for Americans website. Available at: www.dietaryguidelines.gov (Accessed September 9, 2025).

Dipla, K., Kraemer, R. R., Constantini, N. W., and Hackney, A. C. (2021). Relative energy deficiency in sports (RED-S): Elucidation of endocrine changes affecting the health of males and females. *Hormones (Athens, Greece)*, *20*(1), 35–47. doi.org/10.1007/s42000-020-00214-w

Dolara, P., Bigagli, E., and Collins, A. (2012). Antioxidant vitamin and mineral supplementation, life span expansion, and cancer incidence: A critical commentary. *European Journal of Nutrition*, *51*, 769–781.

Edwards, L., Holloway, C., Murray, A., Knight, N., Carter, E., et al. (2011). Endurance exercise training blunts the deleterious effect of high-fat feeding on whole body efficiency. *American Journal of Physiology: Regulatory, Integrative, and Comparative Physiology*, *301*, R320–R326.

Emmerich, S. D., Fryar, C. D., Stierman, B., and Ogden, C. L. (2024). Obesity and severe obesity prevalence in adults: United States, August 2021–August 2023. *NCHS Data Brief*, 508, 10.15620/cdc/159281. https://doi.org/10.15620/cdc/159281

Erlenbusch, M., Haub, M., Munoz, K., MacConnie, S., and Stillwell, B. (2005). Effect of high-fat or high-carbohydrate diets on endurance exercise: A meta-analysis. *International Journal of Sport Nutrition and Exercise Metabolism*, *15*, 1–14.

Escobar, K. A., McLain, T. A., and Kerksick, C. M. (2015). Protein application in sports and nutrition – part II: Timing and protein patterns, fat free mass accretion, and fat loss. *Strength and Conditioning Journal*, *37*(3), 22–34.

FDA. (n.d.a). Dietary supplements. Available at: www.fda.gov/food/dietary-supplements (Accessed September 9, 2025).

FDA. (n.d.b). Label claims for conventional foods and dietary supplements. Available at: www.fda.gov/food/nutrition-food-labeling-and-critical-foods/label-claims-conventional-foods-and-dietary-supplements (Accessed September 9, 2025).

FDA. (n.d.c). Nutritional facts label. Available at: www.FDA.gov/NutritionFactsLabel (Accessed September 9, 2025).

Ferguson, L. R., De Caterina, R., Gorman, U., Hooman, A., Kohlmeier, M., et al. (2016). Guide and position of the International Society of Nutrigenetics/Nutrigenomics on personalized nutrition: Part 1 – fields of precision nutrition. *Journal of Nutrigenetics and Nutrigenetics*, *9*, 12–27.

Fink, H. H., and Mikesky, A. E. (2025). *Practical applications in sports nutrition* (7th ed.). Boston, MA: Jones & Bartlett Learning.

Fishman, E. I., Steeves, J. A., Zipunnikov, V., Koster, A., Berrigan, D., Harris, T. A., and Murphy, R. (2016). Association between objectively measured physical activity and mortality in NHANES. *Medicine and Science in Sports and Exercise*, *48*(7), 1303–1311.

Fleming, J., Sharman, M., Avery, N., Love, D., Gomez, A., et al. (2003). Endurance capacity and high-intensity exercise performance responses to a high-fat diet. *International Journal of Sport Nutrition and Exercise Metabolism*, *13*, 466–478.

Framingham Heart Study. (n.d.). Framingham Heart Study website. Available at: www.framinghamheartstudy.org (Accessed September 9, 2025).

Gioia, S., Vlasac, I. M., Babazadeh, D., Fryou, N. L., Do, E., Love, J., Robbins, R., Dashti, H. S., and Lane, J. M. (2023). Mobile apps for dietary and food timing assessment: Evaluation for use in clinical research. *JMIR Formative Research*, *7*, e35858. https://doi.org/10.2196/35858

Hasler, C. M., Brown, A. C., and Burns, J. A. (2009). Position of the American Dietetic Association: Functional foods. *Journal of the American Dietetic Association*, *109*(4), 735–746.

Havemann, L., West, S., Goedecke, J., Macdonald, I., et al. (2006). Fat adaptation followed by carbohydrate-loading compromises high intensity sprint performance. *Journal of Applied Physiology*, *100*, 194–202.

Heydenreich, J., Kayser, B., Schutz, Y., and Melzer, K. (2017). Total energy expenditure, energy intake, and body composition in endurance athletes across the training season: A systematic review. *Sports Medicine – Open*, *3*(1), 8. https://doi.org/10.1186/s40798-017-0076-1

Holick, M. (2007). Vitamin D deficiency. *New England Journal of Medicine, 357,* 266–281.

Institute of Medicine. (2005). *Dietary Reference Intakes for Energy, Carbohydrates, Fiber, Fatty Acids, Cholesterol, Protein, and Amino Acids (Macronutrients).* Food and Nutrition Board. Washington, DC: National Academies Press.

IOC. (n.d.). IOC Diploma in Sports Nutrition. Available at: www.iocsportsnutrition.com (Accessed September 9, 2025).

Isaak, C. K., and Siow, Y. L. (2013). The evolution of nutrition research. *Canadian Journal of Physiology and Pharmacology*, *91*, 257–267.

ISSN. (n.d.). International Society of Sports Nutrition website. Available at: www.sportsnutritionsociety.org (Accessed September 9, 2025).

Jacobs, K. A., Paul, D. R., Geor, R. J., Hinchcliff, K. W., and Sherman, W. M. (2004). Dietary composition influences short-term endurance training-induced adaptations of substrate partitioning during exercise. *International Journal of Sport Nutrition and Exercise Metabolism, 14*(1), 38–61.

Kavalukas, S., and Barbul, A. (2011). Nutrition and wound healing: An update. *Plastic and Reconstructive Surgery*, *127*(Suppl.), 38S–43S.

Keys, A., Brozek, J., Henschel, A., Mickelsen, O., and Taylor, H. (1950). *The biology of human starvation*, Vols. I and II. Minneapolis, MN: University of Minnesota Press.

Lambert, E. V., et al. (2001). High-fat diet versus habitual diet prior to carbohydrate loading: Effects on exercise metabolism and cycling performance. *International Journal of Sport Nutrition and Exercise Metabolism*, *11*, 209–225.

Leveille, G. A. (2016). 2015 Trailblazer Lecture: A journey through the past and a perspective on the future of nutrition, food science, and health. *Journal of the Academy of Nutrition and Dietetics*, *116*(6), 1031–1034.

Loucks, A. B., Kiens, B., and Wright, H. H. (2011). Energy availability in athletes. *Journal of Sports Sciences*, *29 Suppl 1*, S7–S15. https://doi.org/10.1080/02640414.2011.588958

Marsh, K., Barclay, A., Colagiuri, S., and Brand-Miller, J. (2011). Glycemic index and glycemic load of carbohydrates in the diabetes diet. *Current Diabetes Reports*, *11*(2), 120–127. https://doi.org/10.1007/s11892-010-0173-8

McCardle, W. D., Katch, F. I., and Katch, V. L. (2023). *Exercise physiology: Energy, nutrition, and human performance* (9th ed.). Wolters Kluwer.

Mifflin, M. D., St Jeor, S. T., Hill, L. A., Scott, B. J., Daugherty, S. A., and Koh, Y. O. (1990). A new predictive equation for resting energy expenditure in healthy individuals. *The American Journal of Clinical Nutrition*, *51*(2), 241–247. https://doi.org/10.1093/ajcn/51.2.241

MyPlate®. (n.d.). MyPlate® website. Available at: www.myplate.gov (Accessed January 23, 2026).

Nazem, T. G., and Ackerman, K. E. (2012). The female athlete triad. *Sports Health*, *4*(4), 302–311. https://doi.org/10.1177/1941738112439685

Neeha, V. S. and Kinth, P. (2013) Nutrigenics research: A review. *Journal of Food Science and Technology*, *50*(3), 415–428.

NCI. (n.d.). Automated Self-Administered 24-Hour (ASA24®) Dietary Assessment Tool. Available at: www.epi.grants.cancer.gov/asa24/ (Accessed September 9, 2025).

NDC. (n.d.). National Dairy Council website. Available at: www.nationaldairycouncil.org (Accessed September 9, 2025).

NIH. (n.d.). National Institutes of Health: Office of Dietary Supplements. Available at: http://ods.od.nih.gov (Accessed September 9, 2025).

Nolte, S., Krüger, K., Hollander, K., and Carlsohn, A. (2024). Approaches to prevent iron deficiency in athletes. *German Journal of Sports Medicine*, *75*, 195–202. doi:10.5960/dzsm.2024.607

Okano, G., Sato, Y., Takumi, Y., and Sugawara, M. (1996). Effect of 4 h pre-exercise high carbohydrate and high fat meal ingestion on endurance performance and metabolism. *International Journal of Sports Medicine*, *17*, 530–534.

Okano, G., Sato, Y., and Yoshihisa, M. (1998). Effect of elevated blood FFA levels on endurance performance after a single fat meal ingestion. *Medicine and Science in Sports and Exercise*, *30*(5), 763–768.

O'Sullivan, T. A., Hafekost, K., Mitrou, F., and Lawrence, D. (2013). Food sources of saturated fat and the association with mortality: A meta-analysis. *American Journal of Public Health*, *103*(9): e31–e42.

Powers, S., Howley, E., and Quindry, J. (2024). *Exercise physiology: Theory and application to fitness and performance* (12th ed.). New York: Wolters Kluwer.

Prichett, K., Bishop, P., Prichett, R, Green, M., and Katica, M. (2009). Acute effects of chocolate milk and a commercial recovery beverage on post-exercise recovery indices and endurance cycling performance. *Applied Physiology, Nutrition and Metabolism*, *34*, 1017–1022.

Rawson, E., Branch, D., and Stephenson, T. (2023). *Williams' nutrition for health, fitness, and sport* (13th ed.). New York: McGraw-Hill.

Roberts, C. K., and Barnard, R. J. (2005). Effects of exercise and diet on chronic disease. *Journal of Applied Physiology*, *98*(1), 3–30. https://doi.org/10.1152/japplphysiol.00852.2004

Seth, I., Lim, B., Cevik, J., Gracias, D., Chua, M., Kenney, P. S., Rozen, W. M., and Cuomo, R. (2024). Impact of nutrition on skin wound healing and aesthetic outcomes: A comprehensive narrative review. *JPRAS open*, *39*, 291–302. https://doi.org/10.1016/j.jpra.2024.01.006

Sherman, W. M., Costill, D. L., Fink, W. J., and Miller, J. M. (1981). Effects of exercise-diet manipulation on muscle glycogen and its subsequent utilization during performance. *International Journal of Sports Medicine*, 2, 1–15.

Shivappa, N., Blair, C. K., Prizment, A. E., Jacobs Jr., D. R., Steck, S. E., and Herbert, J. R. (2016). Associations between inflammatory potential of diet and mortality in the Iowa Women's Health study. *European Journal of Nutrition*, 55, 1491–1502.

Solberg, A., and Reikvam, H. (2023). Iron status and physical performance in athletes. *Life*, *13*(10), 2007. https://doi.org/10.3390/life13102007

Smith, D., Plowman, S., and Ormsbee, M. (2022). *Exercise physiology for health, fitness, and performance* (6th ed.). New York: McGraw-Hill.

Smith, G. I., Atherton, P., Reeds, D. N., Mohammed, B. S., Rankin, D., Rennie, M. J., and Mittendorfer, B. (2011). Dietary omega-3 fatty acid supplementation increases the rate of muscle protein synthesis in older adults: A randomized controlled trial. *The American Journal of Clinical Nutrition*, *93*(2), 402–412. https://doi.org/10.3945/ajcn.110.005611

Tang, B. M., Eslick, G. D., Nowson, C., Smith, C., and Bensoussan, A. (2007). Use of calcium or calcium in combination with vitamin D supplementation to prevent fractures and bone loss in people aged 50 years and older: A meta-analysis. *Lancet*, *370*(9588), 657–666. https://doi.org/10.1016/S0140-6736(07)61342-7

The Food and Nutrition Board of the National Academies of Sciences, Engineering, and Medicine. (n.d.) Nutrient recommendations: Dietary Reference Intakes (DRI). Available at: https://ods.od.nih.gov/HealthInformation/nutrientrecommendations.aspx (Accessed September 9, 2025).

The University of Sydney. (n.d.). Glyemic index research and GI news. Available at: www.glycemicindex.com (Accessed September 9, 2025).

Thomas, D. T., Erdman, K. A., Burke, L. M., and MacKillop, M. (2016). Position of the Academy of Nutrition and Dietetics, Dietitians of Canada, and the American College of Sports Medicine: Nutrition and athletic performance. *Journal of the Academy of Nutrition and Dietetics*, *116*, 501–528.

Tieland, M., Dirks, M. L., van der Zwaluw, N., Verdijk, L. B., van de Rest, O., de Groot, L. C., and van Loon, L. J. (2012). Protein supplementation increases muscle mass gain during prolonged resistance-type exercise training in frail elderly people: A randomized, double-blind, placebo-controlled trial. *Journal of the American Medical Directors Association*, *13*(8), 713–719. https://doi.org/10.1016/j.jamda.2012.05.020

Tipton, K. D. (2015). Nutritional support for exercise induced injuries. *Sports Medicine*, *45*(Suppl 1), S93–S104.

Tipton, K. D., Elliott, T. A., Cree, M. G., Wolf, S. E., Sanford, A. P., and Wolfe, R. R. (2004). Ingestion of casein and whey proteins result in muscle anabolism after resistance exercise. *Medicine and Science in Sports and Exercise*, *36*(12), 2073–2081.

Trumbo, P., Schlicker, S., Yates, A. A., Poos, M., and Food and Nutrition Board of the Institute of Medicine, The National Academies (2002). Dietary reference intakes for energy, carbohydrate, fiber, fat, fatty acids, cholesterol, protein and amino acids. *Journal of the American Dietetic Association*, *102*(11), 1621–1630. https://doi.org/10.1016/s0002-8223(02)90346-9

Upshaw, A. U., Wong, T. S., Bandegan, A., and Lemon, P. W. R. (2016). Cycling time trial performance 4 hours after glycogen lowering exercise is similarly enhanced by recovery nondairy chocolate beverages versus chocolate milk. *International Journal of Sport Nutrition and Exercise Metabolism*, 26, 65–70.

van Zonneveld, S. M., van den Oever, E. J., Haarman, B. C. M., Grandjean, E. L., Nuninga, J. O., van de Rest, O., and Sommer, I. E. C. (2024). An anti-inflammatory diet and its potential benefit for individuals with mental disorders and neurodegenerative diseases—a narrative review. *Nutrients*, *16*(16), 2646. https://doi.org/10.3390/nu16162646

Weaver, C. M., Gordon, C. M., Janz, K. F., Kalkwarf, H. J., Lappe, J. M., Lewis, R., O' Karma, M., Wallace, T. C., and Zemel, B. S. (2016). The National Osteoporosis Foundation's position statement on peak bone mass development and lifestyle factors: a systematic review and implementation recommendations. *Osteoporosis International*, 27(4), 1281–1386. https://doi.org/10.1007/s00198-015-3440-3

World Health Organization. (1985). *Energy and protein requirements. Report of a joint FAO/WHO/UNU expert consultation. Technical report series 724.* Geneva: World Health Organization.

Yeo, W., Carey, A., Burke, L., Spriet, S., and Hawley, J. (2011). Fat adaptation in well-trained athletes: Effects on cell metabolism. *Applied Physiology, Nutrition, and Metabolism*, *36*, 12–22.

Zhang, L., Misir, A., Boshuizen, H., and Ocké, M. (2021). A systematic review and meta-analysis of validation studies performed on dietary record apps. *Advances in Nutrition*, *12*(6), 2321–2332. https://doi.org/10.1093/advances/nmab058

5 Exercise Physiology

Loree L. Weir

LEARNING OBJECTIVES

After studying this chapter, the student will be able to:

- understand the development of the field of exercise physiology, tracing its roots back to the seemingly disparate fields of math, chemistry, physiology, medicine, and physical education, and finally to modern molecular biology
- understand the difference between an exercise response and an exercise adaptation and be able to give examples of each
- make connections between select research topics in exercise physiology as they relate to health, performance, and clinical applications
- identify the research tools and technology that are integral to the study of exercise physiology
- describe career opportunities related to exercise physiology and understand the educational pathway to careers of interest
- list prominent professional organizations, journals, and certifications relevant to the field of exercise physiology

INTRODUCTION

Exercise physiology is a specialized area of study within the broader field of physiology that examines how single and repeated bouts of exercise affect cells, tissues, and organ systems of the human body (Powers, Howley, and Quindry, 2024). The job of an exercise physiologist can vary from a research scientist to a fitness professional and/or clinician working with clients of all ages to help them meet their health and performance goals through exercise. As an example, see Exhibit 5.1 for general job descriptions for exercise physiologists who are certified to work with healthy individuals, individuals with disease, and with athletes (more on career opportunities and certifications at the end of the chapter).

Essentially, the field of exercise physiology is interested in the short-term (acute) **responses** that happen right before, during, or after a bout of exercise and in the longer-term (chronic) **adaptations** that occur with consistent exercise training. If the readers of this book were to run up four flights of stairs, many changes would occur; for instance, their heart rate and breathing would rapidly increase in response to the physiological challenge. However, if these individuals were to run up the stairs three times per day for six weeks, they would find that they were no longer as out of breath

DOI: 10.4324/9781032697185-5

Exhibit 5.1 Sample job descriptions for exercise physiologists certified to work with athletes, healthy populations, and individuals with disease

Certification	*Job Description*
NSCA – CSCS*	A Certified Strength and Conditioning Specialist® is a professional who applies scientific knowledge to train athletes for the primary goal of improving athletic performance. The NSCA-CSCS conducts sport-specific testing sessions, designs and implements safe and effective strength training and conditioning programs and provides guidance regarding nutrition and injury prevention. Recognizing that their area of expertise is separate and distinct, a CSCS consults with and refers athletes to other professionals when appropriate.
ACSM – EP**	An ACSM Certified Exercise Physiologist® (ACSM-EP®) works with apparently healthy clients and those with medically controlled diseases to establish safe and effective exercise and healthy lifestyle behaviors to optimize both health and quality of life. The ACSM-EP® conducts preparticipation health screenings, submaximal graded exercise tests, strength, flexibility, and body composition assessments.
ACSM – CEP***	An ACSM Certified Clinical Exercise Physiologist® (ACSM-CEP®) is a health professional who utilizes prescribed exercise and basic health behavior interventions, as well as promotes physical activity for individuals with chronic diseases or conditions. The ACSM-CEP® provides primary and secondary prevention strategies designed to improve, maintain or attenuate declines in fitness and health in populations ranging from children to older adults. The ACSM-CEP® provides exercise screening, exercise and fitness testing, exercise prescriptions, exercise and physical activity counseling, exercise supervision, exercise and health education/promotion, and measurement and evaluation of exercise and physical activity-related outcome measures.

*NSCA-CSCS = NSCA Certified Strength and Conditioning Specialist®
**ACSM-EP = ACSM Certified Exercise Physiologist®
***ACSM-CEP = ACSM Certified Clinical Exercise Physiologist®

Source: American College of Sports Medicine. Copyright ©2024 by ACSM. Reprinted by permission; National Strength and Conditioning Association (2025, p. 2)

and that their heart rate would not rise as high as when they started. Their bodies are adapting to the consistent challenge placed on them. Students in exercise physiology learn to describe these changes and dive deep into the cellular **mechanisms** (physiological processes) that are responsible for the short-term responses and longer-term adaptations that occur.

Other terms that are sometimes used synonymously with exercise physiology include **sports physiology**, **environmental physiology**, and **work physiology.** Although these terms are closely related, they each have a different focus, i.e., working with athletes to maximize performance, studying exercise done in hot, cold, humid climates or at altitude, and focusing on work and fatigue in industrial workers and jobs requiring manual labor. In summary, exercise physiologists are interested in how the body responds and adapts to various types of exercise (e.g., resistance, aerobic, or sprint training) and how this knowledge can be applied in a practical way to health, fitness, performance, and clinical settings.

HISTORICAL PERSPECTIVES

Exercise physiology is a relatively new discipline that, although its roots stretch back to ancient Greece, started to coalesce in the work of physical educators and physiologists in the early 20th century (Chapter 1). **Physiology** (Chapter 3) involves the study of the function of the body and is based on other disciplines such as anatomy, biochemistry, and cellular biology. **Physical education (PE)** is concerned with the development of the human body through movement and, as early as the 1890s, included a study of exercise physiology as part of the curricula (Buskirk, 1996; Weir and Weir, 2017). For example, PE teachers design programs that will develop neuromuscular coordination, agility, strength, and physical fitness in children.

Researchers from many different backgrounds, but with a common desire to understand the effects of movement on the human body, applied their expertise to further the body of knowledge that would become known as exercise physiology. For example, two pioneering exercise physiologists, A.V. Hill and Otto Meyerhof, won the 1922 Nobel Prize for their work studying heat production and muscle metabolism during exercise. They were able to combine what they knew about thermodynamics and biochemistry to work out the difference between **aerobic** (with oxygen) and **anaerobic** (without oxygen) metabolism (Bassett Jr, 2002). Hill was from Britain with training in mathematics and physics, whereas Meyerhof was from Germany and trained in medicine. Both of their careers were interrupted by WWI and WWII, with Meyerhof fleeing with his family when the Nazis invaded France (Nobel Prize, n.d.a.). These two researchers, along with many others, had a common interest in understanding the physiological **mechanisms** (i.e., the how and why things happen, or the sequence of cause and effect) underlying the responses and adaptations associated with human movement. History buffs interested in a more comprehensive overview of the development of the field of exercise physiology are referred to Tipton (2014).

FUNDAMENTAL CONCEPTS

Exercise physiology may have emerged from the fields of physiology and physical education, but the discipline has grown rapidly over the last 100 years and matured into an essential field of study for anyone interested in health, sport, and/or medicine. As exercise physiology has evolved into its own discipline, it has integrated scientific breakthroughs and technologies from many other disciplines, most notably from molecular biology.

Moving from Descriptive to Mechanistic Physiology

To exercise physiologists, physical activity is used as a stressor, thereby serving as a useful tool to challenge an organism and study its responses and adaptations to the stressor (Brooks, 1987). In an undergraduate exercise physiology course, students will initially learn to describe changes associated with the stress of exercise. For example, students will learn that muscles get bigger (**hypertrophy**) and stronger with resistance training, longer with flexibility training, and have more blood vessels (capillaries) and **mitochondria** (a cellular organelle involved in aerobic energy production) with aerobic training. They will discover that there are different types of **muscle fibers** (i.e., skeletal muscle cells), **fast-twitch** and **slow-twitch**, and they will learn that fiber type can change with training. However, as they go on to more advanced classes, begin reading articles in professional journals, and get involved in research projects, students will soon realize how essential it is that exercise physiologists learn more about topics within molecular biology and genetics, so that they can train their brains to think more mechanistically and be able to grasp the interconnectedness of cells and tissues in the body.

Understanding Muscle Crosstalk

Exercise physiologists are trained to understand how the various systems of the body function and interact during exercise and how they adapt to exercise training. The reader would probably be able to guess that exercise affects the heart, blood vessels, bone, and skeletal muscle, but it might not be as obvious that hundreds of chemicals released by muscle during exercise communicate with other organs and systems such as the brain, gut, liver, and immune system. Exercise initiates a cascade of events, where signaling molecules called **myokines** (chemicals released by muscle) allow **crosstalk,** that is, communication, between organ systems (Thyfault and Bergouignan, 2020). For example, many people have heard of a molecule called lactate which is produced in muscles during exercise, and they may have heard (erroneously) that it is a harmful substance that causes muscle soreness. Lactate is actually a very useful molecule with many positive roles in metabolism and can communicate with other parts of the body. Exhibit 5.2 (Brooks et al., 2023) illustrates the far-reaching influence lactate can have in the body and is an example of how exercising muscle, through the many chemicals that are released from the muscle and other

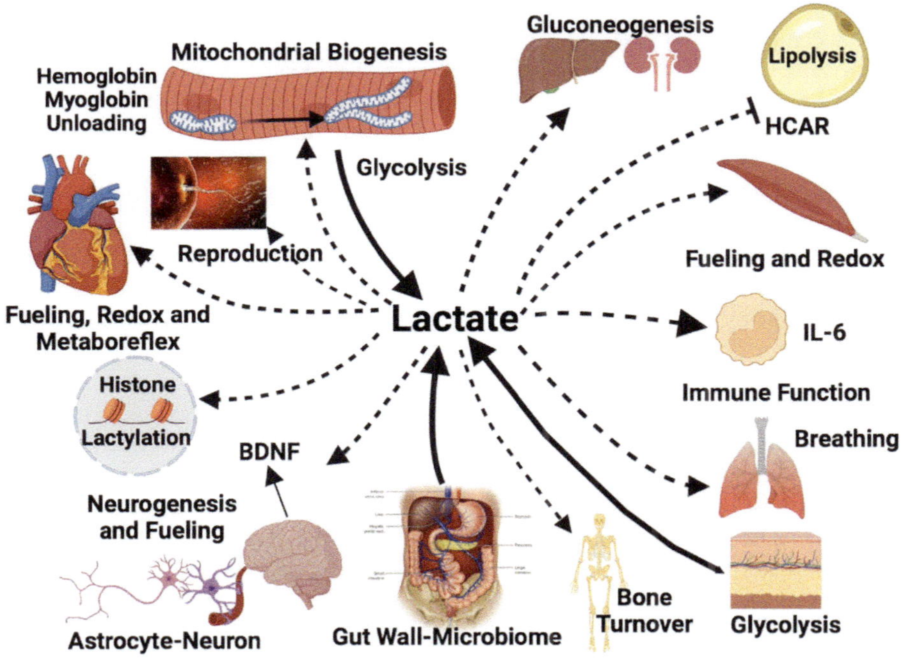

Exhibit 5.2 Lactate as a myokine and its influence on diverse tissues. Lactate is an example of a molecule that communicates with, and influences the function of, many different tissues, including the heart and blood vessels, lungs, liver, and brain. Tissues that produce lactate are shown with solid lines, including lactate generated through glycolysis in skeletal muscle during exercise. Tissues that consume lactate are shown by dashed lines. Lactate turns on diverse signaling pathways in tissues throughout the body

Source: Adapted from Brooks, Osmond, Arevalo, Duong, Curl, Moreno-Santillan, and Leija (2023)

tissues, can "talk" to every organ system in the body (Brooks et al., 2023; Severinsen and Pedersen, 2020), including cancer cells (Brooks et al., 2022; San-Millan et al., 2020).

Exercise Physiology Expands Its Scope

Over the past few decades, the study of the cellular, molecular, and genetic aspects of exercise have become an integral part of research and practice in exercise physiology and sport science (Kim, Wheeler, and Ashley, 2022; Noone et al., 2024; Tanisawa et al., 2020). To that end, exercise science students can expect to be introduced to the exciting areas of **genomics, epigenetics, transcriptomics, proteomics, metabolomics** and **fluxomics**. These terms will be defined in the technology section of this chapter.

APPLICATIONS TO EXERCISE SCIENCE

Exercise physiology is an important pillar in the field of exercise science. As previously mentioned, it answers the how and why questions. However, before taking an exercise physiology class, a firm foundation of scientific knowledge is essential. That is why students who major in exercise science will take classes in biology, anatomy, physiology, and chemistry before they take higher level classes in their major such as exercise physiology. Chapter 3 outlined the basic areas of study in anatomy and physiology which include the cardiovascular, pulmonary, skeletal, nervous, and muscular systems. A working knowledge of the endocrine and immune systems is also important. In addition, Chapter 4 explained the importance of understanding basic biochemistry and nutrition in exercise science, as these areas explain how the body generates energy (in the form of ATP) for muscular work via the breakdown of fat, protein, and carbohydrates from food. By building a strong knowledge base, learning to think critically, and gradually integrating this knowledge as they prepare for careers as fitness, sport, and healthcare professionals, students will realize the importance of asking questions, knowing where to go for evidence-based answers, and being able to understand and explain to their clients the "why" of the assessment and prescription tools that they are using in the field. Even the most basic observations, that heart rate increases during exercise, for example, are quite complex. What makes one's heart rate go up in anticipation of a race or athletic event, even before one step has been taken? Why does heart rate increase when one starts walking at a certain speed and then level-out only to gradually drift upward over time (Coyle and Gonzalez-Alonso, 2001)? Why does heart rate increase with increasing workloads and what makes it level off at a certain maximal value for that individual? Why does it take a while for the heart rate to come back to resting levels after exercise? Why is resting heart rate substantially lower in individuals that consistently exercise? The list could go on. If the reader is not able to answer the questions above, hopefully they are feeling curious to know the answers and looking forward to taking an exercise physiology class. A warning, though: the process of "knowing the answers" is a lifelong quest, and the exercise science student can look forward to endless discoveries as they progressively increase their understanding with their curiosity never being fully satisfied.

HEALTH/CLINICAL ASPECTS

A few students reading this chapter will go on to graduate school and become research scientists in exercise physiology and make discoveries that will guide practitioners in the field. However, most exercise science students want to work in applied settings and will go on to pursue careers in health/fitness or healthcare related fields. Whether students end up working in a strength and conditioning facility, fitness center, corporate wellness center, clinic, or hospital, they will have a common goal of helping each individual client meet their health, fitness, and/or performance related goals. Chapter 6 introduces the process of exercise prescription (designing exercise programs) for individual clients.

There are many areas of applied study in exercise physiology. Exercise physiologists can be found working with individuals interested in improving athletic performance (sports physiologists), healthy individuals that want to maintain or improve their health, as well as individuals with disease (see career opportunities section). Some exercise physiologists work in very specialized areas such as studying the effect of microgravity and spaceflight on bone and muscle health or working with individuals who have experienced a spinal cord injury (Weir and Weir, 2017). For instance, one study showed that during one month of spaceflight, postmenopausal women lost as much bone mass as they would in one year on Earth (Cavanagh, Licata, and Rice, 2005). Exercise physiologists can help design exercise programs that will minimize this bone loss. For spinal cord patients, exercise physiologists are involved in discovering ways to mitigate the risk of developing cardiovascular disease and other issues associated with varying degrees of paralysis. The reader might be surprised to find that exercise guidelines for most clinical populations (e.g., individuals with cardiovascular and pulmonary disease, Parkinson's disease, multiple sclerosis), are very similar to those for the general population (Liguori and ACSM, 2022). For example, the recommendations for individuals who have experienced a spinal cord injury include at least two days/week of aerobic exercise and two days/week of resistance exercise (Evans et al., 2015).

While exercise physiologists are shedding light on many fascinating areas of study with application to healthy and clinical populations, this section will focus on two areas of research that will give the reader a glimpse into how researchers in exercise physiology contribute to helping exercise professionals keep their clients healthy, avoid chronic disease, and ultimately live longer without disability. We will look at the simple idea of taking frequent breaks to move during the day (exercise snacks) and then consider the more complex phenomena of muscle loss (sarcopenia) with age and how to mitigate the associated loss of function. To best understand these examples, the ideas of chronic inflammation and the dangers of the dual pandemics of lack of exercise and sedentary behavior will be introduced.

Chronic Inflammation Leads to Chronic Diseases

The development of most chronic diseases (e.g., cardiovascular, type II diabetes, cancer, non-alcoholic fatty liver disease) are related to low-level, systemic **chronic inflammation** (SCI) in the human body. While acute inflammation is essential to healing from an infection or injury, ongoing SCI can damage body tissues. The widespread lack of physical activity contributes to this chronic, inflammatory environment and leads to dysfunction, disability, and death. Exhibit 5.3 illustrates the connection between physical exercise and healthy aging (El Assar et al., 2022).

Physical Inactivity and Sedentary Behavior Pandemics

Exercise physiology is closely related to **sedentary physiology**, the study of what happens to a human body that does not move off and on throughout the day. Less than a quarter of adults meet the minimum physical activity guidelines, and the majority of

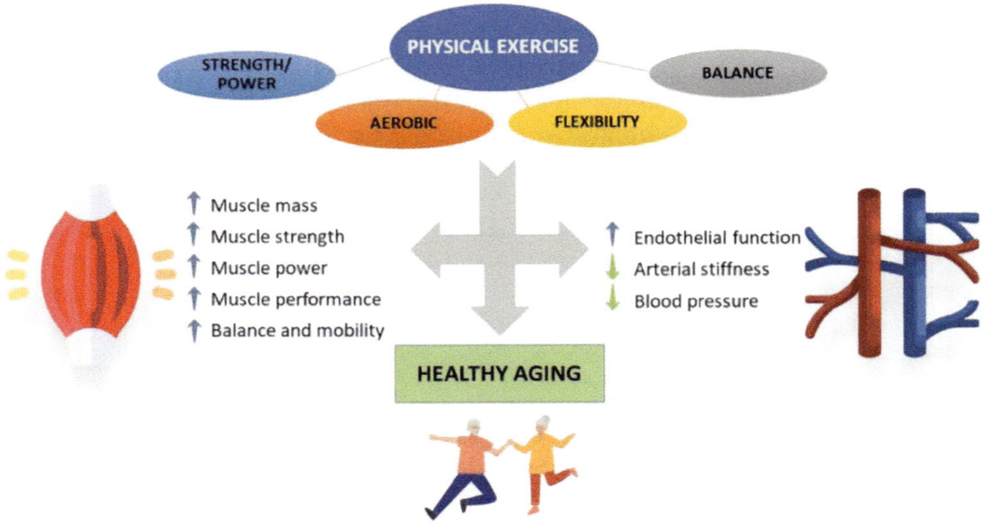

Exhibit 5.3 Physical exercise reduces chronic inflammation and promotes healthy aging. Different modalities of physical exercise (strength/power, aerobic, flexibility, and balance) exert benefits on multiple clinical variables through improving muscular and vascular functions. The expression of these benefits is associated with disease prevention and healthy aging

Source: Adapted from El Assar, Alvarez-Bustos, Sosa, Angulo, and Rodriguez-Manas (2022)

individuals sit for much of their waking hours (Liguori and ACSM, 2021). This lack of activity contributes to the development of the major causes of death (e.g., cardiovascular disease, cancer) and was declared a pandemic in 2012 (Kohl et al., 2012), with Hall and colleagues emphasizing that there is a simultaneous **sedentarism** pandemic (Hall et al., 2021). Therefore, a two-pronged approach to sit less and move more is essential for health. In other words, all individuals should engage in regular, consistent exercise that includes both an aerobic and resistance training component and should also break up their sedentary time with frequent activity breaks during the day. For example, a college student could go to the fitness center and run on a treadmill or swim for 30 minutes, five times per week, but if the rest of the week is spent sitting while at work, school, or on electronic devices, then they could still be at risk for developing chronic disease.

Example: Breaking up Sedentary Behavior with Exercise Snacks

Recently, a small body of research has developed around the idea of **exercise snacks**, defined as "isolated bouts of vigorous exercise lasting < 1 min and performed periodically throughout the day" (Islam, Gibala, and Little, 2022). Similarly to people taking a break from what they are doing to get a cup of tea or eat a granola bar, it appears that developing a habit of breaking up the day with short bouts of exercise can help counteract too much sedentary time. For instance, a college student who is studying could get up once every hour or two and do a very quick bout of high-intensity work such as walking up three flights of stairs or doing a set of body weight squats. Rafiei et al. (2021) showed that, for overweight or obese adults who sat for 9 hours but took a 30-second stair climbing break each hour, there was a lower insulin and free fatty acid response following a meal compared to subjects who did not perform these "snacks." Exercise snacks are also being studied in clinical populations to investigate whether they can improve health and possibly treat disease. See Exhibit 5.4 to read an abstract of a study that used brief, high intensity exercise bouts in cancer patients and found that, in addition to improving cardiovascular and metabolic health, exercise snacks may suppress tumor growth (Jenkins et al., 2023).

Exhibit 5.4 Abstract of a research review that examined the benefits of very brief bouts of exercise (i.e., exercise snacks) in cancer patients

Jenkins, D.G., Devin, J.L., Weston, K.L., Jenkins, J.G., and Skinner, T.L. (2023). Benefits beyond cardiometabolic health: the potential of frequent high intensity "exercise snacks" to improve outcomes for those living with and beyond cancer. *The Journal of Physiology*, *601*(21), 4691–4697. https://doi.org/10.1113/JP284985

Abstract

High intensity interval training (HIIT) has been shown to consistently elicit rapid and significant adaptations in a number of physiological systems, across many different healthy and clinical populations. In addition, there is increasing interest in how some acute, yet transient responses to high intensity exercise potentially reduce the risks of particular diseases. Recent work has shown that discrete, brief bouts of high intensity exercise (termed "exercise snacks") can improve glucose control and vascular health and thus counter the negative cardiometabolic consequences of prolonged, uninterrupted periods of inactivity. In this brief review, we advance the case, using evidence available from pre-clinical studies in the exercise oncology literature, that brief, frequently completed bouts of high intensity exercise embedded within an individual's overall daily and weekly physical activity schedule, may transiently impact the tumor microenvironment and improve the health outcomes for those who have been diagnosed and treated for cancer.

Example: Inactivity and Sarcopenia

Human bodies thrive on movement and a body that does not move regularly will not enjoy optimal health. Exercise physiologists have demonstrated the "use it or lose it" principle clearly in fascinating research into the loss of muscle function with age (Chen, Datzkiw, and Rudnicki, 2020; Wiedmer et al., 2021; Yang and Chan, 2022). In general, as people age, they become less active. It is critical to understand that being less active means that muscles are activated (i.e., turned on) less frequently, and usually at a lower intensity, meaning that a decrease in physical activity with aging means the powerful fast-twitch muscle fibers are rarely required. The point is that as individuals age and move less in general and do less vigorous activity in particular, they lose muscle mass (**sarcopenia**), gain body fat, and lose muscle strength and power (**dynapenia**). There are many reasons why this happens (Yang and Chan, 2022) but only two will be introduced below.

Before discussing the implications of these age-related changes, there are two terms the reader needs to understand: motor units and satellite cells. Muscle is typically made up of both slow-twitch and fast-twitch muscle fibers that are organized into motor units. A **motor unit** is defined as one motor neuron (think nerve cell to skeletal muscle) and all the muscle fibers that it innervates. Motor units that are made up of slow-twitch muscle fibers are activated (i.e., recruited) first at low intensities of exercise and the fast-twitch fibers are activated with higher intensities of exercise (Hu, Rymer, and Suresh, 2013). Motor unit firing rates are lower in older adults (Kirk et al., 2021) and abnormal firing patterns of motor units can be seen in older adults who are losing muscle mass but are not yet classified as being sarcopenic (Hirono et al., 2024). **Satellite cells** are stem cells that are normally dormant (i.e., inactive) and are located around the periphery of muscle fibers. Satellite cells can be activated through physical activity and are important for muscle repair and growth (Chen, Datzkiw, and Rudnicki, 2020). As people age and are less active, they rarely activate their fast-twitch fibers or their satellite cells and without use, they will lose the fast-twitch motor units and the ability to activate satellite cells. This contributes to sarcopenia and potentially harmful results. For example, if individuals can't react quickly when they trip over the corner of a rug or a crack in the sidewalk, they will likely fall and may break a hip or other bones, which many individuals never recover from (Sing et al., 2023).

Exercise Is Medicine

At this point the reader may begin to see how important frequent movement is to health and wonder why there isn't more emphasis placed on the double pandemics of physical inactivity and sedentarism. Therefore, it may not be surprising that there is currently a strong push for healthcare providers to routinely ask clients about their physical activity and prescribe exercise as part of the treatment plan, referring clients to qualified exercise professionals for follow-up. There is ample evidence that exercise, in the proper dose, can prevent and/or treat dozens of diseases (Thompson et al., 2020), including cancer, osteoporosis, and brain disorders (e.g., depression, dementia). The American College of Sports Medicine (ACSM) manages a program called Exercise is Medicine (EIM®), which demonstrates the strong connection between regular physical activity and optimal health and encourages healthcare providers to include exercise when designing treatment plans. Explore the EIM® website (Exercise is Medicine, n.d.) to learn more about this important initiative, how it is being implemented, and to check out the resources and helpful tools that are available such as the Cancer Exercise App which is available for download (Cancer Exercise App, n.d.).

SPORTS/PERFORMANCE ASPECTS

This section focuses on the contribution exercise physiologists make to optimize training for individuals interested in improving athletic performance. Most athletes train to improve qualities such as muscle size (**hypertrophy**), strength, power, speed, agility, endurance, and maximal aerobic capacity (**VO_2Max**). The difference between winning and losing is very small at the elite level. Therefore, even seemingly small improvements from exercise training can translate to athletic success. The following are two examples of research topics in exercise physiology that focus on understanding the science behind the pursuit of athletic excellence.

Example: Specificity of Training and Muscle Growth

To begin the first example, readers should think about their own training habits and ask themselves some questions (and hopefully think of some more!). What is my training goal? To reach that goal, what needs to happen? Do I need to get stronger? Bigger? Faster? For example, let's assume the reader wants to put on more muscle mass. What would they have to do to gain muscle through training? It may be obvious that starting a long-distance running program or focusing on balance or flexibility are probably not the answer. Resistance training (e.g., exercises with body weight, resistance bands, dumbbells, and barbells) would be a lot more effective than running for building muscle, but why? What is it about resistance training that stimulates muscle growth? The reader may be thinking about a lot of other questions by now about the specific type of resistance training protocol such as what exercises to do, how often to do them, how many sets and repetitions, and many others. Those are all questions that sport scientists are answering and that exercise science students can begin learning about in Chapter 6. However, as the reader thinks more about building muscle, eventually, the questions will focus on what is happening inside the muscle fibers themselves. What is it about doing sets of squats and lunges that will cause the thigh muscles to get bigger? There are multiple answers to that question but, for our example, we will focus on the mechanical stress involved. In other words, the shortening and lengthening of the cell membrane triggers a signaling pathway that ultimately turns on a molecule called mammalian target of rapamycin (mTOR). Activating mTOR leads to events in the nucleus of the cell, where genes are turned on that code for the synthesis of specific proteins (Wang and Proud, 2006). If protein synthesis is greater than protein breakdown, with consistent training, the muscle will grow. Exercise science students will have the opportunity to learn exactly how this works (there are lots of molecules involved) and how to influence this pathway, for example, by consuming enough protein, and even specific types of amino acids (e.g., leucine) in addition to the workout itself, to maximize muscle growth (Ely et al., 2023). By studying muscle growth, it is clear how exercise physiology researchers and practitioners (e.g. personal trainers, strength and conditioning coaches) work in partnership to optimize athletic performance.

Importance of Following the Evidence

Exercise physiologists enjoy the process of discovery and are willing to change their minds when scientific evidence accumulates in a specific direction. In fact, many ideas that used to be accepted dogma have since been refined and occasionally have undergone substantial revision. An example is a recent paper entitled "Resistance Training Recommendations to Maximize Muscle Hypertrophy in an Athletic Population: Position Stand of the IUSCA" (Schoenfeld et al., 2021), which discusses the evidence for controversial topics such as whether resistance training sets should be done to momentary muscle failure, whether the magnitude of the load or a specific repetition range (e.g., 6–12 reps) is required to maximize hypertrophy, and whether an **interference effect** exists with **concurrent** training. In other words, if an athlete performs resistance and endurance training in the same session, will that interfere with optimal protein synthesis? This relates to the discussion of mTOR above because it is possible that signaling pathways initiated by endurance training could inhibit the activation of mTOR (e.g., activation of the adenosine monophosphate protein kinase [AMPK] pathway). Hopefully, these questions pique the readers' interest, and they look forward to learning about the science behind them and how to integrate that knowledge with what athletes and strength and conditioning coaches do in practice. Exhibit 5.5 contains an abstract from a research article which integrates information from 23 different studies (i.e., a meta-analysis) to determine the best resistance training load for improving strength and muscle hypertrophy (Lacio et al., 2021).

Exhibit 5.5 Abstract of a systematic review article

Lacio, M., Vieira, J.G., Trybulski, R., Campos, Y., Santana, D., Filho, J.E., Novaes, J., Vianna, J., and Wilk, M. (2021). Effects of Resistance Training Performed with Different Loads in Untrained and Trained Male Adult Individuals on Maximal Strength and Muscle Hypertrophy: A Systematic Review. *International Journal of Environmental Research and Public Health*, *18*(21), 11237. https://doi.org/10.3390/ijerph182111237

Abstract

The load in resistance training is considered to be a critical variable for neuromuscular adaptations. Therefore, it is important to assess the effects of applying different loads on the development of maximal strength and muscular hypertrophy. The aim of this study was to systematically review the literature and compare the effects of resistance training that was performed with low loads versus moderate and high loads in untrained and trained healthy adult males on the development of maximal strength and muscle hypertrophy during randomized experimental designs. The Preferred Reporting Items for Systematic Reviews and Meta-Analyses guidelines (2021) were followed with the eligibility criteria defined according to participants, interventions, comparators, outcomes, and study design (PICOS): (P) healthy males between 18 and 40 years old, (I) interventions performed with low loads, (C) interventions performed with moderate or high loads, (O) development of maximal strength and muscle hypertrophy, and (S) randomized experimental studies with between- or within-subject parallel designs. The literature search strategy was performed in three electronic databases (Embase, PubMed, and Web of Science) on 22 August 2021. Results: 23 studies with a total of 563 participants (80.6% untrained and 19.4% trained) were selected. The studies included both relative and absolute loads. All studies were classified as being moderate-to-high methodological quality, although only two studies had a score higher than six points. The main findings indicated that the load magnitude that was used during resistance training influenced the dynamic strength and isometric strength gains. In general, comparisons between the groups (i.e., low, moderate, and high loads) showed higher gains in 1RM and maximal voluntary isometric contraction when moderate and high loads were used. In contrast, regarding muscle hypertrophy, most studies showed that when resistance training was performed to muscle failure, the load used had less influence on muscle hypertrophy. The current literature shows that gains in maximal strength are more pronounced with high and moderate loads compared to low loads in healthy adult male populations. However, for muscle hypertrophy, studies indicate that a wide spectrum of loads (i.e., 30 to 90% 1RM) may be used for healthy adult male populations.

Example: Power, Jumping, and Reflexes

One of the most important skills that a student can acquire during their education is the ability to think critically. In the previous section, the readers were encouraged to ask questions about how to stimulate muscle growth; curiosity is the starting point. By asking questions, students will discover that they don't always have the answers and will understand the importance of learning foundational knowledge and using reliable sources of information to use appropriate terminology and grasp the basic concepts needed to think critically about their questions. In the second example, related to sport performance, the reader is asked to think critically about another physiological concept related to developing **power** (i.e., the ability to exert force quickly).

Many athletes perform plyometric drills to improve their explosiveness and power. **Plyometric exercises** are sometimes called jumping exercises. Examples include skipping rope, depth jumps, jumping side to side over a hurdle, and medicine ball throws/catches against a wall. For this example, a series of vertical jumps will be used to illustrate the physiology behind plyometric training. It is probably easy to imagine that if the goal is to jump as high as possible with each jump, that the person jumping will need to do two things: 1) activate as many motor units as possible, including the large, fast-twitch motor units, to voluntarily produce as much force as possible, as quickly as possible; and 2) harness the reciprocal "bounce" as the elastic nature of the connective tissue in the muscle allows it to stretch upon landing and rebound on the subsequent jump. There is another important mechanism that athletes can use to maximize their vertical jump and it involves the **stretch** (or myotatic) **reflex** which was described over 100 years ago (Liddell and Sherrington, 1924). Focusing on the quadriceps muscles (the large muscle group on the anterior thigh that extends the leg or straightens the knee), the muscle fibers will stretch upon the landing of the vertical jump and cause sensory receptors within the muscle, called **muscle spindles,** that are sensitive to the length of the muscle, to stretch too. When the nerve endings in the muscle spindles fire, a signal is sent to the spinal cord, where the sensory neuron will **synapse** (i.e., connect) with and stimulate a motor neuron that innervates the same muscle that was stretched (Reschechtko and Pruszynski, 2020). This series of events cause the quadriceps muscle that was initially elongated, or stretched, to reflexively contract or shorten in response.

Importance of Critical Thinking Skills

When trainers or coaches understand the science behind the practice of plyometric training, they are able to think critically about the proper technique to maximize results. Using our example, if a coach asks an athlete to perform a series of bounding jumps, timing is very important, and they would need to use the three points outlined above to help the athlete get the most from this training drill. The athlete would be instructed to try to jump as high or far as possible and absorb the shock on landing, which would stretch the muscle and tendon at the knee (and across the back of the hip and ankle) and, using the elastic recoil, to voluntarily jump again. If the timing is right, the stretch reflex would act to recruit additional muscle fibers for a more powerful jump (Komi, 2000). This may sound simple, but it can be difficult to bridge the gap between science and practice, i.e., the research recommendations and what practitioners are doing with athletes in the field in terms of optimizing plyometric programs (Watkins et al., 2021).

TECHNOLOGY AND RESEARCH TOOLS

There are many tools used by exercise physiology researchers and practitioners. This section describes several of the most common tools, technology, and equipment used in research and or clinical environments.

Treadmills and Ergometers

The most common exercise modalities used to stress the human body are treadmills and cycle **ergometers**, devices that measure the work done during exercise. Exercise intensity on a treadmill can be adjusted by either changing the speed of the belt and/or the steepness of the grade. Work on a cycle ergometer is determined by changing the resistance to pedaling the bike. This can be done by changing either the tension on the belt or the pedaling rate (in revolutions per minute or rpm). There are also more expensive electronically braked cycle ergometers that have the advantage of using an electromagnet to provide the resistance and thereby allow the pedaling speed to vary during the work bout. Many other exercise modalities can also be used for testing, such as arm crank ergometers to measure work done by the upper body, ergometers for measuring work done during activities like rowing and cross-country skiing, and swim flumes for determining swimming performance diagnostics (Weir and Weir, 2017). Just like a mechanic who must choose the right tools to fix each vehicle brought into the shop, the exercise physiologist must choose the most appropriate tool to use for each situation, considering the client characteristics (e.g., a cardiac rehabilitation client versus an elite athlete), the purpose of the testing, cost, and equipment available.

Metabolic Measurements

Maximal oxygen consumption (VO_2Max) is a very common physiological measure in exercise physiology that is used to assess an individual's aerobic fitness level. Metabolic testing using indirect calorimetry involves determining the amount of oxygen consumed and the amount of carbon dioxide produced by analyzing the composition of the air going into and out of the lungs with each breath and can be done during rest or exercise. Exhibit 5.6 shows a subject hooked up to a computerized metabolic cart while running on a treadmill. Sensors in the mask detect the amount of oxygen and carbon dioxide in the air that the subject breathes out (i.e., exhales). A person who is more fit will be able to deliver more oxygen to the working muscles and the active muscle tissue will be able to use oxygen at a higher rate. This type of testing also allows for the calculation of energy expenditure (i.e., caloric expenditure) and the type of fuel (fat versus carbohydrate) being used (Weir and Weir, 2017). Portable metabolic units are also available that allow for metabolic measurements outside the laboratory in more natural environments, such as a sprinter running on a track or a cyclist training outdoors (see Exhibit 5.7 for an example).

Wearable Technology

The development of wearable technology has exploded in recent years. There are many devices that can be carried or attached to the body (e.g., smart phones and watches) or integrated into clothing. Accelerometers are very popular and are used to monitor physical

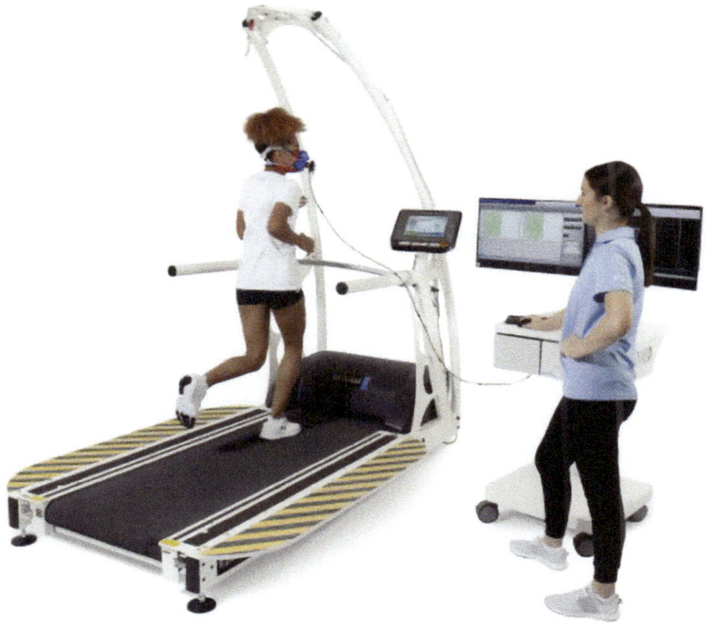

Exhibit 5.6 Individual running on a treadmill wearing a mask used for metabolic testing
Source: Photo courtesy of COSMED USA

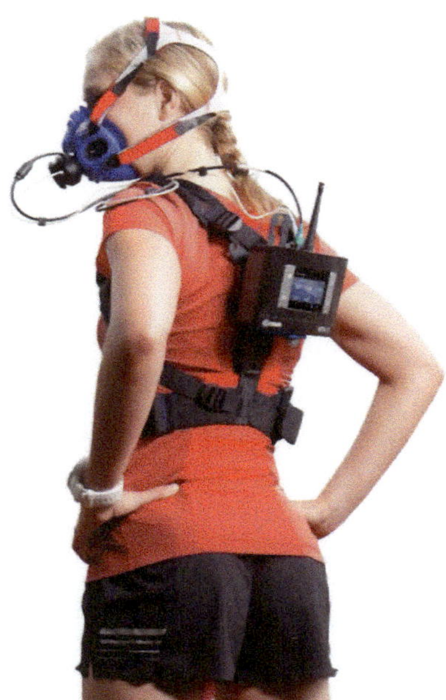

Exhibit 5.7 Individual wearing a portable metabolic system
Source: Photo courtesy of COSMED USA

activity in everyday situations. They allow the accurate counting of how long (i.e., duration) and how hard (i.e., intensity) an individual exercises and can track movement patterns throughout the day, including time spent in sedentary behaviors. This is important because, on average, people are not very accurate at self-reporting, with most overestimating their physical activity and underestimating their sedentariness (Meh et al., 2023).

Other wearable technologies allow researchers to look inside the human body. For example, continuous glucose monitors can sense the amount of glucose in the interstitial fluid and sample it at regular intervals, in both a fasted state and after a meal. Glucose levels could be followed and compared after different kinds of meals such as a high fat versus a high carbohydrate meal, or during and after exercise (Kent and Hayes, 2021). Wearables have become more sophisticated since pedometers were first conceptualized by Leonardo da Vinci in the 15th century (Tudor-Locke, 2002) and this trend will continue.

Muscle Biopsies

Muscle biopsy measurements involve using a specialized needle to extract a small piece of tissue from a muscle from which many different biomarkers can be determined (Weir and Weir, 2017). A local anesthetic is used to numb the tissue before the procedure that involves multiple injections around the biopsy site. This technique is typically performed in research labs because of the invasiveness of the procedure and the high level of technical expertise required. Earlier in this chapter, the cell signaling pathway that involved the activation of the enzyme mTOR was discussed in relation to building muscle mass. A researcher studying muscle growth could take a muscle sample before and after a training session and measure the effectiveness of the session in activating the molecules involved in the mTOR pathway. Or perhaps the researcher is studying the effects of various types of nutritional supplements on protein synthesis and takes a biopsy to see the degree to which a particular supplement upregulates the mTOR pathway. For instance, would a whey-based protein shake or a drink that contains both protein and carbohydrate such as chocolate milk be more effective in stimulating muscle synthesis? Would plant-based protein be as effective as animal-based protein? What is the effect of these supplements alone and in combination with resistance exercise in stimulating increases in strength and/or muscle mass? This area of investigation has had much attention (Morgan et al., 2021; Nunes et al., 2022) and is of practical importance for healthy adults, athletes, and clinical populations such as cancer patients and frail, elderly individuals.

Another use for muscle biopsies could involve researchers who are interested in tracking fiber type changes that occur with different types of training. Although the terms slow-twitch and fast-twitch have been used up to this point to classify muscle fibers based on their contraction velocity, the reader may have guessed that it is more complicated than that. Fiber types exist on a spectrum from **slow-twitch oxidative (SO or Type I) fibers** that are very aerobic, having a good blood supply, lots of mitochondria, and are fatigue resistant, to **fast-twitch oxidative glycolytic (FOG or Type IIa) fibers** that are both aerobic and anaerobic, to **fast-twitch glycolytic (FG or Type IIx) fibers** that are very powerful but fatigue very quickly (Powers, Howley, and Quindry, 2024). There are also hybrid fibers that have characteristics between these three main types (Tobias and Galpin, 2020). Interestingly, these fiber types are not fixed, and an individual's fiber composition can change with training. There are many other uses for muscle biopsies that cannot be covered here, such as examining metabolite accumulation and glycogen depletion during exercise (Weir and Weir, 2017).

Electromyography

Electromyography (EMG) is a technique used to measure the electrical activity associated with the activation of motor units and subsequent muscle contraction. EMG measurements are performed using either surface electrodes placed on the skin over the contracting muscle or more invasive needle electrodes that are inserted into the muscle. Exhibit 5.8 shows a series of muscle contractions that are progressive in intensity. As more motor units are recruited, more muscle fibers are activated, producing more force, and exhibiting more electrical activity. EMG has been used to study how the nervous system adapts to resistance training (Moritani and deVries, 1979) and to investigate the mechanisms of fatigue. For example, the reader may guess that as a muscle fatigues and produces less force, there is also less electrical activity detected by EMG, and this is often the case. However, EMG can also stay the same or even increase with fatigue, demonstrating the importance of avoiding assumptions and taking careful measurements (Bigland-Ritchie, 1981; Moritani, Muro, and Nagata, 1986). More advanced signal processing techniques that use multiple surface electrodes are also being used to investigate the activity of individual motor units. For instance, Herda et al. (2015) showed that motor unit behavior varied between endurance-trained versus resistance-trained individuals.

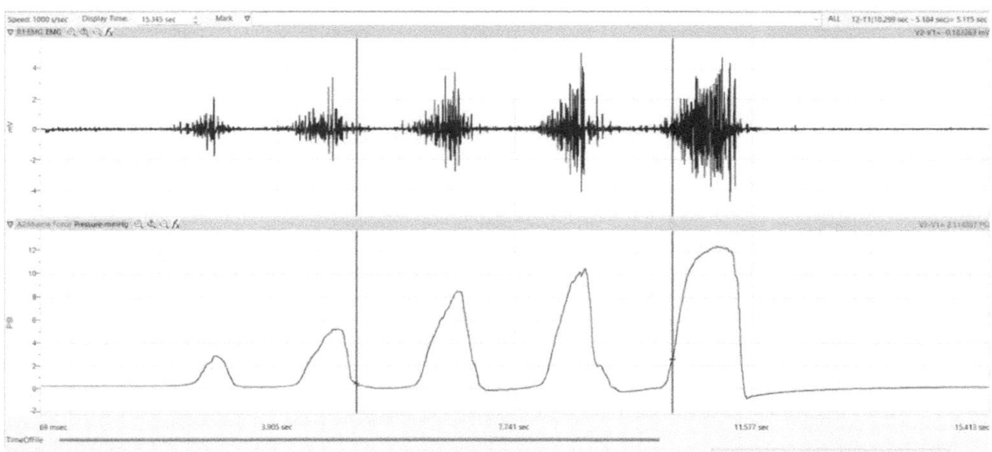

Exhibit 5.8 Relationship between muscle EMG activity and force production. The top row of the graph shows EMG activity, and the bottom row shows muscle force production. The data were obtained from a handgrip dynamometer test where the subject performed a series of progressively harder muscle contractions with a brief rest between each contraction

Source: iWorx

Imaging: Visualizing the Human Body

Imaging technologies vary in terms of what they are measuring and their specific application. For instance, body composition assessment, discussed in Chapters 2 and 6, is important in quantifying the amount of adipose tissue (i.e., fat tissue), muscle mass, bone mass, and water content in an individual's body. This information is helpful when working with clients that want to either gain or lose body weight and reflects the effectiveness of exercise and nutritional programs for weight management. The current "gold standard" or reference method for body composition measurements is **dual-energy X-ray absorptiometry** or DXA (Gibson, Wagner, and Heyward, 2018). This method is associated with a small amount of radiation, but it allows the exercise physiologist or healthcare provider to see where the subject is carrying their fat, under the skin (subcutaneously) versus internally (viscerally). This is important in quantifying how risky the fat is as visceral fat is more closely associated with chronic inflammation and the development of chronic metabolic diseases. DXA also measures bone mineral density. This can be used to follow the decline which occurs with aging, especially in postmenopausal females, or the improvements seen with resistance training and/or other weight bearing exercise.

In addition to DXA, there are many other tools available for visualizing internal structures in the body. Readers of this book are probably familiar with some of these imaging technologies. They may have used a microscope in a biology class to look at different types of cells or perhaps someone has had an X-ray for a broken bone or a magnetic resonance imaging (MRI) scan for a torn ligament in their knee or shoulder. X-rays and computed tomography (CT) scans involve radiation, whereas MRI scans and nuclear magnetic resonance spectroscopy (MRS) use powerful electromagnets to create images of the tissue. Other scanning technologies include positron emission tomography (PET) which is based on radioactive tracers and near-infrared spectroscopy (NIRS). In clinical settings, these tools are typically used for diagnostic purposes but are also used by researchers in exercise physiology. For example, Pilotto et al. (2022) used NIRS as a noninvasive method to study the oxidative capacity (VO_2) and diffusion capacity of muscle during exercise which allowed them to measure the amount of oxygen bound to hemoglobin, which carries oxygen in the blood. As a note, these authors (Pilotto et al., 2022) also used the muscle biopsy technology discussed earlier to obtain samples of the vastus lateralis (one of the quadricep muscles mentioned earlier). A discussion of the scientific basis of each test listed above and their specific applications is beyond the scope of this chapter; however, the point is that these technologies allow for the visualization of anatomical structures, processes, and molecules that enable scientists to identify different types of cells, proteins, and metabolites. Examples of specific variables of interest to exercise physiologists include the identification of cells that have been activated through exercise, tissue oxygenation and blood flow, and metabolites such as ATP, lactate, and glucose (Kent and Hayes, 2021).

The "Omics"

There has been an explosion of new technologies in molecular biology over the past three decades. Starting with the Human Genome Project and rapidly evolving as new technologies become available, our understanding of cells, genes, proteins, and the molecules generated during exercise is continually growing. **Genomics** is a field of biology focused on studying the genome, which includes all the genes encoded by deoxyribonucleic acid (DNA). Much work has gone into identifying the DNA sequence of the human genome and identifying the function of each gene and how it interacts with the others (Collins and McKusick, 2001). **Epigenomics** is the study of the changes or modifications that can occur to one's DNA due to environmental and behavioral factors and how these modifications can be passed on to one's children. The DNA sequence itself does not change, but the expression, i.e., whether a gene is turned on or off, does. **Proteomics** is the study of the proteins coded for by the genome and produced by an organism. **Metabolomics** is the study and analysis of metabolites in the human body (Owens and Bennett, 2024).

Metabolites are small molecules that are generated by cells during metabolic processes. Visit The Human Metabolome Database (n.d.) to gain an appreciation for the thousands of metabolites that have been studied. Lastly, there is the emerging field of **fluxomics,** which allows for an "understanding of the rate at which metabolites move through a metabolic pathway (i.e., metabolic flux)," and provides "context for the interpretation of metabolomics data" (Owens and Bennett, 2024). As a group, these new technologies have provided new opportunities for exercise physiologists to study and describe the effects of exercise on the body and to understand, at a molecular level, what is happening and why.

CAREER AND EMPLOYMENT OPPORTUNITIES

Students can use an undergraduate exercise science degree as a jumping off point to many career pathways. As is true of many college degrees, the exercise science student will be served best by their degree if they are motivated to study hard and gain the skills and knowledge that will open future educational and career opportunities. Employment opportunities may include working as an exercise physiologist in a health/wellness/fitness center, as a clinical exercise physiologist in a hospital or outpatient clinic, or working with athletes as a strength and conditioning or performance coach. This section will discuss career pathways in exercise science, followed by the educational requirements for each pathway, as well as professional organizations, certifications, and journals.

Clinical Settings

Most clinical exercise physiologists work in cardiopulmonary rehabilitation settings with individuals who have cardiovascular or pulmonary disease and may have undergone surgery, have heart failure, chronic obstructive pulmonary disease (COPD), or other related conditions. However, clinical exercise physiologists are increasingly working in a wider range of settings with a variety of clients who may have osteoarthritis, multiple sclerosis, diabetes mellitus, cancer, or Parkinson's disease, to name a few examples. They may also work with Alzheimer's disease patients or clients with intellectual disabilities. Working with special populations requires advanced training (more on that later) and extensive experience working in clinical settings. In general, the clinical exercise physiologist performs exercise testing and designs and/or supervises exercise programs for special populations. Clinical exercise testing (also called stress testing) is commonly used for individuals who have cardiopulmonary disease. Testing normally starts at a light intensity, which then gradually increases until the client develops symptoms or is unable to continue the test. For instance, at rest an individual may not exhibit any signs or symptoms of disease, but at higher workloads, the client may be very out of breath and experience chest pain and/or dizziness that may indicate cardiac ischemia. **Cardiac ischemia** means that the heart is not getting enough oxygen due to fatty plaques in the walls of the blood vessels (atherosclerosis), occluding blood flow to the heart (Ligouri and ACSM, 2020). During testing, the client's blood pressure and electrocardiogram (ECG) are monitored for abnormalities and a metabolic cart may be used to monitor ventilation and gas exchange parameters during the test. The results of a stress test can help diagnose disease, indicate how severe it is, determine the client's exercise capacity, and be used to design an appropriate exercise program for the client (Weir and Weir, 2017). Exhibit 5.9 gives a detailed job description for a clinical exercise physiologist position in the area of cardiopulmonary rehabilitation.

Position Summary

The Clinical Exercise Physiologist in Cardiopulmonary Rehabilitation is responsible for designing, implementing, and supervising exercise programs for patients with cardiovascular and pulmonary conditions. This role involves assessing patient needs, developing individualized rehabilitation plans, and collaborating with a multidisciplinary healthcare team to promote recovery, improve functional capacity, and enhance quality of life.

Key Responsibilities

- **Patient Assessment**: Conduct comprehensive evaluations of patients' medical history, physical fitness, and cardiopulmonary function to determine appropriate exercise prescriptions.
- **Exercise Program Development**: Design and implement safe, evidence-based exercise plans tailored to individual patient needs, including aerobic, strength, and flexibility training.
- **Program Supervision**: Monitor patients during exercise sessions, ensuring safety and adherence to protocols, and adjusting plans as needed based on patient progress or complications.
- **Patient Education**: Educate patients and families on exercise benefits, lifestyle modifications, risk factor management, and strategies for long-term health maintenance.
- **Collaboration**: Work closely with cardiologists, pulmonologists, nurses, dietitians, and other healthcare professionals to coordinate care and optimize patient outcomes.
- **Documentation**: Maintain accurate records of patient assessments, progress, and treatment plans in compliance with hospital policies and regulatory standards (e.g., HIPAA)
- **Equipment Management**: Ensure proper use and maintenance of rehabilitation equipment, such as treadmills, stationary bikes, and telemetry monitors.
- **Research and Quality Improvement**: Stay current with research and best practices in clinical exercise physiology, participate in program development, and quality improvement initiatives to enhance rehabilitation services.

Qualifications

- **Education**: Bachelor's degree in Exercise Physiology, Kinesiology, or a related field required; Master's degree preferred.
- **Certification**:
    - Certified Clinical Exercise Physiologist (CEP) through the American College of Sports Medicine (ACSM) or equivalent.
    - Basic Life Support (BLS) and Advanced Cardiac Life Support (ACLS) certifications required.
- **Experience**:
    - Experience with telemetry monitoring and stress testing.
    - Minimum of 1-2 years of experience in cardiopulmonary rehabilitation or a related clinical setting preferred.
- **Skills**:
    - Strong knowledge of cardiopulmonary pathophysiology and exercise physiology.
    - In-depth knowledge of exercise testing, prescription, and chronic disease management.
    - Ability to interpret ECGs and recognize abnormal responses to exercise.
    - Excellent communication and interpersonal skills for patient education and team collaboration.
    - Proficiency in electronic medical record (EMR) systems.

Exhibit 5.9 A sample job description for a clinical exercise physiologist in cardiopulmonary rehabilitation

Source: Adapted from response to "Write a job description for a hospital based clinical exercise physiologist in cardiopulmonary rehabilitation" (xAI, Grok 3, April 30, 2025)

Health and Fitness Settings

Exercise physiologists frequently work with generally healthy populations in health and fitness settings, such as health clubs, fitness centers, corporate fitness centers, and community wellness centers. They may also work directly for a company, organization, or have their own business. For instance, an individual could have a personal training business and contract with a health club to provide services. The job description in these settings typically involves performing pre-participation health screenings with clients, performing fitness testing and interpretation, designing individualized exercise programs, supervising training sessions, and developing educational materials to support the client's health and/or fitness goals. Although exercise physiologists primarily work with healthy adults between 18–65 years, they may also work with healthy populations with special considerations, which includes children and adolescents, pregnant women, and older clients. Exercise prescription guidelines for these populations are generally the same as for healthy adults as described in Chapter 6, but there are special considerations with these populations (Ligouri and ACSM, 2020). For example, pregnant women should avoid activities that may involve contact or an increased chance of falling such as mountain biking and martial arts, and young, old, and pregnant populations should take extra care to stay hydrated when they are exercising in hot and/or humid environments. Older adults may be very healthy and fit. However, they also may be extremely deconditioned and have multiple chronic diseases. Therefore, there is often some overlap with clinical populations and the exercise physiologist must determine if they are qualified to work with a specific individual and be willing to refer clients to the appropriate professional when necessary. A typical example might be a client who experiences chronic low back pain, has high blood pressure, high cholesterol, and is taking multiple medications, but may still be able to work with an exercise physiologist in a community wellness center if the client is not currently experiencing signs and symptoms of disease and has clearance from a healthcare provider to engage in an exercise program.

Sports Performance Settings

There are many opportunities for exercise physiologists in the world of sport science, working with individuals and sport teams in many different venues. They may work in high school, college, and professional settings designing and implementing strength and conditioning programs for athletes and coordinating with athletic trainers and sports medicine personnel in the rehabilitation of injured athletes. They may work with groups such as a local swim club or soccer team or do one-on-one training such as working with a high school cross-country athlete or professional cyclist. The focus of sports and conditioning coaches, performance coaches, and personal trainers working with athletes is not only on helping athletes develop the capacities (e.g., mobility, speed, agility, coordination, muscular strength and endurance, anaerobic capabilities, aerobic endurance and/or capacity, and technical skills) they need to excel in their specific sports or positions, but also on their long-term athletic development. This includes injury prevention and a holistic concern for their health and well-being. There are opportunities for entrepreneurial individuals to develop specialty gyms (e.g., working with baseball players or master's athletes) and consulting businesses. The education, experience, and certification needed to be competitive in this area are discussed in the next sections.

EDUCATION REQUIREMENTS

The academic training for any of the career pathways in exercise physiology outlined above is not standardized in the way it would be for a nurse or elementary school teacher. There is no agreement on the level of education required (bachelor's, master's, or doctoral degree) to be an exercise physiologist or exactly what classes and experiences are necessary (Weir and Weir, 2017). In addition, different programs stress different competencies. For instance, some programs have a clinical focus, others have a sports science focus, some stress research experience, and some are a combination of the above.

Undergraduate Programs

Undergraduate exercise science programs vary in terms of their emphasis and tend to fall into two tracks: 1) an applied course of study focused on practical knowledge and skills and 2) a pre-professional track for those planning on going to graduate school, which generally requires more science classes.

Food for Thought

A typical first year student may not know what they want their future to be; that is why they take an introduction to exercise science class, so they can explore their options. It is quite common for exercise science students to choose the major because they enjoy exercising, are an athlete, or have experienced rehabilitation after an injury, but they haven't thought through what they want to do with their degree after college. In general, effective strategies for beginning exercise science students include keeping their career options open by getting good grades, developing a disciplined mind, and taking full advantage of opportunities that come their way. As they begin to develop a clear career goal, it is advisable for students to also consider backup plans and pivot as needed, because sometimes life is unpredictable. Exercise science is a valuable degree to those who understand how it can contribute to their professional preparation and success, but, like many other college degrees, it may not be useful to students that lack clear goals. Students should also realize that merely checking off course requirements does not mean that there will be a job awaiting them upon graduation, so, in addition to classwork, students should be intentional about gaining job experience, volunteering, shadowing, doing an internship, and planning on taking one or more certification tests upon graduation (Weir and Weir, 2017).

Coursework

This chapter has stressed the importance of developing critical thinking skills and has made the case that students interested in pursuing degrees in exercise physiology need a strong science background. A recent review by Kent and Hayes (2021) stated that "a solid foundation in biochemistry, physics, molecular biology, and computer sciences will be increasingly important for future exercise physiologists who want to contribute to generating new knowledge about how humans and other animals respond to acute and chronic exercise." That is why undergraduate exercise science programs generally require classes in biology, anatomy, physiology, chemistry, math, statistics, and physics. These subjects provide a solid foundation so that the student is prepared to take more advanced science classes, such as biochemistry, genetics, and biomechanics, as well as upper-division courses in their major. Exercise science majors typically take only one course in exercise physiology, plus additional courses in applied kinesiology, nutrition, exercise testing and prescription, and other subjects that form the basis for their degree.

Graduate Programs: Master's

Many exercise science students will use their degree as a stepping stone to an advanced degree. For instance, students that want to pursue careers in physical therapy, occupational therapy, athletic training, or medicine will go on to professional programs in those areas. Other students may want to get a master's or doctoral degree in exercise physiology. To gain the knowledge and skills they need to be confident and competent professionals and be competitive in the job market, students that are interested in clinical exercise physiology will likely need to pursue a master's degree and gain further knowledge about pathophysiology, exercise testing and programming for special populations, how to interpret ECGs, and clinical internship experiences. Similarly, students interested in sport science pursue graduate programs that have a strong emphasis on the science of training and include classes related to athletic populations, including tactical athletes (firefighters, warfighters), and emphasize internships. The importance of hands-on internship experiences cannot be overstated for those students who are preparing to enter the workforce. Master's level students who want to pursue careers as research scientists and go on to get their doctoral degree (PhD or EdD), typically choose a thesis option (i.e., a research project), whereas others choose a non-thesis option and focus on gaining clinical experience.

Graduate Programs: Doctoral

Doctoral programs train students to conduct research in exercise physiology and develop their critical thinking, problem solving, and writing skills. Students take coursework in advanced statistical techniques and data analysis and processing, as well as courses in the biological sciences, such as endocrinology, immunology, and neurophysiology (Weir and Weir, 2017). They also take advanced exercise physiology classes and work closely with a faculty mentor to learn how to conduct research, culminating in a dissertation project. As part of this project, the student will propose their research question, design the study, collect and analyze the data, write up the results, and defend their dissertation before a faculty committee. When applying for research positions at universities, hospitals, or in private industry, having a strong research record is necessary. Therefore, much of a graduate student's time is invested in multiple research projects and in preparing articles to submit to scientific journals (see description of journals in exercise physiology later in this chapter). Students should educate themselves regarding the application process to graduate school, including the importance of identifying a mentor who has compatible research interests and the availability of assistantships, so that they can fund their education and get the teaching and research experience they need.

CERTIFICATIONS AND LICENSURE

Unlike other health professions, such as physical therapy and medicine, there are no licensure requirements for exercise physiologists. Instead, exercise physiologists typically obtain certifications relevant to the client populations they will be working with. Three professional organizations that offer certifications are discussed below, although there are many other organizations that also offer certifications. Students should spend time educating themselves about which certifications are considered legitimate by prospective employers. If a certificate or certification seems easy to get and does not require a background in exercise science, think twice about its professional value.

American College of Sports Medicine® (ACSM)

The ACSM was founded in 1954 and started its certification program in 1975 with over 32,000 exercise professionals currently holding at least one of several available ACSM certifications (American College of Sports Medicine Committee on Certification and Registry Boards, 2023). The ACSM Certified Personal Trainer® (ACSM-CPT) and the ACSM Certified Group Exercise Instructor® (ACSM-GEI) do not require a college degree. The ACSM-Certified Exercise Physiologist® (ACSM-EP) requires a bachelor's degree in exercise science and is recommended for students who want to work with apparently healthy clients and those with medically controlled diseases (Exhibit 5.1). The ACSM Certified Clinical Exercise Physiologist® (ACSM-CEP) exam can only be taken by individuals with a bachelor's degree in exercise science and 1,200 hours of clinical experience or a master's degree in clinical exercise physiology plus 600 hours of clinical experience and is the highest certification level offered by the ACSM. The ACSM also offers the EIM® credential discussed earlier and offers certificate courses for the ACSM/ACS Certified Cancer Exercise Specialist, ACSM/NCHPAD Inclusive Fitness Specialist Certificate, Physical Activity and Public Health Specialist, and ACSM/NYSHSI Youth Fitness Specialist. For detailed, up-to-date information on any of these certifications, refer to the ACSM Certification website (ACSM, n.d.).

National Strength and Conditioning Association® (NSCA)

The NSCA began offering their first certification in 1985, and the focus for many of their current certifications is very different compared to the ACSM. NSCA certifications that can be earned with a high school diploma are the NSCA Certified Personal Trainer® (NSCA-CPT) and Tactical Strength and Conditioning Facilitator® (TSAC-F). Three certifications require a bachelor's degree in exercise science or related field: the Certified Strength and Conditioning Specialist® (CSCS), the Certified Special Population Specialist® (CSPS), and NSCA's newest certification, the Certified Performance and Sport Scientist (CPSS) which is for "experienced professionals who apply data and research to train athletes to top levels of performance" (NSCA, n.d.).

American Council on Exercise® (ACE)

The ACE offers Personal Trainer, Group Fitness Instructor, Health Coach, and Medical Exercise Specialist certifications that are accredited by the National Commission for Certifying Agencies (NCCA) (ACE, n.d.) and specialty certificates in a wide array of topics, including Fitness Nutrition, Senior Fitness, Corrective Exercise, Functional Training, Weight Management, Behavior Change, Sports Performance, Youth Fitness, Pilates Mat, Pain-Free Movement, Size Inclusive Fitness, Cancer Exercise, and the Biomechanics Method Corrective Exercise Program.

A Note on Accreditation of Exercise Science Programs

Exercise science students should be aware that beginning in 2027 for the ACSM-EP and ACSM-CEP exams, candidates will be required to have graduated from a program accredited by the Commission on Accreditation of Allied Health Education Programs (CAAHEP), and starting in 2030, to be eligible to take the NSCA-CSCS exam, students will need to have graduated from a program accredited by the Council on Accreditation of Strength and Conditioning Education (CASCE). This is meant to ensure that students who are ACSM-EP or ACSM-CEP certified have gone through a program that focuses on working with healthy and/or clinical populations (Ward-Ritacco and Magal, 2020), and those that are CSCS certified have gone through an academic program that focuses on strength and conditioning (NSCA, n.d.b.). These changes may affect student choices regarding where to go to college and/or which certifications they wish to pursue.

PROFESSIONAL ORGANIZATIONS

Professional organizations support members through education, networking, conferences, advocacy, and certification opportunities. Many of these organizations have student memberships available, offer grants for student research projects, and organize student-friendly events at regional and national conferences. Students are encouraged to take advantage of these opportunities since the costs for student membership and conference registration fees are substantially below those for professional members.

American Association of Cardiovascular and Pulmonary Rehabilitation® (AACVPR)

The AACVPR is an organization for healthcare providers, such as nurses and physicians, who specialize in cardiac and pulmonary rehabilitation. Exercise physiologists who are on a clinical exercise physiology career pathway will find valuable information and opportunities through the AACVPR. More information can be found at their website (AACVPR, n.d.).

American College of Sports Medicine® (ACSM)

The ACSM, with over 50,000 members, is the leading organization in the world for those interested in the advancement and dissemination of scientific research in exercise science and sports medicine. This is reflected in their vision statement, which aims to "extend and enrich lives through the power of movement" (ACSM, n.d.). National meetings are held each year, where participants can attend research presentations, tutorials on specific topics, and other lectures and events. There are also 12 regional chapters which hold their own conferences and events and are very student focused. Student membership is available. Go to their website for more information (ACSM, n.d.).

American Physiological Society® (APS)

The APS was founded in 1887 and is made up of over 10,000 members, most of whom are scientists who do research in the physiological sciences. Specifically, the APS is "Empowering scientists to understand life and improve health by advancing and communicating discoveries in physiology and medicine" (APS, n.d.). The organization publishes 16 journals, including the Journal of Applied Physiology, and offers a student membership. More information can be found at their website (www.aps.org).

National Strength and Conditioning Association® (NSCA)

The NSCA was founded in 1978 and currently has over 60,000 members (NSCA, n.d.a). Their mission is to "disseminates research-based knowledge and its practical application to elevate athletic performance and fitness for all people" (NSCA, n.d.a). They do this through both national and regional meetings and events, publishing journals, and providing educational resources. Students interested in working with athletes may enjoy the NSCA Coaching Podcast. This and other information can be found on their website (NSCA, n.d.a).

JOURNALS

The professional organizations discussed in the previous section publish original research in exercise physiology. Many publish multiple journals, so the following is not a comprehensive list. The APS began publishing the *American Journal of Physiology* in 1898 and *Journal of Applied Physiology* in 1948. Influential European journals include the *European Journal of Applied Physiology* and *Acta Physiologica Scandinavia*. The ACSM's primary journal is *Medicine and Science in Sports and Exercise*. They also publish a quarterly journal, *Exercise and Sport Sciences Reviews*, which is a very useful resource for those who want to get up to date on the latest research in exercise physiology. The AACVPR publishes the *Journal of Cardio-pulmonary Rehabilitation*, which contains research relevant to clinical exercise physiologists. The NSCA publishes the *Journal of Strength and Conditioning Research*, which focuses on research relevant to strength and conditioning, as well as *Strength and Conditioning* which contains practical articles relevant to practitioners. There are many other scientific journals that frequently publish high-quality research in exercise physiology that are not mentioned here, including open access journals such as one of the journals from the Public Library of Science entitled *PLOS One*. Open access journals are free and available to anyone and are part of a trend to make scientific information accessible to everyone. A word of caution to students in exercise science: with so many journals available and new journals being published every year, readers will want to learn how to identify low quality, and often predatory journals who may have questionable publishing practices, so that they cannot be misled by incorrect information and unwittingly be a part of propagating bad science in their own writing. Some journals offer a combination of open access and traditional articles that cost the user money, although many are in the process of transitioning to the open access model. For instance, the *European Journal of Applied Physiology* began a series of excellent articles in 2021, called "A Century of Exercise Physiology." If readers search for these articles in PubMed or Google Scholar, they will notice that a pdf can be downloaded immediately for some articles, but others are behind a paywall. Fortunately, students are often able to access articles through their institution, which will help reduce their cost.

FUTURE DIRECTIONS

In the previous edition of this textbook (Weir and Weir, 2017), it was predicted that the high incidence of obesity and the aging of the population would impact both practitioners and researchers in exercise physiology. The importance of an integrative approach, utilizing the tools of molecular biology as well as advances in data analysis software and processing techniques, was stressed. All of these are still relevant; therefore, the future is bright for the field of exercise physiology. Metabolic dysfunction associated with high levels of insulin resistance, obesity, and diabetes continues to impact health and quality of life for too many people and, while new anti-obesity medications are helping many people lose weight, the role of exercise for improving metabolic health cannot be overemphasized and will continue to be an important area for exercise physiology research in the future. The role of regular exercise in helping people age well, avoiding chronic disease and loss of muscle mass and function, will continue to be a hot topic for exercise professionals and scientists. The technological innovations that have made advances in wearable technology possible and the "Omics" discussed earlier in the chapter will provide research questions for the foreseeable future. Readers may be interested in ACSM's annual report on worldwide health and fitness trends (A'Naja et al., 2024), with wearable technology at the top of the list, and fitness programs for older adults and exercise for weight loss coming in third and fourth. Other trends include high-intensity interval training, lifestyle medicine, data-driven training technology, EIM®, and exercise for mental health, all of which are fertile areas of inquiry and practice for exercise physiologists.

SUMMARY

Exercise physiologists are interested in how the body responds and adapts to exercise and how this knowledge can be applied in health, fitness, performance, and clinical settings. Undergraduate exercise science students take a course in exercise physiology because this topic will help them understand the how and why behind the exercise tests they perform and the exercise programs they write for clients, with the goal of improving their clients' health, fitness, and performance. Without a knowledge of exercise physiology, a personal trainer wouldn't be able to explain to a client why it is perfectly normal for a muscle not to grow in size very much during the first month of a resistance training program even though the client is getting stronger, a conditioning coach would not have a coherent explanation as to why they are having an athletic team perform specific exercises and drills, and a health coach would be unable to explain how exercise can get glucose into muscle cells, without the need for insulin, leading to improved metabolic health. Exercise physiology is one of the fundamental sciences included as part of an exercise science curriculum ranging from undergraduate to doctoral level.

STUDY QUESTIONS

1. Explain how an exercise response is different than an exercise adaptation and give five examples of each.
2. Discuss what the words mechanism, process, and cause-and-effect have to do with understanding the purpose of research in exercise physiology.
3. Contrast the terms physiology, exercise physiology, sedentary physiology, sports physiology, work physiology and environmental physiology. Explain what these terms have in common.
4. What is meant by the term crosstalk and how are myokines involved in this process?
5. Explain who could benefit from taking frequent exercise snack breaks and explain your reasoning.
6. Differentiate the terms atrophy, sarcopenia, and dynapenia. How are they related to healthy aging and fall prevention in elderly people?
7. Briefly describe the role of the molecule mTOR and satellite cells in skeletal muscle hypertrophy.

8. Outline the various muscle fiber types and the characteristics of each and explain what a muscle biopsy is.
9. Describe the variety of "Omic" technologies outlined in this chapter.
10. Discuss the role of professional organizations and certifications for aspiring exercise physiologists.
11. In addition to coursework, what other activities should an exercise science student engage in to maximize their ability to proceed in their chosen career path after college? Explain your answer.

LEARNING ACTIVITIES

1. Two health-related and two sports-related examples were given to help the reader understand the breadth of research topics studied by exercise physiologists. Summarize these two sections and explain the practical implications of these lines of research to practice in exercise physiology.
2. Look up the Human Genome Project and explain its impact on the types of research studies that can be done in exercise physiology.
3. Go to the ACE website and look for the requirements for each certification exam. How are the requirements different from those for the NSCA-CSCS exam or the ACSM-EP exam?
4. Find a job description for a university strength and conditioning coach, a personal trainer at a fitness center, an exercise physiologist at a corporate fitness center, and a clinical exercise physiologist working with bariatric or cancer clients. Compare and contrast the job descriptions and responsibilities of the four jobs identified.
5. Read the banquet speech delivered by A.V. Hill (Nobel Prize, n.d.b.) and the award ceremony speech for the Nobel prize (Nobel Prize, n.d.c.). Dr. Hill refers to the "romance and adventure of discovery," and the "brotherhood of science." Explain what he meant by integrating these two speeches with the content of this chapter.
6. Reflect on the importance of developing a disciplined mind that can think and problem solve effectively and where you are in this process.
   a. Explain why critical thinking is, arguably, the most important skill a student can develop during college.
   b. Interview two people that you consider competent exercise professionals and ask them their advice on how to develop these skills and why they are essential to their professional practice.

SUGGESTED READING AND WEBSITES

American College of Sports Medicine. (n.d.). Exercise is Medicine Website. https://www.exerciseismedicine.org/

Hoffman, N.J. (2017). Omics and exercise: global approaches for mapping exercise biological networks. *Cold Spring Harbor Perspectives in Medicine*, *7*(10), a029884.

Lavin, K.M., Coen, P.M., Baptista, L.C., Bell, M.B., Drummer, D., Harper, S.A., Lixandrão, M.E., et. al. (2022). State of knowledge on molecular adaptations to exercise in humans: historical perspectives and future directions. *Comprehensive Physiology*, *12*(2), 3193.

Pedersen, B.K. (2019). The physiology of optimizing health with a focus on exercise as medicine. *Annual Review of Physiology*, *81*(1), 607–627.

Tipton, C.M. (2014). *History of exercise physiology*. Champaign, IL: Human Kinetics.

REFERENCES

AACVPR. (n.d.). American Association of Cardiovascular and Pulmonary Rehabilitation Website. www.aacvpr.org

American College of Sports Medicine (ACSM). (n.d.). *About our brand*. ACSM Website. https://www.acsm.org/about/our-brand

American College of Sports Medicine Committee on Certification and Registry Boards. (2023). *Annual Report 2023*. ACSM Certification Website. https://www.acsm.org/docs/default-source/certification-documents/acsm-certification-2023-annual-report.pdf

American College of Sports Medicine. (2024). *ACSM Certification Guidebook*. ACSM Certification Website. https://acsm.org/acsm-candidate-handbook-july-2024/

American Council on Exercise. (n.d.). ACE Certification Website. https://www.acefitness.org/

American Physiological Society. (n.d.). APS Website. https://www.physiology.org/about/welcome?SSO=Y

A'Naja, M.N., Reed, R., Sansone, J., Batrakoulis, A., McAvoy, C., and Parrott, M.W. (2024). 2024 ACSM worldwide fitness trends: future directions of the health and fitness industry. *ACSM's Health and Fitness Journal*, *28*(1), 14–26.

Bassett Jr, D.R. (2002). Scientific contributions of A.V. Hill: exercise physiology pioneer. *Journal of Applied Physiology*, *93*(5), 1567–1582.

Bigland-Ritchie, B. (1981). EMG/force relations and fatigue of human voluntary contractions. *Exercise and Sport Sciences Reviews*, *9*, 75–117.

Brooks, G.A. (1987). The exercise physiology paradigm in contemporary biology: to molbiol or not to molbiol—that is the question. *Quest*, *39*(3), 231–242.

Brooks, G.A., Arevalo, J.A., Osmond, D.A., Leija, R.G., Curl, C.C., and Tovar, A.P. (2022). Lactate in contemporary biology: a phoenix risen. *Journal of Physiology*, *600*(5), 1229–1251.

Brooks, G.A., Osmond, A.D., Arevalo, J.A., Duong, J.J., Curl, C.C., Moreno-Santillan, D.D., et. al. (2023). Lactate as a myokine and exerkine: drivers and signals of physiology and metabolism. *Journal of Applied Physiology*, *134*(3), 529–548. https://doi.org/10.1152/japplphysiol.00497.2022

Buskirk, E.R. (1996). Exercise physiology. Part I. Early history in the United States. In J.D. Massengale and R.A. Swanson (Eds.), *History of exercise and sport science*, pp. 367–396. Champaign, IL: Human Kinetics.

Cancer Exercise App. (n.d.). Cancer Exercise App Website. https://www.cancerexerciseapp.com/

Cavanagh, P.R., Licata, A.A., and Rice, A.J. (2005). Exercise and pharmacological countermeasures for bone loss during long-duration space flight. *Gravit. Space Biol. Bull.*, Jun, *18*(2), 39–58.

Chen, W., Datzkiw, D., and Rudnicki, M.A. (2020). Satellite cells in ageing: use it or lose it. *Open Biology*, *10*(5), 200048.

Collins, F.S. and McKusick, V.A. (2001). Implications of the Human Genome Project for medical science. *JAMA*, *285*(5), 540–544.

Coyle, E.F. and Gonzalez-Alonso, J. (2001). Cardiovascular drift during prolonged exercise: new perspectives. *Exercise and Sport Sciences Reviews*, *29*(2), 88–92.

El Assar, M., Álvarez-Bustos, A., Sosa, P., Angulo, J., and Rodríguez-Mañas, L. (2022). Effect of physical activity/exercise on oxidative stress and inflammation in muscle and vascular aging. *International Journal of Molecular Sciences*, *23*(15), 8713. https://doi.org/10.3390/ijms23158713

Ely, I.A., Phillips, B.E., Smith, K., Wilkinson, D.J., Piasecki, M., Breen, L., et. al. (2023). A focus on leucine in the nutritional regulation of human skeletal muscle metabolism in ageing, exercise and unloading states. *Clinical Nutrition*, *24*, 1849–1865.

Evans, N., Wingo, B., Sasso, E., Hicks, A., Gorgey, A.S., and Harness, E. (2015). Exercise recommendations and considerations for persons with spinal cord injury. *Archives of Physical Medicine and Rehabilitation*, *96*(9), 1749–1750.

Exercise is Medicine. (n.d.). Exercise is Medicine Website. https://www.exerciseismedicine.org

Gibson, A.L., Wagner, D., and Heyward, V. (2018). *Advanced fitness assessment and exercise prescription* (8th ed.). Champaign, IL: Human Kinetics.

Hall, G., Laddu, D.R., Phillips, S.A., Lavie, C.J., and Arena, R. (2021). A tale of two pandemics: how will COVID-19 and global trends in physical inactivity and sedentary behavior affect one another? *Progress in Cardiovascular Diseases*, *64*, 108.

Herda, T.J., Siedlik, J.A., Trevino, M.A., Cooper, M.A., and Weir, J.P. (2015). Motor unit control strategies of endurance-versus resistance-trained individuals. *Muscle and Nerve*, *52*(5), 832–843.

Hirono, T., Takeda, R., Nishikawa, T., Okudaira, M., Kunugi, S., Yoshiko, A., et. al. (2024). Motor unit firing patterns in older adults with low skeletal muscle mass. *Archives of Gerontology and Geriatrics*, *116*, 1–7.

Hu, X., Rymer, W.Z., and Suresh, N.L. (2013). Motor unit pool organization examined via spike-triggered averaging of the surface electromyogram. *Journal of Neurophysiology*, *110*(5), 1205–1220.

Islam, H., Gibala, M.J., and Little, J.P. (2022). Exercise snacks: a novel strategy to improve cardiometabolic health. *Exercise and Sport Sciences Reviews*, *50*(1), 31–37.

Jenkins, D.G., Devin, J.L., Weston, K.L., Jenkins, J.G., and Skinner, T.L. (2023). Benefits beyond cardiometabolic health: the potential of frequent high intensity "exercise snacks" to improve outcomes for those living with and beyond cancer. *The Journal of Physiology*, *601*(21), 4691–4697. https://doi.org/10.1113/JP284985

Kent, J.A. and Hayes, K.L. (2021). Exercise physiology from 1980 to 2020: application of the natural sciences. *Kinesiology Review*, *10*(3), 238–247.

Kim, D.S., Wheeler, M.T., and Ashley, E.A. (2022). The genetics of human performance. *Nature Reviews Genetics*, *23*(1), 40–54.

Kirk, E.A., Christie, A.D., Knight, C.A., and Rice, C.L. (2021). Motor unit firing rates during constant isometric contraction: establishing and comparing an age-related pattern among muscles. *Journal of Applied Physiology*, *130*(6), 1903–1914.

Kohl, H.W., Craig, C.L., Lambert, E.V., Inoue, S., Alkandari, J.R., Leetongin, G., et. al. (2012). The pandemic of physical inactivity: global action for public health. *The Lancet*, *380*(9838), 294–305.

Komi, P. V. (2000). Stretch-shortening cycle: a powerful model to study normal and fatigued muscle. *Journal of Biomechanics*, *33*(10), 1197–1206.

Lacio, M., Vieira, J.G., Trybulski, R., Campos, Y., Santana, D., Filho, J.E., et. al. (2021). Effects of resistance training performed with different loads in untrained and trained male adult individuals on maximal strength and muscle hypertrophy: a systematic review. *International Journal of Environmental Research and Public Health*, *18*(21), 11237. https://doi.org/10.3390/ijerph182111237

Liddell, E.G.T. and Sherrington, C.S. (1924). Reflexes in response to stretch (myotatic reflexes). *Proceedings of the Royal Society of London. Series B, Containing Papers of a Biological Character*, *96*(675), 212–242.

Liguori, G. (Ed.), and American College of Sports Medicine. (2020). *ACSM's guidelines for exercise testing and prescription* (11th ed., pp. 7–9). Philadelphia, PA: Lippincott Williams & Wilkins.

Meh, K., Sember, V., Sorić, M., Vähä-Ypyä, H., Rocha, P., and Jurak, G. (2023). The dilemma of physical activity questionnaires: fitter people are less prone to over reporting. *PLOS One*, *18*(8), 1–16.

Morgan, P.T., Harris, D.O., Marshall, R.N., Quinlan, J.I., Edwards, S.J., Allen, S.L., et. al. (2021). Protein source and quality for skeletal muscle anabolism in young and older adults: a systematic review and meta-analysis. *The Journal of Nutrition*, *151*(7), 1901–1920.

Moritani, T. and deVries, H.A. (1979). Neural factors versus hypertrophy in the time course of muscle strength gain. *American Journal of Physical Medicine and Rehabilitation*, *58*(3), 115–130.

Moritani, T., Muro, M., and Nagata, A. (1986). Intramuscular and surface electromyogram changes during muscle fatigue. *Journal of Applied Physiology*, *60*(4), 1179–1185.

National Strength and Conditioning Association. (2025). NSCA Certification Handbook (v.010825). https://www.nsca.com/certification/cscs/

National Strength and Conditioning Association (NCSA). (n.d.a). *About the NSCA*. NSCA Website. https://www.nsca.com/about-us/about-us/

National Strength and Conditioning Association (NCSA). (n.d.b). CASCE Accreditation Webpage. https://www.nsca.com/education/casce/

Nobel Prize. (n.d.a.). *Nobel Prize in Physiology or Medicine 1922.* NobelPrize.org. https://www.nobelprize.org/prizes/medicine/1922/meyerhof/biographical/

Nobel Prize. (n.d.b.). *A.V. Hill banquet speech, Nobel Prize in Physiology or Medicine 1922.* NobelPrize.org. https://www.nobelprize.org/prizes/medicine/1922/hill/speech/

Nobel Prize. (n.d.c.). *A.V. Hill ceremony speech, Nobel Prize in Physiology or Medicine 1922.* NobelPrize.org. https://www.nobelprize.org/prizes/medicine/1922/ceremony-speech/

Noone, J., Mucinski, J.M., DeLany, J.P., Sparks, L.M., and Goodpaster, B.H. (2024). Understanding the variation in exercise responses to guide personalized physical activity prescriptions. *Cell Metabolism, 36*(4), 702–724.

Nunes, E.A., Colenso-Semple, L., McKellar, S.R., Yau, T., Ali, M.U., Fitzpatrick-Lewis, D., et. al. (2022). Systematic review and meta-analysis of protein intake to support muscle mass and function in healthy adults. *Journal of Cachexia, Sarcopenia and Muscle, 13*(2), 795–810.

Owens, D.J., and Bennett, S. (2024). An exercise physiologist's guide to metabolomics. *Experimental Physiology*, 109, 1066–1079.

Pilotto, A.M., Adami, A., Mazzolari, R., Brocca, L., Crea, E., Zuccarelli, L., et. al. (2022). Near-infrared spectroscopy estimation of combined skeletal muscle oxidative capacity and O2 diffusion capacity in humans. *The Journal of Physiology, 600*(18), 4153–4168.

Powers, S.K., Howley, E.T., and Quindry, J. (2024). *Exercise physiology: Theory and application to fitness and performance* (12th ed.). New York: McGraw-Hill.

Rafiei, H., Omidian, K., Myette-Cote, E., and Little, J.P. (2021). Metabolic effect of breaking up prolonged sitting with stair climbing exercise snacks. *Medicine and Science in Sports and Exercise, 53*(1), 150–158.

Reschechtko, S. and Pruszynski, J.A. (2020). Stretch reflexes. *Current Biology, 30*(18), R1025–R1030.

San-Millan, I., Julian, C.G., Matarazzo, C., and Brooks G.A. (2020). Is lactate an oncometabolite? Evidence supporting a role for lactate in the regulation of transcriptional activity of cancer-related genes in MCF7 breast cancer cells. *Frontiers in Oncology*, 9, 1–10.

Schoenfeld, B., Fisher, J., Grgic, J., Haun, C., Helms, E., Phillips, S., et. al. (2021). Resistance training recommendations to maximize muscle hypertrophy in an athletic population: position stand of the IUSCA. *International Journal of Strength and Conditioning, 1*, 1–30.

Severinsen, M.C.K., and Pedersen, B.K. (2020). Muscle–organ crosstalk: the emerging roles of myokines. *Endocrine Reviews, 41*(4), 594–609.

Sing, C.W., Lin, T.C., Bartholomew, S., Bell, J.S., Bennett, C., Beyene, K., et. al. (2023). Global epidemiology of hip fractures: secular trends in incidence rate, post-fracture treatment, and all-cause mortality. *Journal of Bone and Mineral Research, 38*(8), 1064–1075.

Tanisawa, K., Wang, G., Seto, J., Verdouka, I., Twycross-Lewis, R., Karanikolou, A., et. al. (2020). Sport and exercise genomics: the FIMS 2019 consensus statement update. *British Journal of Sports Medicine, 54*(16), 969–975.

The Human Metabolome Database. (n.d.). The Human Metabolome Database. https://hmdp.ca.

Thompson, W.R., Sallis, R., Joy, E., Jaworski, C.A., Stuhr, R.M., and Trilk, J.L. (2020). Exercise is medicine. *American Journal of Lifestyle Medicine, 14*(5), 511–523.

Thyfault, J.P. and Bergouignan, A. (2020). Exercise and metabolic health: beyond skeletal muscle. *Diabetologia, 63*(8), 1464–1474.

Tipton, C.M. (2014). *History of exercise physiology*. Champaign, IL: Human Kinetics.

Tobias, I.S. and Galpin, A.J. (2020). Moving human muscle physiology research forward: an evaluation of fiber type-specific protein research methodologies. *American Journal of Physiology: Cell Physiology, 319*(5), C858–C876.

Tudor-Locke, C. (2002). Taking steps toward increased physical activity: using pedometers to measure and motivate. *President's Council on Physical Fitness and Sports Research Digest*, Jun; *3*(17).

Wang, X. and Proud, C.G. (2006). The mTOR pathway in the control of protein synthesis. *Physiology*, *21*(5), 362–369.

Ward-Ritacco, C. and Magal, M. (2020). American College of Sports Medicine. *Adopting CAAHEP / CoAES Accreditation as a Requirement for ACSM-EP and ACSM-CEP Certifications*. ACSM Website. https://www.acsm.org/blog-detail/acsm-certified-blog/2020/11/04/caahep-coaes-accreditation-requirement-acsm-ep-acsm-cep-certification

Watkins, C.M., Storey, A.G., McGuigan, M.R., and Gill, N.D. (2021). Implementation and efficacy of plyometric training: bridging the gap between practice and research. *The Journal of Strength and Conditioning Research*, *35*(5), 1244–1255.

Weir, J.P. and Weir L.L. (2017). Exercise physiology. In T.J. Housh, D.J. McCanlies, and G.O. Johnson (Eds.), *Introduction to exercise science*, pp. 86–130. Routledge.

Wiedmer, P., Jung, T., Castro, J.P., Pomatto, L.C., Sun, P.Y., Davies, K.J., et. al. (2021). Sarcopenia–Molecular mechanisms and open questions. *Ageing Research Reviews*, *65*, 1–17.

Winter, G. and Krömer, J.O. (2013). Fluxomics–connecting 'omics analysis and phenotypes. *Environmental Microbiology*, *15*(7), 1901–1916.

xAI. (2025) Prompt: "Write a job description for a hospital based clinical exercise physiologist in cardiopulmonary rehabilitation". Grok, Version 3, Accessed April 30, 2025, https://grok.com/

Yang, Q. and Chan, P. (2022). Skeletal muscle metabolic alternation develops sarcopenia. *Aging and Disease*, *13*(3), 801.

ACKNOWLEDGEMENT

Grok (Version 3) was used to generate an example job description based on the prompt "Write a job description for a hospital based clinical exercise physiologist in cardiopulmonary rehabilitation". This output was adapted by the author to inform the content of Exhibit 5.9.

6 Exercise Prescription for Health and Sports Performance

David J. Cornell and Kyle T. Ebersole

LEARNING OBJECTIVES

After studying this chapter, the student will be able to:

- define the principles and techniques of exercise prescription and training, including key components such as frequency, intensity, time, and type (FITT), and their role in improving health and fitness
- describe the tools and assessments associated with health, fitness, and performance, including their applications in evaluating physical capacity, identifying risk factors, and developing individualized exercise prescriptions
- identify and describe career pathways for professionals who apply principles of exercise prescription in various fields, including fitness, rehabilitation, sports science, and clinical settings

INTRODUCTION

Exercise prescription is the process of creating a personalized exercise program tailored to the specific health needs, fitness goals, and physical capabilities of an individual (Zhu et al., 2024). Key components of exercise prescription include aerobic exercise to enhance cardiovascular endurance, resistance training for building muscular strength and endurance, flexibility exercises to improve range of motion, and balance exercises to enhance stability and coordination. The process begins with a comprehensive assessment of the health status and fitness level of the individual, followed by goal setting to establish measurable and achievable objectives. By applying the FITT-VP (Frequency, Intensity, Time, Type, Volume, and Progression) principles, discussed in detail later in this chapter, exercise prescription ensures a well-rounded program that facilitates continuous improvement, promotes better physical health, reduces risk factors associated with chronic diseases, and improves mental well-being, all of which contribute to a higher quality of life (Liguori et al., 2021).

Although the formal science of exercise prescription initially emerged from exercise physiology laboratories and medical settings and was first applied by professionals in physical education, more specialized disciplines and practitioners have evolved over time. Today, three primary fields integrate exercise prescription as a central component of practice: health and fitness, human performance, and allied health.

DOI: 10.4324/9781032697185-6

Health and Fitness Professions

Practitioners in the health and fitness sector use exercise and other wellness strategies to improve their clients' physical fitness and overall well-being (Gallo, 2020). A key consideration in this setting is that clients are generally medically stable and free from serious health conditions that might make exercise unsafe, such as cardiovascular disease, diabetes, or mental health disorders like depression or substance abuse. In cases where such conditions exist, medical clearance from a healthcare provider is typically required before beginning an exercise program. While there are many roles within this field, this chapter focuses on three common career paths: group exercise instructors, personal trainers, and health and wellness coaches.

Human Performance Professions

Practitioners in the human performance sector apply exercise and training principles to enhance athletic performance. This career path originally evolved from traditional sport coaching, where coaches were responsible for all aspects of an athlete's training, including strength and conditioning (Shurley, Todd, and Todd, 2017). Today, clients include a wide range of individuals from recreational and collegiate athletes to elite professionals and tactical athletes such as military personnel, firefighters, and law enforcement officers. These professionals may work with people of all ages, including children, adolescents, adults, and older adults. As exercise science has advanced, more clearly defined career pathways have emerged, particularly for strength and conditioning specialists and sport scientists.

Allied Health Professions

Professionals in the allied health sector use exercise and training strategies not only to improve health and fitness but also to help manage or treat diseases and medical conditions. They often work with patients who may have stable or unstable health issues. Some of these professionals hold clinical licenses and can bill for their services using medical reimbursement codes. Depending on their role and training, they may work independently as healthcare providers or under the supervision of a physician (Gallo, Ward-Ritacco, and Lynch, 2022). While these individuals may utilize other non-exercise-based interventions in addition to their structured exercise programming, they do not deliver medical interventions, such as administering pharmacotherapies or conducting surgical procedures. This sector encompasses a wide range of professionals; however, this chapter will focus on exercise physiologists, clinical exercise physiologists, athletic trainers, and physical therapists, as these individuals most often utilize exercise prescription within their practice.

HISTORICAL PERSPECTIVES

The history of exercise prescription has evolved over the centuries, reflecting changes in our understanding of health, fitness, and medicine. In ancient civilizations, such as Greece and Rome, figures like Hippocrates and Galen emphasized the importance of physical activity for overall health and well-being, and their knowledge of the human body persisted over a thousand years. The Renaissance (14th to 17th centuries) marked a major turning point in the history of exercise when advances in anatomy and physiology, driven by scholars like Andreas Vesalius and physicians such as William Harvey, laid the foundation for a more structured and scientific understanding of human movement and health. The Industrial Revolution in the 19th century began to call to attention health issues arising from sedentary lifestyles, prompting the emergence of physical education programs that promoted regular physical activity and led to the founding of the "American Association for Health, Physical Education, and Recreation" (AAHPER) around 1885 (Berryman, 2010). The AAHPER (currently known as SHAPE America) is widely considered the first professional organization dedicated to advancing professional practice and research related to physical activity. Therefore, much of the early application of structured exercise prescription grew from physical education programming.

Significant advancements in exercise prescription occurred during the 20th century. For example, Thomas L. DeLorme, a physician and US Army surgeon during World War II, introduced the concept of progressive resistance training as a rehabilitation technique for injured soldiers (Todd, Shurley, and Todd, 2012). His work in the 1940s showed that heavier resistance stimulated muscle growth and recovery and laid the foundation for modern resistance training principles used not only in rehabilitation, but also in athletic and fitness training. Another influential study was the 1953 London Bus Study by British epidemiologist Jeremy N. Morris whose research established a link between physical activity and cardiovascular health by comparing the health outcomes of sedentary bus drivers and physically active conductors (Zhu et al., 2024). This study demonstrated that the conductors who climbed many stairs daily had a significantly lower incidence of heart attacks.

Exercise prescription within the context of exercise science also advanced during the 20th century, as formal exercise physiology research laboratories and centers such as the Harvard Fatigue Laboratory (1927–1947) and the Thomas K. Cureton Physical Fitness Research Laboratory (founded in 1944 at the University of Illinois Urbana-Champaign) started to develop (Berryman, 2010). The development of these institutions contributed to the formation of several professional organizations such as the American College of Sports Medicine (ACSM) and the National Strength and Conditioning Association (NSCA) to disseminate knowledge and advance the science of exercise and physical activity. In addition, specialized subsections were developed within larger physiology organizations, such as the American Physiological Society, which expanded the scope and influence of exercise science (Berryman, 2010).

In the 1960s, Dr. Kenneth H. Cooper's promotion of aerobic exercise, including the popularization of the 12-minute run test, led to greater awareness of the benefits of aerobic fitness. The Cooper Center Longitudinal Study (CCLS) is a long-term research project focusing on the relationship between physical fitness, health behaviors, and various health outcomes. Started in 1970 by the Cooper Institute in Dallas, TX, it is one of the largest and longest-running studies of its kind. The CCLS has produced numerous findings that have demonstrated the importance of regular physical activity in reducing the risk of chronic diseases and early mortality (Tipton, 2014). The publication of the ACSM *Guidelines for Graded Exercise Testing and Exercise Prescription* in 1975 became a seminal resource, reflecting decades of research. Further advancements in the 1990s, including the introduction of the metabolic equivalent of task (MET) by Dr. Barbara E. Ainsworth, provided new ways to quantify energy expenditure during different types of physical activity and, in 1996, the first *Surgeon General's Report on Physical Activity and Health* was published, emphasizing the health benefits of 150 minutes of moderate-intensity activity per week, that continues to shape modern guidelines (Zhu et al., 2024).

More recently, the Exercise is Medicine® (EIM®) initiative launched by the ACSM and the American Medical Association in 2007, marked a pivotal moment in public health by integrating exercise into routine clinical practice (Berryman, 2010). Other allied health fields, such as clinical exercise physiology, athletic training, and physical therapy had been incorporating exercise prescription as a core component of their practice since the 1960s (Moore, 2004). Professionals in non-healthcare sectors, such as personal trainers, group exercise instructors, and strength and conditioning specialists, developed their own defined scopes of practice around that same timeframe.

In summary, the development of exercise prescription has been shaped by centuries of progress in our understanding of health and fitness, from early practices in ancient civilizations to modern public health efforts. Milestones such as the introduction of progressive resistance training, recognizing the role of physical activity in cardiovascular health, and the growing emphasis on aerobic fitness have all influenced modern exercise science (see Exhibit 6.1). Professional organizations and research centers have also played a key role in advancing and sharing this knowledge, while initiatives like EIM® reflect the increasing integration of exercise into healthcare systems.

Exhibit 6.1 Key events in the development of exercise prescription during the 20th–21st centuries

Date	*Event/Development*
1927	The **Harvard Fatigue Laboratory,** a pioneering research facility in exercise physiology and human performance established in **1927** by **Lawrence J. Henderson** and **David Bruce Dill.**
1944	Dr. Thomas K. Cureton established the **Physical Fitness Research Laboratory** at the **University of Illinois and conducted groundbreaking research on the effects of physical activity on health and performance.**
1945	Army physician Dr. Thomas L. DeLorme introduced progressive resistance training for rehabilitating soldiers injured in World War II.
1953	The London Bus Study by Jeremy N. Morris, recognized the relationship between physical activity (PA) and health, was published in *The Lancet*
1968	Dr. Kenneth H. Cooper published the book *Aerobics* and developed the 12-minute test to predict maximum oxygen consumption. Cooper's work led to the establishment of the Cooper Clinic and the Cooper Aerobics Research Center, resulting in the world's largest fitness and health database.
1975	The American College of Sports Medicine (ACSM) published the first edition of the *Guidelines for Graded Exercise Testing and Exercise Prescription*, which later evolved into the *ACSM's Guidelines for Exercise Testing and Prescription.* The 12th edition was published in 2025.
1993	Dr. Barbara E. Ainsworth led the publication of the *Compendium of Physical Activity* to provide MET values for activities, with updates published in 1993, 2000, 2011, and 2024.
1994	Dr. William Haskell outlined the direct dose-response relationship between exercise and health outcomes.
1996	*Physical Activity and Health: A Report by the Surgeon General* was published, setting a foundation for exercise prescription.
1996	Research on measuring physical activity objectively began, leading to the publication of key texts on physical activity assessment.
2007	ACSM and the American Medical Association launched the *Exercise is Medicine®* program to integrate exercise into clinical practice.
2008	The US Department of Health and Human Services published the *Physical Activity Guidelines for Americans*, updated in 2018.

FUNDAMENTAL CONCEPTS

Depending on the population, whether patients, clients, or athletes, the focus of an exercise prescription, the tools used to implement it, and the measures used to guide it vary across disciplines. For consistency, the term "client" will be used throughout this chapter to refer to any individual seeking to improve their health or fitness, including athletes and patients. The core foundations of any exercise prescription include **Frequency, Intensity, Time, Type, Volume,** and **Progression** (FITT-VP) (Liguori et al., 2021) and apply to both aerobic and anaerobic exercise, as well as strength training exercise program design (Garber et al., 2011).

Before starting any exercise program, it is important to obtain a client's health history using tools such as the Physical Activity Readiness Questionnaire (see PAR-Q+, n.d.; Warburton et al., 2022), and participate in a brief subjective intake interview with the practitioner to identify any potential safety concerns or health risks that might require medical clearance from their doctor before beginning a formal training program (Riebe et al., 2015). Once cleared for exercise, the practitioner must develop an overall training goal for their client based on their own individual health status and unique performance demands. Training goals could range from general health and fitness promotion, improvements in cardiorespiratory fitness, and weight loss or changes in body composition, to enhancement of strength or muscle hypertrophy, reduction of cardiovascular disease risk factors, improvements in gait or running speed, and many others. To maximize the effectiveness of the training program, it is important that there is a mutual understanding between the practitioner and the client regarding how to accomplish the established goals. After completing these processes, a practitioner can then use the FITT-VP framework to prescribe exercises by utilizing a basic step-by-step process of developing an exercise training program (Schoenfeld and Snarr, 2022).

Frequency (F)

Frequency refers to the number of training sessions per week and depends on several factors, including the current fitness level or training status of the individual (Schoenfeld and Snarr, 2022). Specifically, an individual with limited fitness or who is novice to exercise training, will likely need to be prescribed fewer training sessions when beginning an exercise training program. However, even for a beginner, it is still recommended that an individual engage in aerobic exercise 3–5 days per week (2018 Physical Activity Guidelines Advisory Committee, 2018), and resistance training exercise 2–3 days per week (Garber et al., 2011) to improve or maintain health and fitness. The number of training sessions per week may also depend on the intensity of exercise completed in each training session (Haff and Triplett, 2016). In other words, if the overall intensity of the prescribed exercise sessions is high, the frequency of training may need to be low, depending on the fitness level of the individual.

Intensity (I)

Prescribing exercise intensity can be accomplished in numerous ways depending on the exercise. As shown in Exhibit 6.2, aerobic exercise intensity is typically expressed as a percentage of an individual's maximal oxygen uptake ($\dot{V}O_2max$), percentage of maximal heart rate (%HRmax), or percentage of HR reserve, which is the difference between HRmax and resting HR (%HRR), as well as their rating of perceived exertion (RPE) (Garber et al., 2011).

Exhibit 6.2 Relative intensity prescription of aerobic exercise

Intensity	*%$\dot{V}O_2max$*	*%HRmax*	*%HRR*	*RPE*
Very Light	<37%	<57%	<30%	<9/20
Light	37%–45%	57%–63%	30%–39%	9/20 – 11/20
Moderate	46%–63%	64%–76%	40%–59%	12/20 – 13/20
Vigorous	64%–90%	77%–95%	60%–89%	14/20 – 17/20
Near Maximal	≥91%	≥96%	≥90%	≥18/20

Abbreviations: %$\dot{V}O_2$max, percentage maximal oxygen uptake; %HRmax, percentage maximal heart rate; %HRR, percentage heart rate reserve; RPE, rating of perceived exertion

Source: Adapted from Garber et al. (2011)

$\dot{V}O_2$max testing measures the maximum amount of oxygen an individual can utilize during intense exercise and is typically performed in a laboratory using a graded exercise test (i.e., GXT) on a treadmill or a cycle ergometer. The individual wears a mask connected to a machine called a **metabolic cart** that measures oxygen intake and carbon dioxide output (Exhibit 6.3). The exercise intensity is gradually increased in stages until the person reaches exhaustion or can no longer maintain the required pace. The metabolic cart continuously records the data, and the highest oxygen consumption ($\dot{V}O_2$) level reached during the test is recorded as the $\dot{V}O_2$max. Because $\dot{V}O_2$max testing must be conducted by trained individuals, is time consuming, and requires expensive equipment, most practitioners estimate $\dot{V}O_2$max from HR using submaximal exercise tests, such as cycle ergometry tests, step tests, run/walk tests, or various treadmill tests. Due to the linear relationship between HR and $\dot{V}O_2$ during exercise (Powers, Howley, and Quindry, 2024), $\dot{V}O_2$ can be estimated by simply determining an individual's age-predicted HR-max using the following equation (Liguori et al., 2021):

$$HR_{max} = 208 - \left(0.7 \times age\left[yrs\right]\right)$$

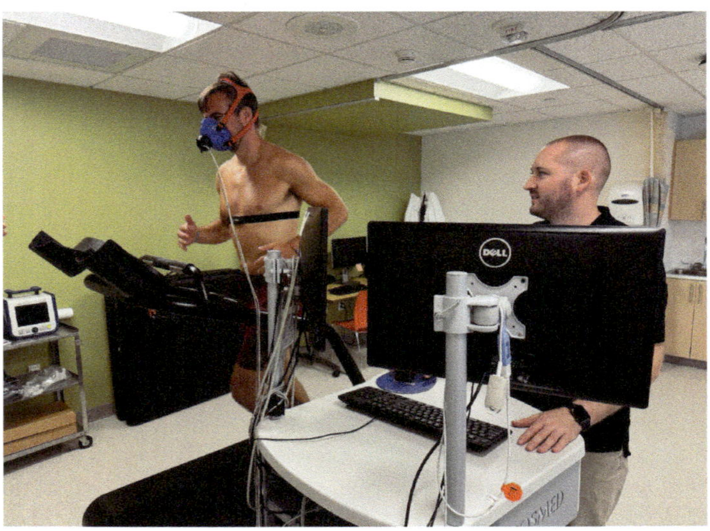

Exhibit 6.3 Graded exercise testing with a metabolic cart

As shown above in Exhibit 6.2, once HRmax ($b \cdot min^{-1}$) is determined, aerobic exercise intensity can be prescribed as %HRmax or %HRR (Liguori et al., 2021).

Aerobic exercise can also be prescribed using METs, which is a way to quantify the energy expenditure associated with an activity and is particularly useful when including recreational activities within exercise programming (Herrmann et al., 2024). In addition, aerobic exercise intensity may be prescribed using RPE, or how strenuous an individual is perceiving a task, which is subjectively rated using the Borg 6–20 scale (Exhibit 6.4) or the modified Borg Category-Ratio (CR)-10 scale (Exhibit 6.5) (Kilpatrick et al., 2020). Other forms of aerobic intensity prescription include the use of work, power, or velocity (Liguori et al., 2021).

Exhibit 6.4 Borg 6–20 Scale

6	No exertion at all
7	Extremely light
8	
9	Very light
10	
11	Fairly light
12	
13	Somewhat hard
14	
15	Hard (heavy)
16	
17	Very hard
18	
19	Extremely hard
20	Maximal exertion

Source: Adapted from Kilpatrick et al. (2020)

Exhibit 6.5 Modified Borg CR-10 Scale

0	Nothing at all
0.3	
0.5	Extremely weak
0.7	
1	Very weak
1.5	
2	Weak
2.5	
3	Moderate
4	
5	Strong
6	
7	Very strong
8	
9	
10	Extremely strong
11	Absolute maximum

Abbreviations: CR-10 Scale, Category-Ratio-10 Scale

Source: Adapted from Kilpatrick et al. (2020)

The intensity of resistance exercise is normally characterized by an individual's one repetition maximum (1RM), which is the maximum amount of weight an individual can lift one time for a given exercise (Kraemer and Ratamess, 2004). The 1RM can be determined directly by having an individual perform a series of attempts using incremental loads separated by 1–5 minutes rest until a 1RM is achieved using proper technique or may be predicted using equations that include the number of repetitions performed for a given load during a particular exercise (Nuzzo et al., 2024).

When prescribing resistance exercise, the number of repetitions and the load used are based on the desired outcome, such as strength, hypertrophy, or muscular endurance. For example, to increase strength, use a lower repetition scheme with heavy loads, such as 1–5 reps per set at 85–100% of the 1RM, and to improve muscular endurance, use a higher repetition scheme with light loads, such as 15 reps at 60% of the 1RM (Exhibit 6.6) (Haff and Triplett, 2016).

Exhibit 6.6 Percent 1RM training continuum

Resistance Training Goal	*%1RM*	*Reps*
Muscular Endurance	≤67%	≥12
Muscular Hypertrophy	67%–85%	6–12
Muscular Strength	≥85%	≤8
Muscular Power		
Single-Effort	80%–90%	1–2
Multiple-Effort	75%–85%	3–5

Abbreviations: %1RM, percent one-repetition maximum; reps, repetitions

Source: Adapted from Haff and Triplett (2016)

Time (T)

Time refers to the duration of exercise performed and applies to a specific exercise (e.g., 30-minutes of jogging) or the overall session (e.g., 60-minute weightlifting routine) (Liguori et al., 2021). In addition, the duration can be adjusted to create short intervals (e.g., 60–360 seconds) of alternating high-intensity and low-intensity exercise (Schoenfeld and Dawes, 2009). This approach establishes a "work-to-rest ratio" based on the alternating periods of high and low intensity.

Type (T)

Based on the training goal(s), the practitioner should employ the **principle of specificity**, which states that the more specific the exercise mode (or type) is to the activity or sport in which the individual participates, the greater likelihood for improved performance (Haff and Triplett, 2016). Potential modes of aerobic exercise include treadmill walking and running (Exhibit 6.7a), cycling (Exhibit 6.7b), elliptical machines (Exhibit 6.7c), stairclimbing (Exhibit 6.7d), and other forms (e.g., calisthenics, swimming/aquatic exercise, etc.).

Potential modes of exercise to increase muscular strength and endurance include barbell weights (Exhibit 6.8a), dumbbell weights (Exhibit 6.8b), resistance bands (Exhibit 6.8c), and resistance machines (Exhibit 6.8d), as well as bodyweight exercises (e.g., push-ups, sit-ups, jump squats, walking lunges) and other modalities (e.g., medicine balls, kettlebells).

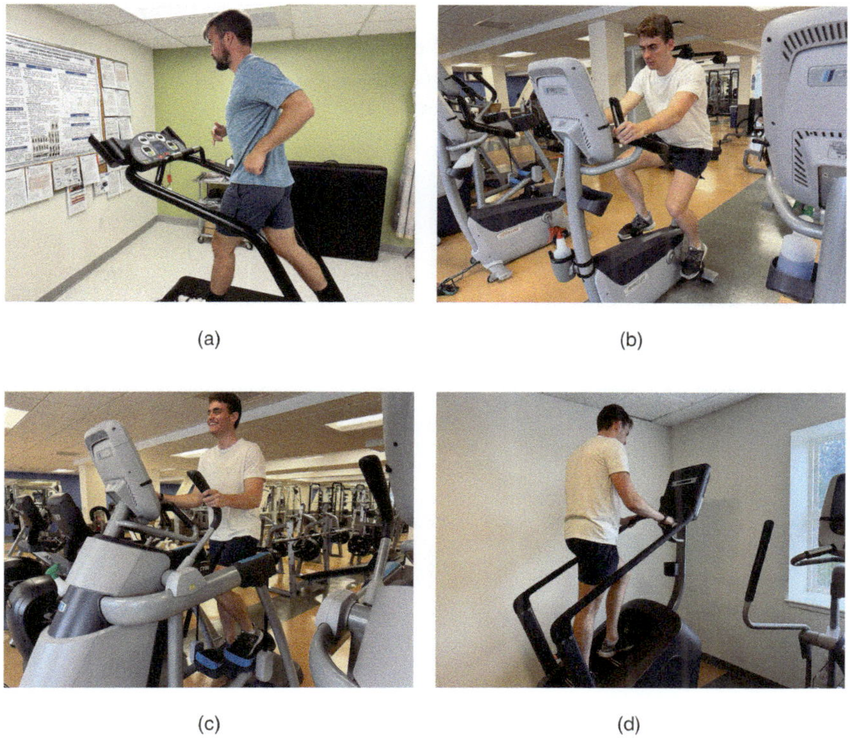

Exhibit 6.7a–d Modes of aerobic exercise

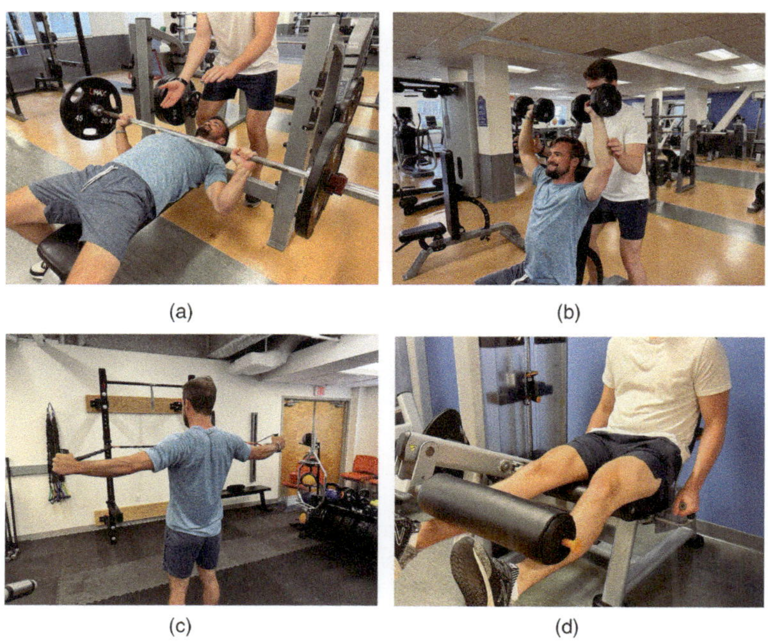

Exhibit 6.8a–d Modes of resistance exercise

Various modes of flexibility and mobility training also exist, including both static stretching (Exhibit 6.9a) and proprioceptive neuromuscular facilitation stretching (Exhibit 6.9b), as well as dynamic range motion exercises (Exhibit 6.9c) and the use of various modalities, such as foam rollers (Exhibit 6.9d).

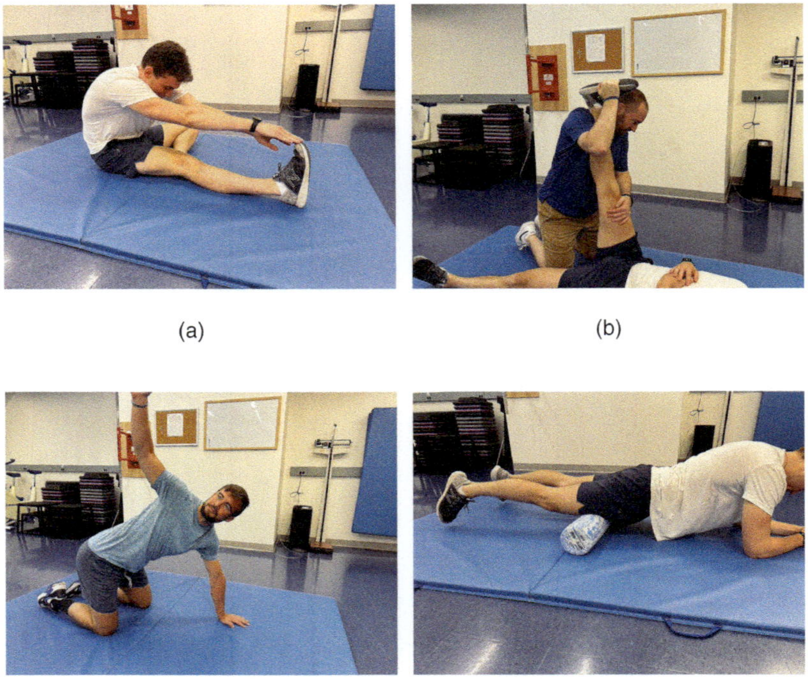

(a) (b)

(c) (d)

Exhibit 6.9a–d Modes of flexibility and mobility training

Functional modes of exercise can also be manipulated to emphasize either aerobic or anaerobic energy systems. For example, running can be aerobic when performed at a lower intensity, such as walking or jogging, or anaerobic when performed at a higher intensity, such as sprinting. Therefore, it is important for practitioners to select and apply exercise modes appropriately based on the desired training outcome.

Volume (V)

As a principle, exercise volume is the product of Frequency (F), Intensity (I), and Time (T) (Liguori et al., 2021). For aerobic exercise, this is often quantified as MET-minutes per week ($\text{MET-min}\cdot\text{wk}^{-1}$). For resistance exercise, it is the product of the load and intensity of a specific exercise or overall exercise session, which could simply be the calculation of repetitions × sets × weight (Kraemer and Ratamess, 2004).

Volume also considers the number of sessions per week and any additional training the individual may be performing (Schoenfeld and Snarr, 2022). For example, a practitioner may manipulate the training volume for an athlete based on the current state of their season (e.g., pre-season, off-season, in-season), which is a concept known as **periodization** (Haff and Triplett, 2016).

Progression (P)

After engaging in an exercise program for a period of time, "**supercompensation**" occurs, and positive physiological adaptations will take place. However, to elicit further physiological adaptations and/or continue to improve performance, the exercise program will need to be progressed. This fundamental concept of progression is the **overload principle,** which refers to gradually increasing the stress placed upon the body during exercise training (American College of Sports Medicine, 2009). Progressive overload could simply be achieved by increasing any of the Frequency, Intensity, or Volume components of the original prescription. Progression could also include the incorporation of additional exercises within a single session. While there are numerous ways an exercise prescription can be progressed, it is generally recommended to slowly progress until an individual has successfully engaged in an exercise program for at least 1-month before a large progression is prescribed to minimize risks of musculoskeletal injury and excessive fatigue or prevent the long-term development of **overtraining** (Liguori et al., 2021).

Another fundamental concept of progression is **variation**, which refers to varying the intensity or load of an exercise prescription (American College of Sports Medicine, 2009). An example of variation within aerobic training is prescribing a high-intensity, low duration session one day of the week, and a low-intensity, long duration session another day. In resistance training, this same principle could refer to changing the type of exercise modality from week-to-week (e.g., dumbbells vs. barbells).

APPLICATIONS TO EXERCISE SCIENCE

Exercise prescription is a vital tool in exercise science, applied across both health and clinical settings as well as in sports performance. It ensures that exercise is safe, effective, and tailored to individual needs, with the goal of optimizing health, rehabilitation, or athletic performance. The following sections highlight how exercise prescription is used in different contexts, providing examples from both clinical and performance-based applications.

HEALTH/CLINICAL ASPECTS

General Health and Fitness Recommendations

Although exercise programs should be tailored to an individual's specific needs, general recommendations have been developed based on evidence from the Department of Health and Human Services (2018 Physical Activity Guidelines Advisory Committee, 2018) and the ACSM (Garber et al., 2011) to promote health and reduce the risk of chronic disease (Liguori et al., 2021).

Aerobic Exercise Prescription

It is recommended that most adults engage in 30–60 minutes of moderate intensity exercise ≥ 5 days per week, or 20–60 minutes of vigorous intensity exercise ≥ 3 days per week, or a combination of moderate and vigorous intensity exercise ≥ 3–5 days per week (Liguori et al., 2021). A weekly target volume of ≥ 500–1,000 MET-minutes is recommended, which can typically be met by accumulating 150 minutes of moderate-intensity exercise, or 75 minutes of vigorous-intensity exercise each week.

Long-term aerobic training provides a wide range of health benefits. These include lowering the risk of premature death, heart disease, and stroke; supporting weight and blood sugar management in individuals with metabolic or cardiovascular conditions; and enhancing mental well-being through improvements in mood, self-esteem, and overall quality of life (Crookham, 2013).

Resistance Exercise Prescription

It is recommended that most adults participate in resistance training at least 2 to 3 days per week (Liguori et al., 2021). For novice-to-intermediate individuals, exercises are typically prescribed within the muscular endurance and hypertrophy ranges of the 1RM continuum (e.g., 60% to 80% of 1RM for 10 to 15 repetitions). When working with sedentary individuals or older adults, it may be more appropriate to begin with lighter loads and higher repetitions, such as 40% to 50% of 1RM for 15 to 20 repetitions, before gradually progressing in intensity. In contrast, highly trained individuals often perform exercises in the muscular strength range of the continuum (e.g., 80% or more of 1RM for 8 to 12 repetitions). Research suggests that completing 2 to 4 sets per exercise can promote neuromuscular strength gains in most adults, while a single set may still be effective for older adults or those new to resistance training (American College of Sports Medicine, 2009).

The prescribed exercises should involve each major muscle group, incorporate both concentric and eccentric muscle actions, and include a combination of multi-joint and single-joint exercises (Kraemer and Ratamess, 2004). Multi-joint (i.e., more muscle groups) and higher intensity exercises should be prescribed first, with single-joint (i.e., less muscle groups) and lower intensity exercises prescribed later in each training session. Further, it is recommended that an equal number of pushing (e.g., bench press; triceps extensions) and pulling exercises (e.g., biceps curls; deadlift) are prescribed across a training week to maintain balance between agonist and antagonist muscle groups in both the upper body and lower body.

Beyond improving neuromuscular performance, long-term resistance training has been associated with several health benefits. These include enhanced physical function (such as walking speed, independence, and quality of life), reductions in visceral fat, cholesterol, triglycerides, and blood pressure, better blood glucose control and bone mineral density, as well as improvements in self-esteem and cognitive function (Westcott, 2012).

Flexibility Exercise Prescription

The recommendation for most adults is to engage in flexibility training at least 2–3 days per week, performing 2–4 repetitions of exercises targeting each major muscle group, ideally at the end of an exercise session (Liguori et al., 2021). Static stretches should be held for at least 30 seconds, with a total stretching time of at least 60 seconds per exercise. Other forms of flexibility training may also be used, as shown in Exhibit 6.9, depending on the individual's needs and goals. Flexibility training has been shown to improve joint range of motion, which can help facilitate other functional activities of daily living and also enhance postural stability and balance (Garber et al., 2011).

Neuromotor Exercise Prescription

It is recommended that most adults engage in neuromotor training at least 2–3 days per week (Liguori et al., 2021). Neuromuscular exercises are commonly used to improve proprioception and motor control, which can help reduce fall risk, fear of falling, and enhance quality of life (Garber et al., 2011). These exercises may include targeted balance training (Exhibit 6.10a), coordination exercises (Exhibit 6.10b), gait training (Exhibit 6.10c), or integrative activities that combine multiple movement skills, such as yoga (Exhibit 6.10d) or tai chi. While specific recommendations for intensity and volume are not well defined, performing neuromotor exercises for at least 20–30 minutes per day may be beneficial for general health and fitness.

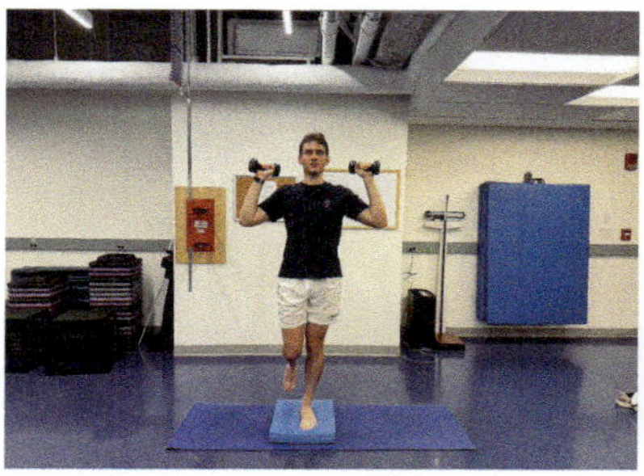

(a)

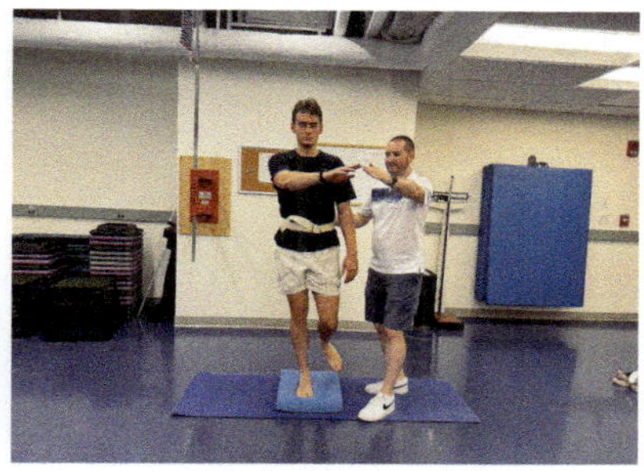

(b)

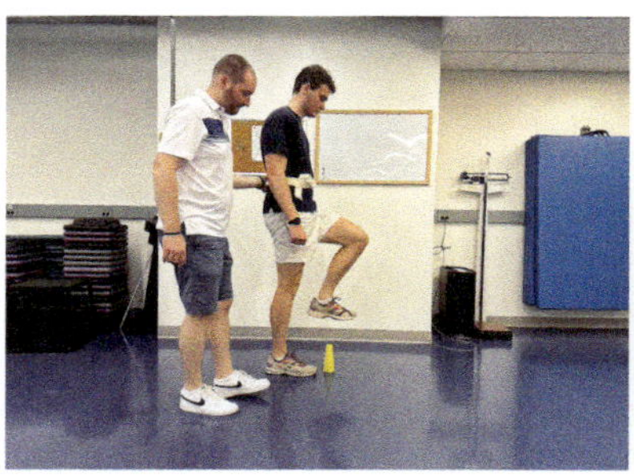

(c)

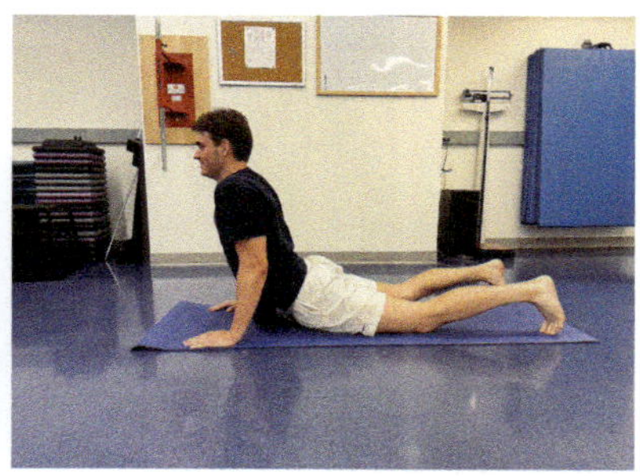

(d)

Exhibit 6.10a–d Examples of neuromotor exercises

Clinical Considerations

While the principles of exercise prescription via the FITT-VP framework remain the same across individuals, clinicians who work with patients who have comorbidities (also known as concomitant diseases) such as diabetes, hypertension, osteoporosis, and heart disease, to name a few, may need to consider some additional factors associated with their condition(s). For example, patients who are taking β-adrenergic antagonist medications (i.e., β-blockers) to treat hypertension often have a blunted HR response to activity. Therefore, using HR measures to monitor and prescribe exercise intensity can be misleading, and the clinician must often rely on other measures such as RPE to guide programming (Kilpatrick et al., 2020). Clinicians may also monitor and manage symptoms that occur before, during, or after exercise, such as dyspnea (shortness of breath) and angina (chest pain) (Liguori et al., 2021). As a result of these considerations, carefully monitoring vitals, such as blood pressure (Exhibit 6.11a) and oxygen saturation (Exhibit 6.11b), is required when guiding patients through exercise.

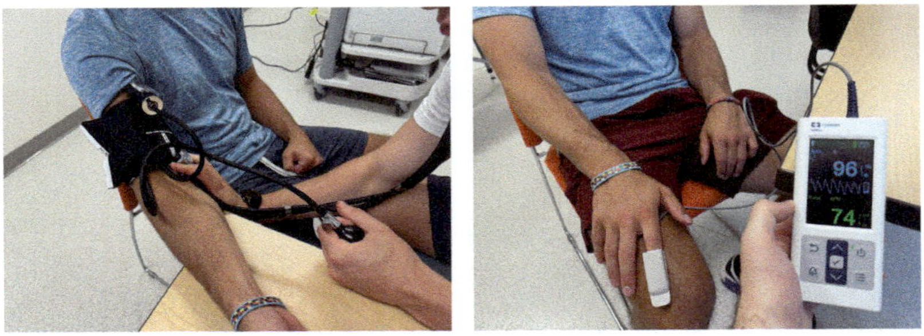

(a) (b)

Exhibit 6.11a–b Monitoring vitals

From an orthopedic perspective, clinicians often need to prescribe exercise based on their current medical state or stage of healing. For example, this may include the use of isometric exercises, gravity eliminated exercises, and passive range of motion exercises, among others. As the patient progresses through the rehabilitative process, the clinician uses the FITT-VP framework to continue progressive overload and improve function during specific tasks (Liguori et al., 2021). Further, the clinician may be able to utilize other exercises, or higher intensity exercises, that stress or strengthen other areas of the body, while still protecting healing tissue.

SPORTS/PERFORMANCE ASPECTS

When designing exercise prescriptions to enhance athletic performance, practitioners often incorporate a broader range of exercise paradigms and specialized training modalities to target sport-specific demands to achieve desired outcomes (Haff and Triplett, 2016). These may include techniques such as Olympic lifting, plyometrics, speed and agility drills, and sport-specific conditioning to enhance power, reaction time, and overall athletic capacity.

Olympic Weightlifting

To enhance maximal power output, practitioners often incorporate Olympic weightlifting movements such as the power clean, clean and jerk, and snatch (see Exhibit 6.12a–c).

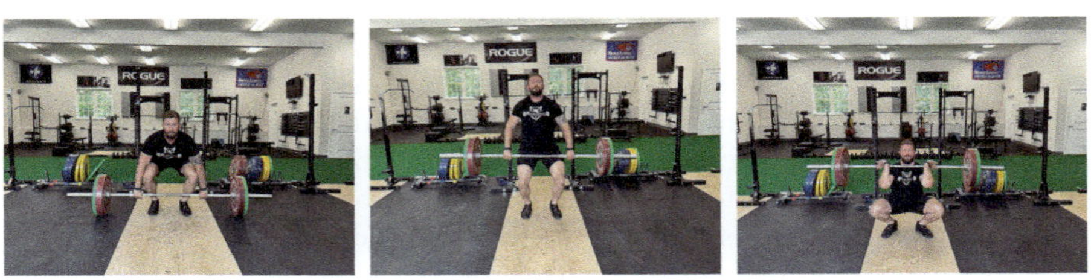

(a) (b) (c)

Exhibit 6.12a–c Example Olympic weightlifting movement

These dynamic, full-body exercises are especially effective for developing explosive strength and are commonly used to improve athletic performance in sports that require rapid force production and change in direction (e.g., volleyball, basketball, football, combat sports, wrestling, track and field).

Plyometrics

Practitioners often incorporate plyometric exercises such as box jumps, bounding, and depth jumps to enhance explosive power and high-velocity force production in athletes (see Exhibit 6.13a–d). Plyometric training is especially beneficial for sports that demand quick, powerful movements, such as basketball, volleyball, track and field (particularly sprints, hurdles, and jumps), soccer, football, gymnastics, and tennis. These exercises improve the stretch-shortening cycle of muscles, which helps athletes generate more force in less time, leading to better speed, agility, and jump performance.

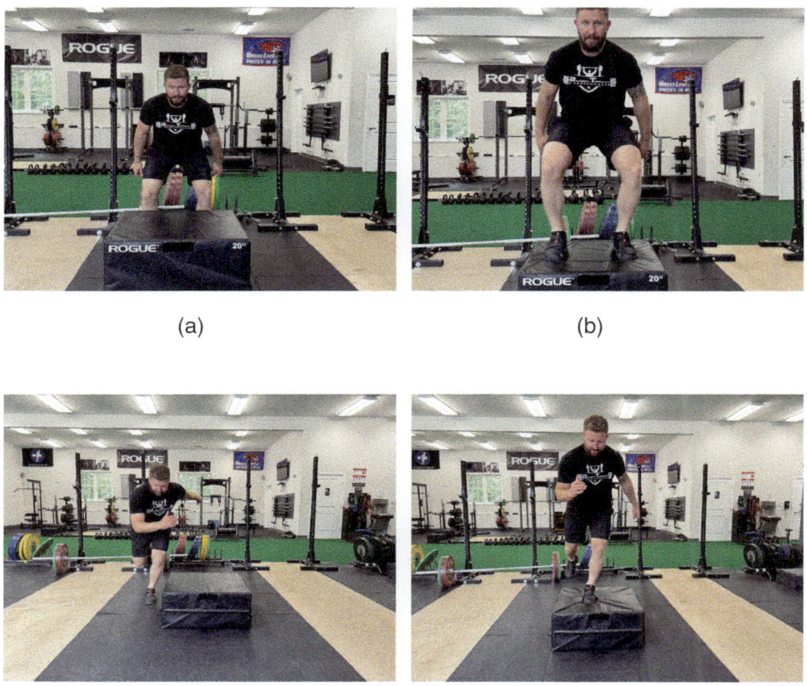

(a) (b) (c) (d)

Exhibit 6.13a–d Example plyometric exercises

Speed and Agility Training

Given the importance of speed and agility in most sports, practitioners will also use targeted techniques to improve these aspects of performance. Common speed training techniques include uphill/downhill running, resisted/assisted towing, and technique training. Common agility training techniques include various ladder drills and hurdle drills (Exhibit 6.14a–b).

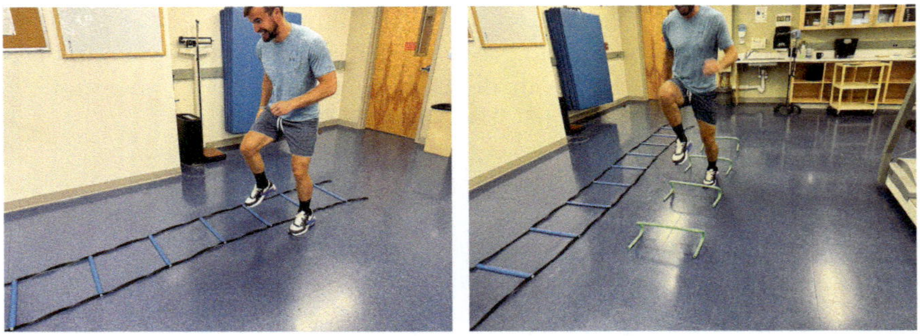

(a) (b)

Exhibit 6.14a–b Example speed and agility training exercises

TECHNOLOGY AND RESEARCH TOOLS

Beyond the various tools used for exercise prescription and training, exercise professionals often use a wide variety of assessment tools to help inform their exercise prescription. Many of these same tools are also used by researchers to evaluate the health, fitness, and performance of study participants (Exhibit 6.15).

Exhibit 6.15 Common exercise tests and fitness assessments

Measures	*Exercise Tests / Fitness Assessments*
Body Composition	• Body Mass Index • Circumferential Assessments • Skinfold Assessments • Bioelectrical Impedance Assessment • Dual Energy X-ray Absorptiometry
Cardiorespiratory Fitness	• Cardiopulmonary Exercise Testing • Treadmill Tests • Step Tests • Bike Tests
Muscular Strength	• Isokinetic Dynamometry • Handheld Dynamometry • Handgrip Dynamometry • 1-Repetition Maximum
Muscular Endurance	• Isokinetic Dynamometry • Push-Up Test • Sit-Up Test • Plank Test
Muscular Power	• Isokinetic Dynamometry • Vertical Jump • Broad Jump • Reactive Strength
Speed / Agility	• Yard Dash • Meter Dash • Pro-Agility Test • T-Test • Hexagon Test
Flexibility	• Sit and Reach • Muscle Length Test Goniometry

(Continued)

Exhibit 6.15 (Continued)

Measures	*Exercise Tests / Fitness Assessments*
Movement Quality	• Functional Movement Screen • Movement Efficiency Screen
Dynamic Balance	• Lower Quarter Y-Balance Test • Upper Quarter Y-Balance Test • Star Excursion Balance Test • Balance Error Scoring System

Body Composition

Body composition can be assessed using a variety of tools and techniques. Common methods include scales and stadiometers to calculate body mass index (BMI) (Exhibits 6.16a–b); tape measures for evaluating circumferential fat distribution (Exhibit 6.16c); skinfold calipers for estimating subcutaneous fat (Exhibit 6.16d); bioelectrical impedance devices for assessing body fat percentage (Exhibit 6.16e); and dual-energy X-ray absorptiometry (DEXA) scans, which provide detailed analysis of body fat and bone mineral density (Exhibit 6.16f).

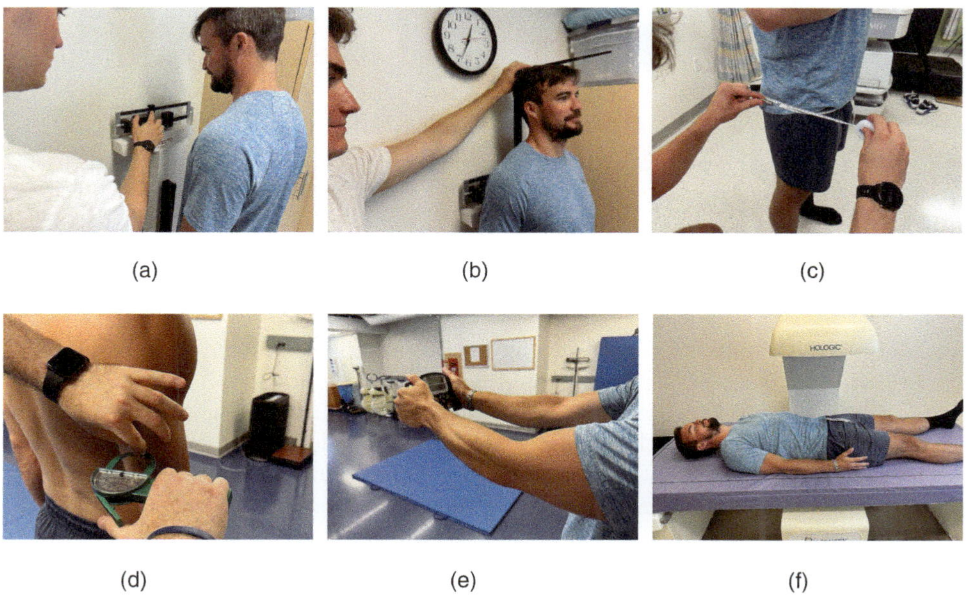

Exhibit 6.16a–f Devices to assess body composition

Cardiorespiratory Fitness

Cardiorespiratory fitness can be evaluated using both laboratory-based and field-based methods. Gold-standard assessments involve the use of metabolic carts for cardiopulmonary exercise testing (Exhibit 6.17a). More accessible field-based options include treadmill tests (Exhibit 6.17b), cycle ergometer tests (Exhibit 6.17c), and step tests (Exhibit 6.17d), which provide estimates of aerobic capacity and endurance.

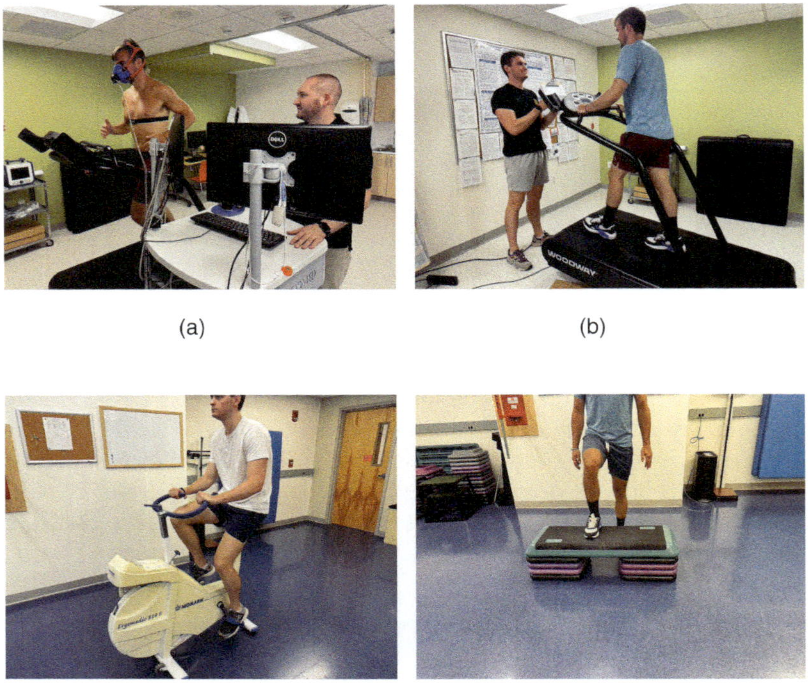

(a) (b) (c) (d)

Exhibit 6.17a–d Assessment of cardiorespiratory fitness

Muscular Strength, Endurance, and Power

Muscular strength may be assessed using gold-standard isokinetic dynamometers (Exhibit 6.18a), which measure peak torque (force) throughout the full range of motion of a joint. These devices are most commonly used in research and clinical rehabilitation settings. However, given the high cost and training needed to operate these machines, muscular strength is routinely assessed via clinic-based handheld dynamometers (Exhibit 6.18b), handgrip dynamometers (Exhibit 6.18c), and barbell weights to determine 1RMs of exercises like the deadlift (Exhibit 6.18d).

Muscular endurance and power can also be assessed using both laboratory and field-based methods. Isokinetic dynamometers are also used in lab settings to measure muscular endurance (Exhibit 6.19a) and power output (Exhibit 6.20a) across a joint's full range of motion. Common field-based tests for muscular endurance include push-ups (Exhibit 6.19b), sit-ups (Exhibit 6.19c), and plank tests (Exhibit 6.19d). For muscular power, field-based assessments include vertical jump stands to measure vertical power (Exhibit 6.20b), timing mats for evaluating reactive power (Exhibits 6.20c–e), and tape-measured broad jumps to assess horizontal power (Exhibits 6.20f–h).

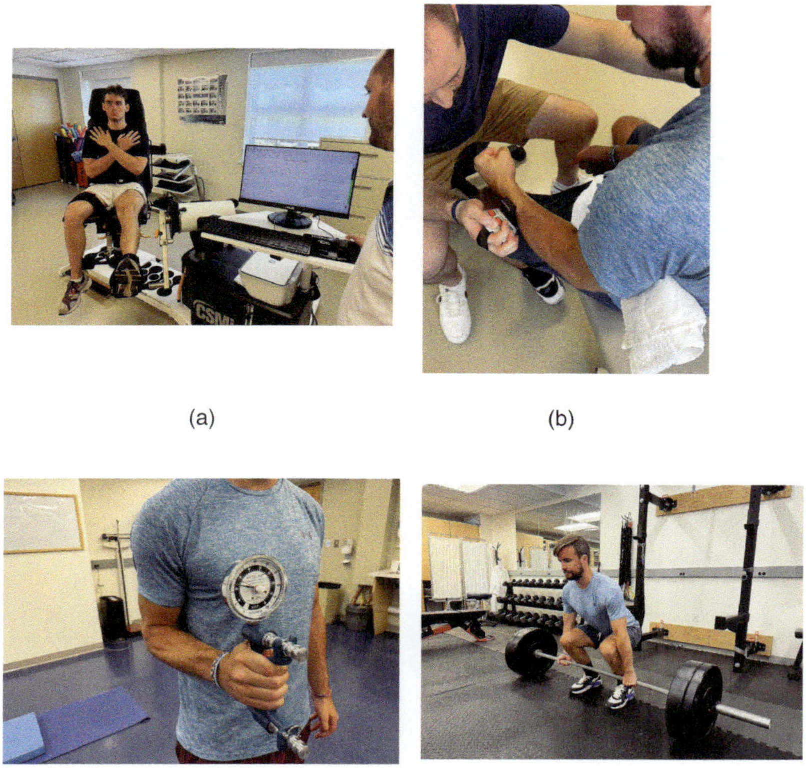

(a) (b) (c) (d)

Exhibit 6.18a–d Assessment of muscular strength

Speed and Agility

Measures of speed are commonly assessed using stopwatches or electronic timing gates during short sprint tests such as the 20- or 40-yard dash and the 100-meter dash. These tests evaluate an individual's ability to accelerate and maintain top-end velocity. Measures of agility, which reflect the ability to rapidly change direction while maintaining speed, balance, and control, are also typically assessed using stopwatches (Exhibit 6.21) or automated timing systems. Common agility tests include the pro-agility test (5–10–5 shuttle), T-test, and hexagon test. These assessments are especially relevant in sports that require frequent changes in direction, such as basketball, soccer, football, and tennis. To ensure accurate and reliable results, standardized protocols and consistent surface conditions are important when administering agility and speed tests.

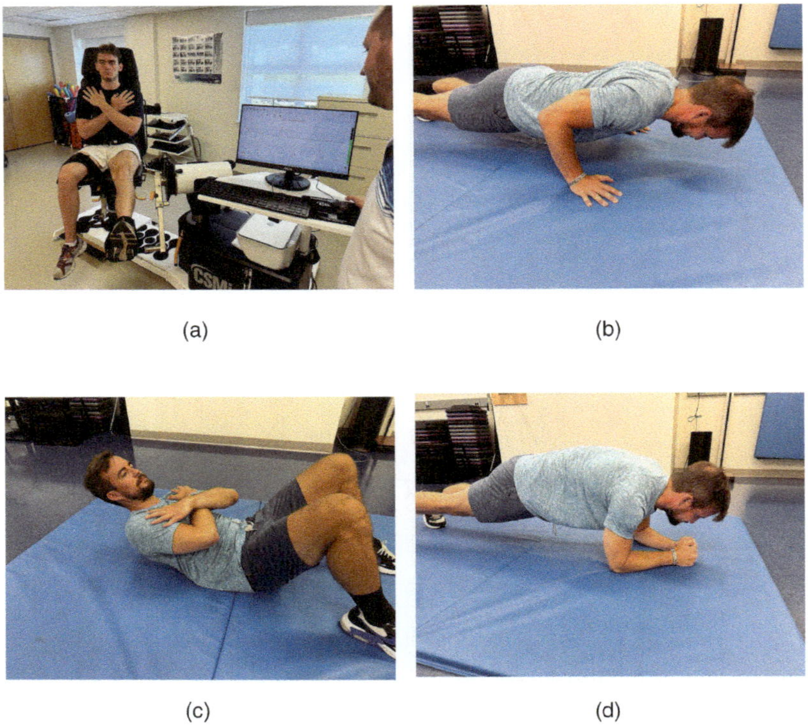

Exhibit 6.19a–d Assessment of muscular endurance

Flexibility

Global flexibility generally refers to the flexibility of multiple muscle groups along the posterior chain, including the hamstrings, lower back, and calves. This is commonly assessed using the sit-and-reach test with a sit-and-reach box (Exhibit 6.22a). In contrast, specific muscle flexibility is measured through muscle length tests using tools like a goniometer or tape measure to evaluate the range of a particular muscle or joint (Exhibit 6.22b).

Movement Quality

The quality of functional movements is often evaluated using standardized movement assessments designed to identify limitations, asymmetries, or compensations that may affect performance or increase injury risk. Common tools include the Movement Efficiency Test and the Functional Movement Screen (FMS), both of which assess movement patterns such as squatting, lunging, and reaching. For example, the FMS uses a test kit to score an individual's ability to perform seven fundamental movements (Exhibit 6.23a–d). These assessments help practitioners develop targeted exercise programs that improve movement quality, enhance performance, and reduce the likelihood of injury (Cornell et al., 2021).

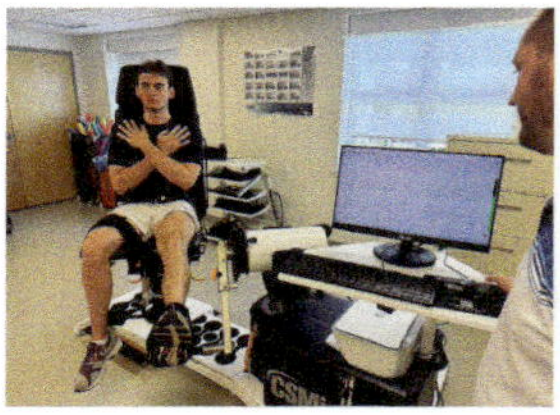

(a)

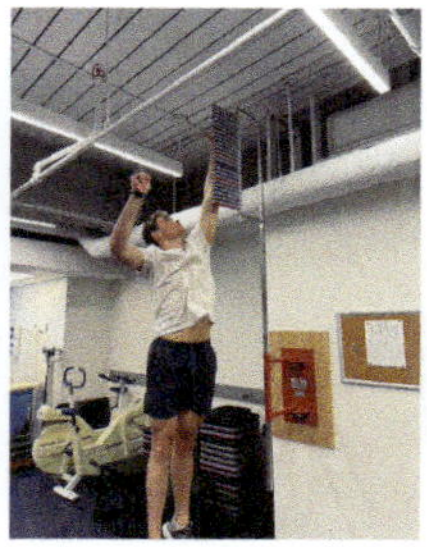

(b)

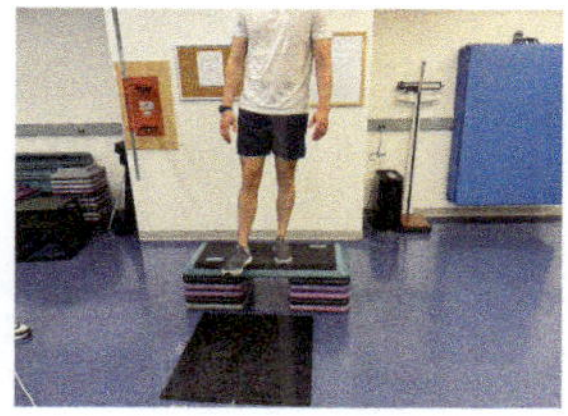

(c)

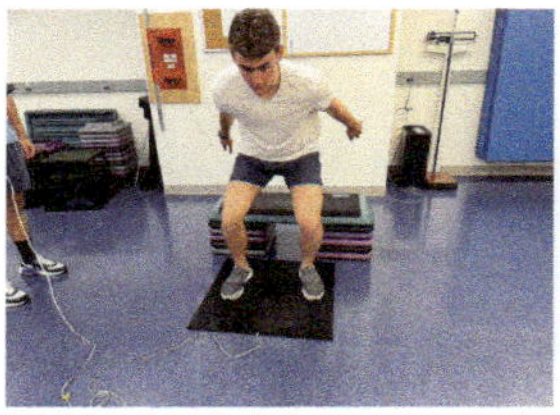

(d)

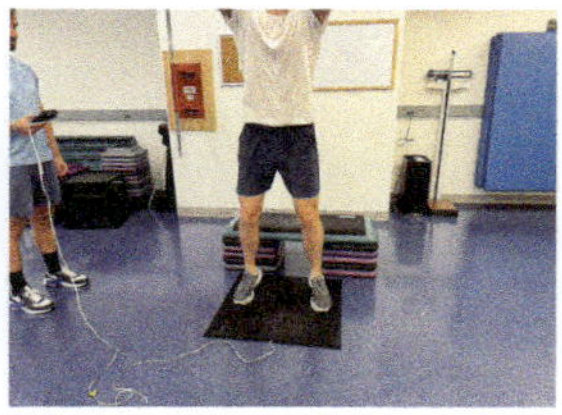

(e)

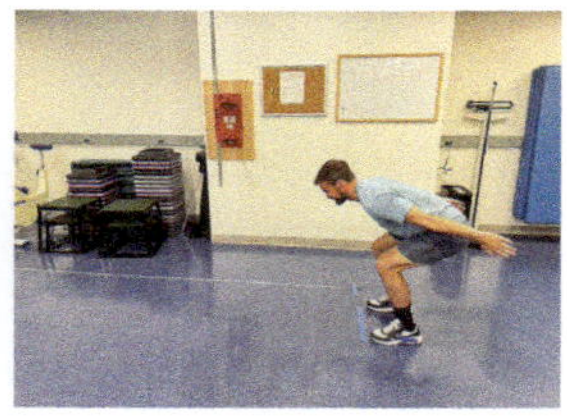

(f)

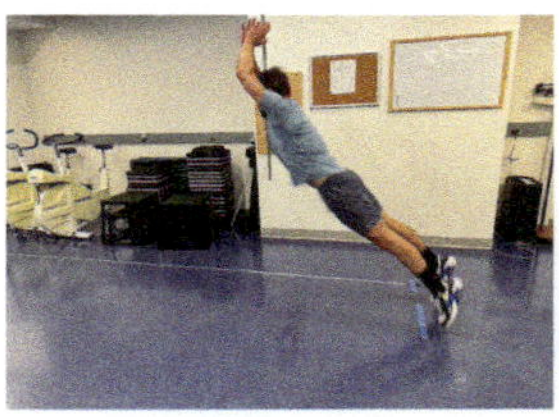

(g)

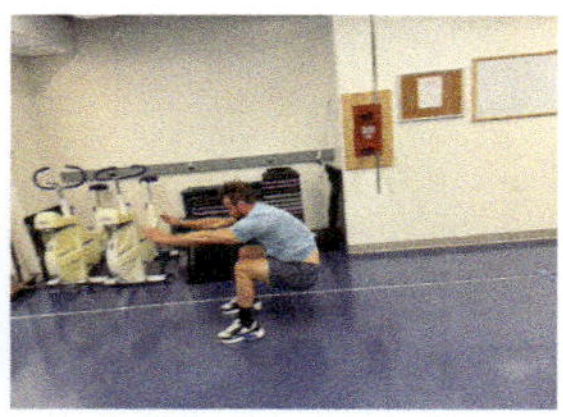

(h)

Exhibit 6.20a–h Assessment of muscular power

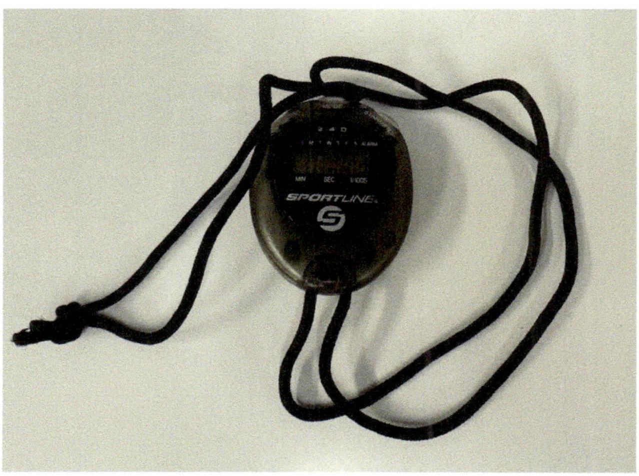

Exhibit 6.21 Stopwatch

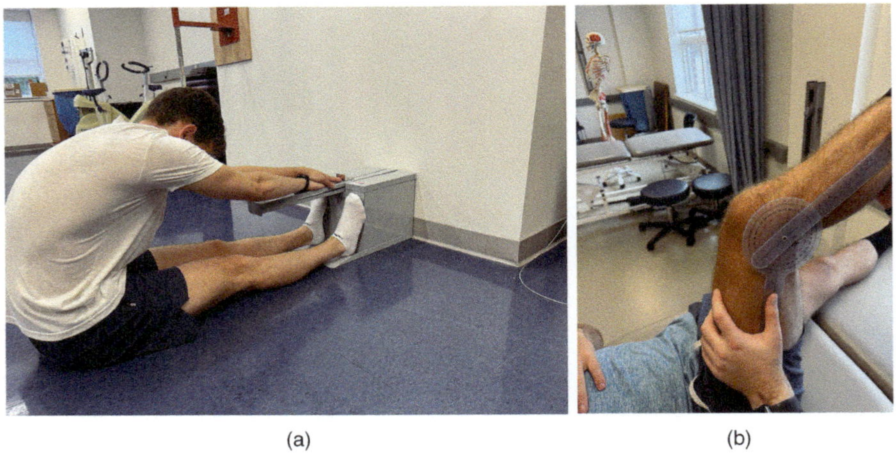

Exhibit 6.22a-b Assessment of flexibility

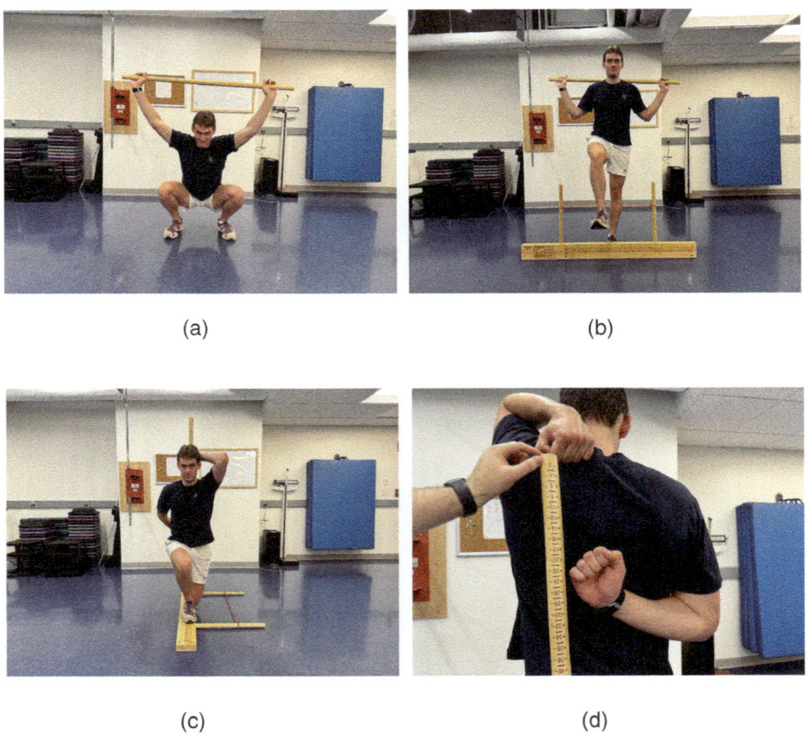

Exhibit 6.23a-d Assessment of movement quality

Balance

Balance is commonly assessed through both static and dynamic tests. Static balance, or the ability to maintain a steady position without movement, is often evaluated using foam balance pads for tests like the Balance Error Scoring System (BESS) Test, shown in Exhibit 6.24a–c, and the Sensory Organization Test. The Romberg Test is another static balance test that requires an individual to stand with their feet together and eyes closed to determine if they can maintain balance without visual input. These tests help assess how well the body's sensory systems work together to keep posture steady (Murray et al., 2014). Dynamic balance, which involves maintaining control while in motion, is typically assessed using either the Star Excursion Balance Test or the Y-Balance Tests for the upper and lower body, using a standardized test kit to help identify balance deficits and potential injury risks. Exhibit 6.24d–f shows an individual performing the Lower Quarter Y-Balance Test (Coughlan et al., 2012).

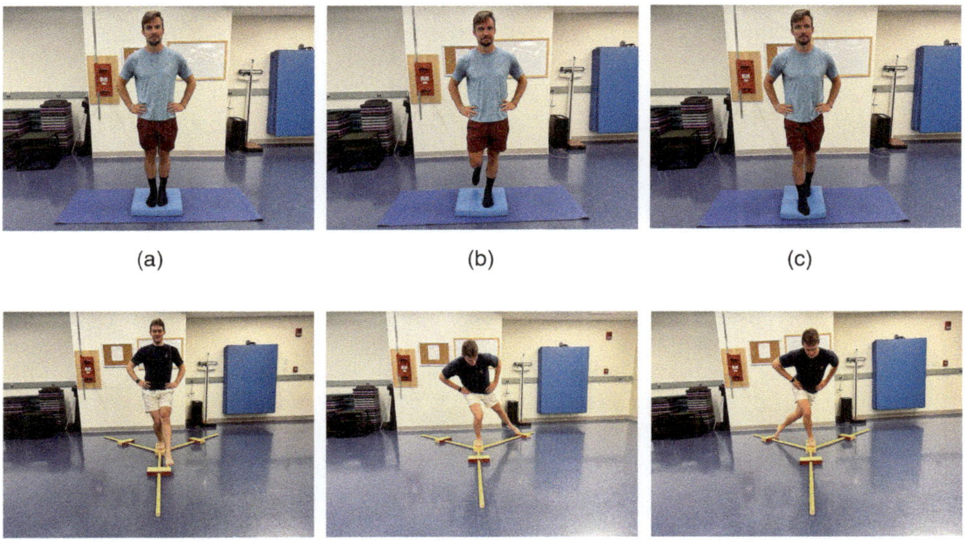

(a) (b) (c)

(d) (e) (f)

Exhibit 6.24a-f Balance assessments

Exhibit 6.25 Abstract of a research study that examined the effect of a corrective exercise program on functional movement quality in firefighters

Cornell, D., and Ebersole, K. (2017). Influence of a corrective exercise program on functional movement quality among active-duty firefighters. *Journal of Strength and Conditioning Research*, *31*(Suppl 1), S90–S91. doi: 10.1519/JSC.0000000000002224.

Due to a link between functional movement quality and musculoskeletal injury (MSKI) risk identified in the literature, practitioners have begun to utilize various assessments, such as the Movement Efficiency (ME) Test, to quantify the functional movement quality of various athletes, including the tactical athlete population of firefighters. However, there is a lack of research examining the influence of a corrective exercise program on functional movement quality among firefighters.

PURPOSE: To examine the influence of a short-term corrective exercise program, known as *The Firefighter-10*, on Overall ME Test scores among active-duty firefighters.

METHODS: 20 male active-duty firefighters were placed into either the experimental (FF-10; $n = 10$) or control (CON; $n = 10$) groups based on their respective suburban fire department (mean ± *SD*, age = 35.5 ± 8.4 yrs; height = 178.2 ± 6.3 cm; weight = 85.8 ± 12.8 kg). Participants in the FF-10 group individually completed corrective exercises associated with *The Firefighter-10* program 3–4 days/week for 4 weeks. *The Firefighter-10* consists of 10 mobility and 10 activation exercises designed to increase the length and strength associated with commonly restricted and weak musculature in the firefighter. Participants in the CON group maintained their current exercise programming for 4 weeks. Functional movement quality data was collected via the ME Test pre- (Week 0), mid- (Week 2), and post-intervention (Week 4). The ME Test consists of 7 sub-tests used to create an Overall ME Test score ranging from 0–100 (worst–best), including a 2-leg squat, a 2-leg squat with a heel lift, bilateral 1-leg squat, a push-up test, 4 shoulder movements, 2 trunk movements, and 2 cervical spine movements. A repeated measures 2 × 3 ANOVA, follow-up main and simple effects, and pairwise analyses were used to identify statistically significant ($p \leq 0.05$) changes in Overall ME Test scores between the FF-10 and CON groups.

RESULTS: A significant group × time interaction was identified ($F_{2,36} = 32.630$, $p < 0.001$) and a significant main effect of time was observed within the FF-10 group ($F_{2,18} = 81.626$, $p < 0.001$). Pairwise analyses indicated that Overall ME Test scores progressively and significantly increased from Week 0 to Week 2 ($p < 0.001$, $d = 1.15$) to Week 4 ($p < 0.001$, $d = 1.46$) within the FF-10 group (49.01 ± 11.10 to 60.79 ± 9.26 to 74.96 ± 10.18, respectively). No changes in Overall ME Test scores were observed in the CON group ($F_{2,18} = 1.062$, $p = 0.367$). In addition, large and significant simple effects were identified at Week 2 ($p < 0.001$, $d = 2.35$) and Week 4 ($p < 0.001$, $d = 3.55$) between the FF-10 and CON groups (60.79 ± 9.26 vs. 41.26 ± 7.20; 74.96 ± 10.18 vs. 44.51 ± 6.61, respectively).

CONCLUSIONS: The results of this study suggest that *The Firefighter-10* corrective exercise program can significantly increase the functional movement quality of active-duty firefighters in just 2 weeks, with further benefits identified at 4 weeks. Future research should examine the influence of *The Firefighter-10* on functional movement quality among other larger cohort populations of firefighters, as well as within other types of fire departments.

PRACTICAL APPLICATIONS: In an effort to maximize the implementation of additional training and/or decrease MSKI risk among firefighters, strength and conditioning professionals can utilize *The Firefighter-10* program to increase functional movement quality in a short time period.

CAREER AND EMPLOYMENT OPPORTUNITIES

Exercise practitioners have a wide range of career opportunities across the fields of health and fitness, human performance, and allied health (Pojednic et al., 2024). The following section highlights several professional roles within these areas, including personal trainers, group exercise/fitness instructors, wellness coaches, strength and conditioning specialists, exercise physiologists, athletic trainers, and physical therapists.

Personal Trainers and Group Exercise Instructors

Personal trainers are health and fitness practitioners who create and deliver safe and effective exercise programs for either apparently healthy individuals or individuals who have been medically cleared to participate in exercise (Schoenfeld and Snarr, 2022). Personal trainers may work in fitness centers (Exhibit 6.26), health clubs, studios, recreation centers, or as independent contractors or sole proprietors. According to the US Bureau of Labor Statistics, there are 329,500 professionals working in this sector, with a projected growth of 14% from 2022 to 2032 (US Bureau of Labor Statistics, 2025a).

Like personal trainers, group exercise instructors are responsible for teaching, leading, and motivating individuals through structured exercise programs. However, their focus is on delivering intentionally designed workouts in a group class format (Gallo, 2020). These instructors lead a range of classes that focus on improving cardiovascular fitness (e.g., spin classes, water aerobics, high-intensity-interval training [HIIT], Zumba), muscular strength and endurance (e.g., circuit training, boot camp, Body Pump, kickboxing), and flexibility (e.g., barre, Pilates, yoga) in various settings, including fitness centers, community recreation facilities, corporate wellness programs, and boutique studios.

Health and Wellness Coaches

Health and wellness coaches incorporate exercise prescription and promote regular physical activity as part of a broader wellness plan. They help clients improve their overall well-being by offering guidance, support, and accountability to make sustainable lifestyle changes. These changes often include better nutrition, increased physical activity, effective stress management, and improved sleep quality. Health and wellness coaches work in a variety of settings, such as corporate wellness programs, healthcare facilities, community health organizations, fitness centers, and private coaching practices.

Strength and Conditioning Specialists

Strength and conditioning specialists use exercise prescription to improve the performance of individual competitive athletes or athletic teams (Haff and Triplett, 2016). As previously discussed, because the focus is on optimizing sport performance, these practitioners incorporate a broader range of exercise strategies and training methods such as Olympic lifts, plyometrics, and speed and agility drills to achieve specific performance outcomes (Durell, Pujol, and Barnes, 2003). Strength and conditioning specialists work in a variety of settings including traditional high schools, collegiate and professional sports teams, military and tactical environments, and private human performance gyms (Exhibit 6.27). Although they do not diagnose or directly treat an injury or medical

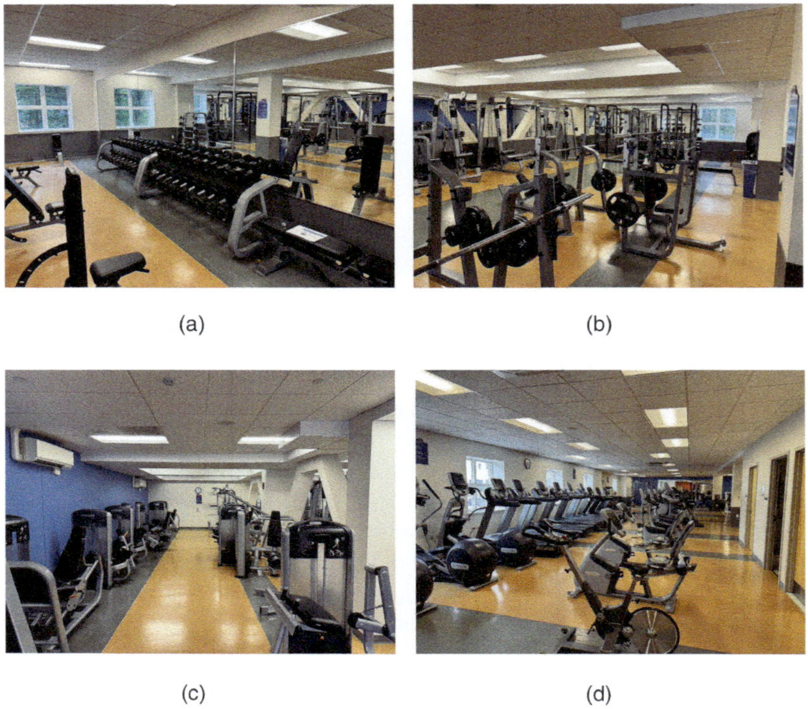

Exhibit 6.26a–d Example of a typical fitness center

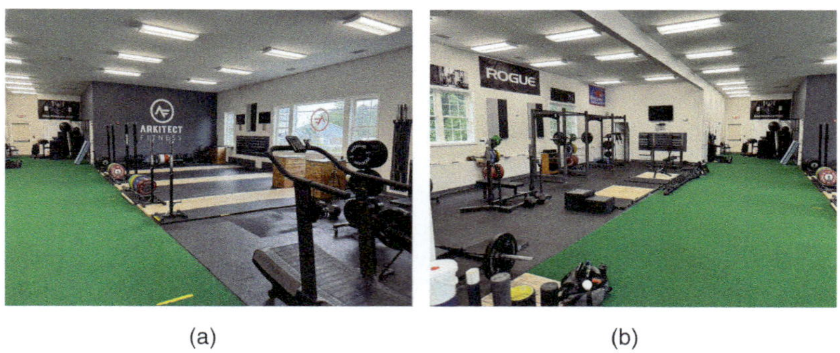

Exhibit 6.27a-b Human performance gym

condition, they often collaborate with the medical team to coordinate return-to-play, as well as modify training programming based on current injuries or medical conditions.

Sport Scientists

Sport scientists are human performance professionals who collect and analyze data to make informed decisions and evidence-based recommendations regarding the training of athletes (Gleason et al., 2024). Therefore, while these individuals are still involved in the delivery of exercise programming, they may coordinate efforts at a higher level and work across multiple sport-related disciplines within the team. Accordingly, sport scientists typically work in elite sport environments (e.g., collegiate athletics, professional teams), but may also contract their services as a sole proprietor or consultant.

Exercise Physiologists and Clinical Exercise Physiologists

Exercise physiologists are allied health professionals who create and deliver safe and effective exercise programs for healthy individuals, as well as individuals with stable medical conditions (e.g., hypertension, diabetes, asthma,) and special populations (e.g., pregnant, older adult, post-rehabilitation) (Cooper et al., 2022). Given their advanced training, these practitioners may coordinate corporate/worksite wellness programs, work in boutique fitness studios or large fitness centers, teach and conduct research at colleges and universities, or work within healthcare teams in hospital systems. According to the US Bureau of Labor Statistics, there are currently about 16,500 exercise physiologists in the US, with a projected growth of 10% from 2022 to 2032 (US Bureau of Labor Statistics, 2025a).

Clinical exercise physiologists are allied health professionals who create and deliver safe and effective exercise programming and other interventions for individuals with active higher risk medical conditions (e.g., heart failure, cardiovascular disease, diabetes, chronic obstructive pulmonary disease), post-medical intervention (e.g., coronary arterial bypass graft, heart transplant, peripheral arterial stent), or post-medical complication (e.g., myocardial infarction, cerebrovascular accident, pulmonary embolism) (Overstreet et al., 2023). These clinicians may also utilize additional equipment to track the progression and ensure the safety of their patients (e.g., electrocardiography telemetry, supplemental oxygen). Therefore, the majority of clinical exercise physiologists report working in specialized facilities that explicitly cater to these types of populations, such as hospital centers (Exhibit 6.28) or cardiac rehabilitation facilities (Hargens et al., 2022).

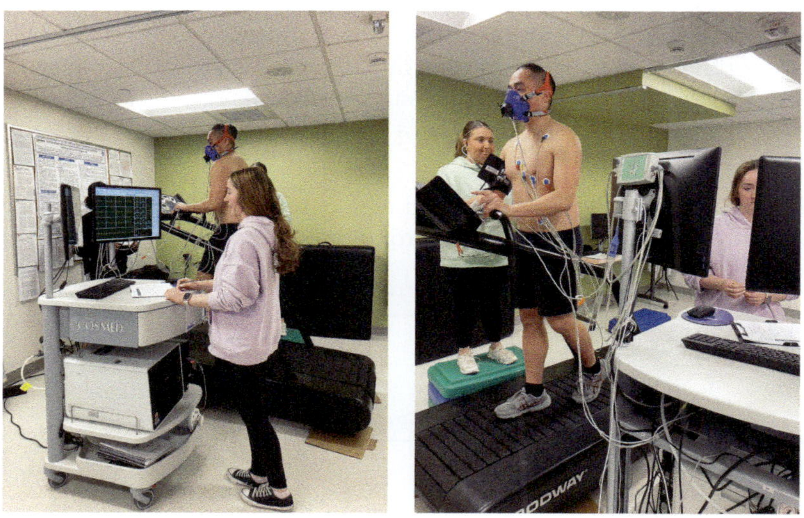

(a) (b)

Exhibit 6.28a–b Example exercise stress testing laboratory

Athletic Trainers

Athletic trainers are allied health professionals who provide service or treatment under the direction of, or in collaboration with, a physician. Athletic trainers provide services in areas such as injury and illness prevention, wellness promotion and education, emergency care, clinical evaluation and diagnosis, therapeutic intervention, and rehabilitation of injuries and medical conditions (Athletic Training Strategic Alliance Inter-Agency Terminology Work Group, 2019). According to the US Bureau of Labor Statistics, there are currently 33,800 athletic trainers in the US, with a projected growth of 14% from 2022 to 2032 (US Bureau of Labor Statistics, 2025b). Athletic trainers work in many settings, ranging from high schools, university/colleges, and professional sports to hospital and healthcare clinics, to tactical settings, such as the military and fire service.

Physical Therapists

Physical therapists are allied health professionals who help individuals maintain, restore, and improve movement, physical activity, and functional ability to support optimal performance, health, and quality of life (American Physical Therapy Association, 2023). Given the large scope of practice of physical therapists as autonomous healthcare providers (American Physical Therapy Association, 2017), these clinicians may treat multiple patient populations impacted by disease, injury, and movement dysfunction, and utilize a very broad range of interventions to treat their patients and clients, including structured exercise programming. However, physical therapists often utilize additional exercise techniques such as manual therapy (joint mobilizations and soft tissue mobilization, for example) and prescribe assistive devices (e.g., walkers, orthotics), which may not be within the scope of practice of other allied health professionals. Physical therapists may also structure their exercise prescriptions to be rehabilitation-focused instead of general fitness or performance-focused.

According to the US Bureau of Labor Statistics, there are currently 246,800 physical therapists in the US, with a projected growth of 15% from 2022 to 2032 (US Bureau of Labor Statistics, 2025c). Physical therapists work in a wide range of settings such as outpatient clinics, inpatient rehabilitation centers, acute care hospitals, or skilled nursing facilities. Accordingly, physical therapists may be employed by large hospital systems, expansive outpatient clinic networks, and small private clinics.

EDUCATION REQUIREMENTS

Education requirements for the career and employment opportunities discussed above range from a high school diploma to a doctoral degree (Exhibit 6.29).

Exhibit 6.29 Training requirements based on career pathways of exercise professionals

Health and Fitness Professionals				
Career	*Education Requirements*	*Program Accreditation*	*State Licensure*	*Certifications*
Personal Trainer	High school diploma	No	No	• Certified Personal Trainer (CPT)
Group Exercise Instructor	High school diploma	No	No	• Certified Group Exercise Instructor (GEI)
Health and Wellness Coach	High school diploma	No	No	• Certified Health Coach • Certified Wellness Coach

(Continued)

Exhibit 6.29 (Continued)

Career	*Education Requirements*	*Program Accreditation*	*State Licensure*	*Certifications*
Human Performance Professionals				
Strength and Conditioning Specialist	At least a bachelor's degree	Upcoming – 2030	No	• Certified Strength and Conditioning Specialist (CSCS) • Strength and Conditioning Coach Certified (SCCC) • Certified Strength Coach (CSC) • Performance Enhancement Specialist (PES) • Tactical Strength and Conditioning – Facilitator (TSAC-F)
Sport Scientist	Bachelor's degree to doctorate	No	No	• Certified Performance and Sport Scientist (CPSS)
Allied Health Professionals				
Exercise Physiologist	At least a bachelor's degree	Upcoming – 2027	No	• Exercise Physiologist (EP)
Clinical Exercise Physiologist	Bachelor's degree to doctorate	Upcoming – 2027	No	• Clinical Exercise Physiologist (CEP) • Certified Cardiac Rehabilitation Professional (CCRP) • Pulmonary Rehabilitation Certificate
Athletic Trainer	Master's degree to doctorate	Yes	Yes (except California)	• Certified Athletic Trainer (ATC)
Physical Therapist	Doctorate	Yes	Yes	• American Board of Physical Therapy Specialties (ABPTS) Board Certifications

Health and Fitness Professions

Generally, the minimum education requirement for entry-level positions in the health and fitness field, such as personal trainers and group exercise instructors, is a high school diploma. However, most professionals also pursue at least one formal certification. Certification not only demonstrates competency in areas like exercise programming and client safety, but it also enhances credibility, improves employment opportunities, and helps ensure the safe and effective delivery of exercise instruction. Many employers and clients expect certification as a standard of professional practice, making it an essential step for those entering the field.

Human Performance Professions

Strength and Conditioning Specialists

The minimum degree requirement for strength and conditioning specialists is a bachelor's degree, but many of these individuals choose to pursue graduate degrees and/or certificates in human performance, strength and conditioning, and sport science. A growing trend in this field is the accreditation of collegiate programs by the Council on Accreditation of Strength and Conditioning Education (CASCE) (Wagner, 2023). These accredited programs ensure that students gain hands-on experience, interact with diverse athlete populations, and demonstrate competency across a standardized set of knowledge, skills, and abilities. This requirement will make the preparation requirements for strength and conditioning specialists more akin to other professionally prepared practitioners, such as physical therapists or athletic trainers, as well as provide a more defined scope of practice compared to other practitioners in the human performance sector (Altiner et al., 2023).

Sport Scientists

Given the need to possess skills in scientific research, statistical analysis, and data science, sport scientists often hold graduate-level degrees, including doctoral degrees such as a Doctor of Philosophy (PhD) or Doctor of Science (ScD/DSc) (Gleason et al., 2024). Their advanced training is typically focused on a specific discipline within exercise science such as biomechanics, sports nutrition, exercise psychology, or strength and conditioning that can then be applied across a range of sports and athletic contexts.

Allied Health Professions

Allied health professionals must hold a college degree in an allied health-related area of study, but this degree could range from a bachelor's degree (e.g., Bachelor of Science in Exercise Science, Bachelor of Science in Kinesiology), to a master's degree (e.g., Master of Science in Athletic Training, Master of Science in Exercise Physiology), to a doctorate (e.g., Doctor of Physical Therapy, Doctor of Clinical Exercise Physiology).

Exercise Physiologists and Clinical Exercise Physiologists

Exercise physiologists typically earn a bachelor's degree in exercise science or a related field, such as kinesiology or health sciences, with many pursuing graduate-level education to expand their expertise (Gallo, 2020). Compared to other health and fitness professionals, their advanced academic training provides them with the qualifications to work with both general and clinical populations. To ensure consistency in training and to promote safety in practice, an increasing number of academic programs are pursuing accreditation through the Commission on Accreditation of Allied Health Education Programs (CAAHEP), which reviews and approves programs based on recommendations from the Committee on Accreditation for the Exercise Sciences (Wagner, 2023). This movement toward accreditation helps better define the professional scope and role of exercise physiologists within the broader allied health workforce (Cooper et al., 2022).

Clinical exercise physiologists have a similar academic foundation but gain advanced training and specialization working with individuals who have chronic diseases and health conditions. While a bachelor's degree is the minimum requirement, the majority (74%) of clinical exercise physiologists hold a master's degree or higher (Hargens et al., 2022). Because of the complexity of clinical practice, accreditation of graduate programs in clinical exercise physiology by CAAHEP is becoming increasingly important to ensure standardized competencies in knowledge, skills, and abilities (Wagner, 2023). This effort may also help support the movement toward professional licensure and reimbursement for services, similar to other recognized allied health professions (Gallo, Ward-Ritacco, and Lynch, 2022). Aligned with efforts to formalize professional standards, the first professional Doctor of Clinical Exercise Physiology (DCEP) program launched in 2022, marking a shift toward doctoral-level preparation similar to that seen in physical therapy and other healthcare professions (Ozemek, 2023; Ozemek et al., 2019).

Athletic Trainers

Athletic trainers are required to complete an athletic training education program accredited by the Commission on Accreditation of Athletic Training Education (CAATE), which sets standards for curriculum content and clinical experience. Starting in spring 2023, all professional athletic training education programs were required to move to master's-level graduate programs (Diakogeorgiou et al., 2021), but there is now a push to elevate athletic training education programs to the doctorate-level, as well (Scifers, 2020).

Physical Therapists

Physical therapists must graduate from a physical therapy program accredited by the Commission on Accreditation in Physical Therapy Education (CAPTE), which sets standards on curricular content and clinical experience requirements for all programs. Starting in 2016, all physical therapy programs were required by CAPTE to be doctorate-level programs (Rapport, Stelzner, and Rodriguez, 2007). Therefore, the only programs that currently exist in the United States are entry-level Doctor of Physical Therapy (DPT) programs.

CERTIFICATIONS AND LICENSURE

Given the wide range of career options in exercise science, many certifications are available as shown in Exhibit 6.29. The certification an individual chooses typically depends on their career goals and the setting in which they plan to work.

Certifications for Health and Fitness Professionals

Personal Trainers

Personal trainers are typically credentialed as a Certified Personal Trainer (CPT) (Gallo, 2020). A variety of professional organizations offer a CPT credential including the American Council on Exercise (ACE), the ACSM, the National Academy of Sports Medicine (NASM), the National Council on Strength and Fitness (NSCF), and the NSCA.

Group Exercise Instructors/Health Wellness Coaches

Group exercise instructors are typically credentialed as a certified Group Exercise Instructor (GEI). GEI certifications exist from a variety of professional organizations, including the ACE, the ACSM, and the NASM. Similarly, health and wellness coaches typically pursue the Certified Health Coach qualification from ACE or a Certified Wellness Coach qualification from NASM.

Certifications for Human Performance Professionals

Since the National College Athletics Association requires strength and conditioning coaches to maintain certification through a nationally accredited strength and conditioning certification program, holding a formal credential in the human performance profession has become standard practice.

Strength and Conditioning Specialists

Common credentials for strength and conditioning specialists include Certified Strength Coach (CSC) from the NCSF, Performance Enhancement Specialist (PES) from the NASM, Strength and Conditioning Coach Certified (SCCC) from the Collegiate Strength and Conditioning Coaches association (CSCCa), and Certified Strength and Conditioning Specialist (CSCS) from the NSCA. Of particular note, starting in 2030, the NSCA will be requiring individuals interested in obtaining the CSCS credential to graduate from a collegiate program accredited by CASCE (Wagner, 2023). The Tactical Strength and Conditioning-Facilitator (TSAC-F) certification also exists from the NSCA for strength and conditioning specialists who work within the tactical sector (i.e., military members, law enforcement, first responders, and other public safety professionals).

Sport Scientists

In addition to potentially holding an advanced graduate degree, sport scientists often earn a credential related to their primary area of specialization (i.e., strength and conditioning, sports nutrition). As the field continues to grow, a formal credential specific to this career path is now available through the NSCA called the Certified Performance and Sport Scientist (CPSS).

Certifications for Allied Health Professionals

Depending on their area of practice, allied health professionals may hold a professional licensure, a professional certification, or a combination of credentials.

Exercise Physiologists and Clinical Exercise Physiologists

The Certified Exercise Physiologist (ACSM-EP) credential from the ACSM is currently the only certification for exercise physiologists recognized in the US Registry of Exercise Professionals (Gallo, 2023). As a result, it is the most commonly pursued credential among exercise physiologists. Beginning in 2027, ACSM will require candidates for the ACSM-EP to graduate from a program accredited by CAAHEP (Wagner, 2023).

Clinical exercise physiologists typically pursue the ACSM clinical exercise physiologist credential (ACSM-CEP) (Overstreet et al., 2023), but individuals specifically working within cardiac rehabilitation or pulmonary rehabilitation programs may choose to pursue the Certified Cardiac Rehabilitation Professional (CCRP) or Pulmonary Rehabilitation Certificate, respectively, from the American Association of Cardiovascular and Pulmonary Rehabilitation (AACVPR). A unique aspect of the ACSM-CEP credential is the eligibility requirement for hands-on work experience with clinical populations. The number of hours needed varies by academic level: 1,200 hours for those with a bachelor's degree and 600 hours for those with a master's degree. Also, starting in 2027, the ACSM will be requiring individuals interested in obtaining the ACSM-CEP credential to graduate from a program accredited by CAAHEP (Wagner, 2023). As mentioned previously, there is a movement toward professional licensure, which would make the credentials of clinical exercise physiologists consistent with other allied health professionals (e.g., athletic trainers, physical therapists).

Athletic Trainers

Athletic trainers are licensed clinicians in 48 of 50 states, as well as the District of Columbia. Their licensure is governed by a health professions board within their state of practice based on the practice act statutes and jurisprudence regulations within that given state. To be eligible for licensure, an individual must pass the national Board of Certification (BOC) examination. However, to be eligible to sit for the BOC exam, a student must first graduate from a CAATE-accredited program.

Physical Therapists

Physical therapists are licensed healthcare professionals in all 50 states and the District of Columbia. Similar to athletic trainers, licensure is regulated by each state's health professions board, and every state establishes its own practice act that defines the scope of practice and legal guidelines, known as jurisprudence, that physical therapists must follow. To be eligible for licensure, an individual must pass the National Physical Therapy Examination (NPTE), which is governed by the Federation of State Boards of Physical Therapy (FSBPT). However, to be eligible to sit for the NPTE, an individual must first graduate from a physical therapy program accredited by the CAPTE. Beyond licensure, a physical therapist may also pursue board certifications within a specialty area of practice, such as orthopedic clinical specialist (OCS), neurological clinical specialist (NCS), pediatric clinical specialist (PCS), and others. These board certifications are governed by the American Board of Physical Therapy Specialties.

PROFESSIONAL ORGANIZATIONS

Numerous organizations are available for exercise professionals to join. Participation in these groups offers opportunities for networking, continuing education, and deeper involvement within the field. While professionals can join more than one organization, they typically align themselves with the organization that most closely matches their area of practice. Examples include:

- American Association of Cardiovascular and Pulmonary Rehabilitation (AACVPR)
- American College of Sports Medicine (ACSM)
- American Physical Therapy Association (APTA)
- Clinical Exercise Physiology Association (CEPA)
- Collegiate Strength and Conditioning Coaches Association (CSCCa)
- National Athletic Trainers' Association (NATA)
- National Strength and Conditioning Association (NSCA)

JOURNALS

A wide variety of journals are available to support exercise professionals. Because some career pathways do not require advanced degrees, many journals present scientific findings in a practical, easy-to-apply format for use in professional settings:

- *ACSM's Health & Fitness Journal*
- *Strength and Conditioning Journal*
- *NSCA Coach*
- *Personal Training Quarterly*
- *TSAC Report*

Given the importance of evidence-based practice, there are also numerous scientific journals that publish original research articles, systematic reviews, meta-analyses, and editorials on relevant topics for exercise professionals:

- *Journal of Strength and Conditioning Research*
- *Medicine and Science in Sports and Exercise*
- *International Journal of Sports Physiology and Performance*
- *Sports Medicine*
- *Scandinavian Journal of Medicine and Science in Sports*

Finally, since defined areas of practice also exist among exercise professionals, there are journals that publish scientific findings specific to an area of practice:

- *Journal of Clinical Exercise Physiology*
- *Journal of Cardiopulmonary Rehabilitation and Prevention*
- *Journal of Athletic Training*
- *Physical Therapy and Rehabilitation*
- *Journal of Orthopedic and Sports Physical Therapy*

FUTURE DIRECTIONS

While the core principles of exercise prescription are unlikely to change, ongoing research continues to refine and expand its application. Emerging areas of interest include the integration of EIM®, the use of HIIT in clinical populations, evaluation of novel training modalities, and the role of exercise for individuals taking weight loss medications (Newsome et al., 2024). As exercise science advances, new opportunities will emerge for professionals to contribute to health promotion, disease prevention, and performance enhancement. At the same time, challenges such as defining scope of practice, establishing licensure pathways, and securing reimbursement for services remain ongoing concerns (Wagner, 2023). To meet these demands, continued emphasis on accreditation and the advancement of educational standards will be critical for preparing competent and informed practitioners.

SUMMARY

Exercise prescription is the process of designing safe and effective physical activity programs to improve health, fitness, or performance. It involves carefully adjusting key training variables such as frequency, intensity, time, and type of exercise, to meet individual needs and goals. While general guidelines help establish a foundation, successful programs require tailoring based on an individual's background, physical condition, and training environment. This is especially important when working with athletes or individuals managing chronic health conditions.

As exercise science continues to grow, so does the need for well-trained professionals who understand not just the science of movement, but how to apply it in real-world settings. Trends like HIIT, exercise for individuals taking weight loss medications, and integration of physical activity into healthcare (e.g., EIM®) are shaping how exercise is used in both fitness and clinical fields. Accreditation standards, certification requirements, and continued research are helping define the role of exercise professionals, making this a dynamic and impactful area of study.

STUDY QUESTIONS

1. What does the acronym FITT-VP stand for?
2. Describe three methods for prescribing aerobic exercise intensity.
3. Define the principle of specificity and provide an example of this principle in practice.
4. Define the principle of progressive overload and provide an example of this principle in practice.
5. What are three different settings in which a personal trainer may work?
6. What careers require a bachelor's degree as an exercise professional?
7. What exercise professionals are licensed practitioners?
8. How does the scope of practice differ between exercise physiologists and clinical exercise physiologists?
9. What differentiates a strength and conditioning specialist from a sport scientist?
10. What is the only certified exercise physiologist credential included in the US Registry of Exercise Professionals?

LEARNING ACTIVITIES

1. Search the websites associated with the AACVPR, ACSM, APTA, CEPA, CSCCa, NATA, and NSCA and write a paper comparing the similarities and differences between these organizations. How do their missions or aims differ?
2. Work with a partner to develop a training goal for each other. Describe what assessments would need to be completed to ensure attainment of that goal.
3. Using the FITT-VP framework, create a one-week training program for yourself that includes aerobic training, resistance training, and flexibility training. Describe how you could utilize the concept of overload to progress your program in four weeks.
4. Using this chapter and the suggested readings, create a video recording of you describing how to administer one of the health and fitness assessments and the tools required to complete that assessment.
5. Pick one of the professional certifications described in this chapter and research specific information about the examination process. Create a brief PowerPoint presentation outlining key elements of the exam, such as the administering organization; eligibility criteria; number of sections; time allotted; number of questions, including number of questions in each topic area.

SUGGESTED READING AND RELATED WEBSITES

Suggested Reading

2018 Physical Activity Guidelines Advisory Committee. (2018). *Physical Activity Guidelines for Americans* (2nd ed.). Washington, DC: US Department of Health and Human Services.

Garber, C. E., Blissmer, B., Deschenes, M. R., Franklin, B. A., Lamonte, M. J., Lee, I. M., Nieman, D. C., Swain, D. P., and American College of Sports, M. (2011). American College of Sports Medicine position stand. Quantity and quality of exercise for developing and maintaining cardiorespiratory, musculoskeletal, and neuromotor fitness in apparently healthy adults: guidance for prescribing exercise. *Medicine & Science in Sports & Exercise*, 43(7), 1334–1359.

Liguori, G., Feito, Y., Fountaine, C., and Roy, B. A. (Eds.). (2021). *ACSM's Guidelines for Exercise Testing and Prescription* (11th ed.). Philadelphia, PA: Lippincott Williams & Wilkins.

Thomas, D. T., Erdman, K. A., and Burke, L. M. (2016). Position of the Academy of Nutrition and Dietetics, Dietitians of Canada, and the American College of Sports Medicine: nutrition and athletic performance. *Journal of the Academy of Nutrition and Dietetics*, *116*(3), 501–528. https://doi.org/10.1016/j.jand.2015.12.006

Related Websites

American Association of Cardiovascular and Pulmonary Rehabilitation (AACVPR)
https://www.aacvpr.org/
American College of Sports Medicine (ACSM)
https://www.acsm.org/
American Council on Exercise (ACE)
https://www.acefitness.org/
American Physical Therapy Association (APTA)
https://www.apta.org/
Board of Certification (BOC) for the Athletic Trainer
https://bocatc.org/
Clinical Exercise Physiology Association (CEPA)
https://www.acsm-cepa.org/
Collegiate Strength and Conditioning Coaches Association (CSCCa)
https://www.cscca.org/
Commission on Accreditation of Athletic Training Education (CAATE)
https://caate.net/
Commission on Accreditation in Physical Therapy Education (CAPTE)
https://www.capteonline.org/
Commission on Accreditation of Allied Health Education Programs (CAAHEP)
https://www.caahep.org/
Council on Accreditation of Strength and Conditioning Education (CASCE)
https://www.nsca.com/casce/
Federation of State Boards of Physical Therapy
https://www.fsbpt.org/
National Academy of Sports Medicine (NASM)
https://www.nasm.org/
National Athletic Trainers' Association (NATA)
https://www.nata.org/
National Council on Strength and Fitness (NCSF)
https://ncsf.org/

National Strength and Conditioning Association (NSCA)
https://www.nsca.com/
US Bureau of Labor Statistics
https://www.bls.gov/

REFERENCES

2018 Physical Activity Guidelines Advisory Committee. (2018). *Physical Activity Guidelines for Americans* (2nd ed.). Washington, DC: U.S. Department of Health and Human Services.

Altiner, B. M. L., Dixon, M. A., Nite, C., and Stock, M. S. (2023). Toward professionalization of the strength and conditioning field. *Strength & Conditioning Journal*, *45*(6), 733–744.

American College of Sports Medicine. (2009). American College of Sports Medicine position stand. Progression models in resistance training for healthy adults. *Medicine & Science in Sports & Exercise*, *41*(3), 687–708.

American Physical Therapy Association. (2017). *Physical Therapist's Scope of Practice* (HOD P06–17–09–16/HOD P06–17–08-07). Alexandria, VA: American Physical Therapy Association.

American Physical Therapy Association. (2023). *APTA Guide to Physical Therapist Practice* (4th ed.). Alexandria, VA: American Physical Therapy Association.

Athletic Training Strategic Alliance Inter-Agency Terminology Work Group. (2019). *Athletic Training Glossary*. Available at: https://www.nata.org/about/athletic-training/terminology

Berryman, J. W. (2010). Exercise is medicine: a historical perspective. *Current Sports Medicine Reports*, *9*(4), 195–201.

Cooper, S. L., Ward-Ritacco, C. L., Maloney, T., and Collins, P. B. (2022). Certified exercise physiologists: educated leaders in fitness and beyond. *ACSM's Health & Fitness Journal*, *26*(4), 23–27.

Cornell, D., and Ebersole, K. (2017). Influence of a corrective exercise program on functional movement quality among active-duty firefighters [abstract]. *Journal of Strength & Conditioning Research*, *31*(Suppl 1), S90–S91.

Cornell, D. J., Ebersole, K. T., Azen, R., Zalewski, K. R., Earl-Boehm, J. E., and Alt, C. (2021). Measures of functional movement quality among firefighters. *Athletic Training and Sports Health Care*, *13*(5), e262–e270.

Coughlan, G. F., Fullam, K., Delahunt, E., Gissane, C., and Caulfield, B. M. (2012). A comparison between performance on selected directions of the star excursion balance test and the Y balance test. *Journal of Athletic Training*, *47*(4), 366–371.

Crookham, J. (2013). A guide to exercise prescription. *Primary Care*, *40*(4), 801–820.

Diakogeorgiou, E., Ray, R. R., Brown, S., Hertel, J., and Casa, D. J. (2021). The evolution of the athletic training profession. *Kinesiology Review*, *10*(3), 308–318.

Durell, D. L., Pujol, T. J., and Barnes, J. T. (2003). A survey of the scientific data and training methods utilized by collegiate strength and conditioning coaches. *Journal of Strength & Conditioning Research*, *17*(2), 368–373.

Gallo, P. M. (2020). A health fitness professional, group exercise instructor, and clinical exercise physiologist walk into a fitness facility… *ACSM's Health & Fitness Journal*, *24*(2), 40–42.

Gallo, P. M. (2023). The United States Registry for Exercise Professionals: how it works and ways it can advance the fitness profession. *ACSM's Health & Fitness Journal*, *27*(2), 51–53.

Gallo, P. M., Ward-Ritacco, C. L., and Lynch, M. (2022). A call to action for clinical exercise physiologists: why you need your national provider identifier and how to get one for free. *ACSM's Health & Fitness Journal*, *26*(2), 54–56.

Garber, C. E., Blissmer, B., Deschenes, M. R., Franklin, B. A., Lamonte, M. J., Lee, I. M., Nieman, D. C., Swain, D. P., and American College of Sports Medicine. (2011). American College of Sports Medicine position stand. Quantity and quality of exercise for developing and maintaining cardiorespiratory, musculoskeletal, and neuromotor fitness in apparently healthy adults: guidance for prescribing exercise. *Medicine & Science in Sports & Exercise*, *43*(7), 1334–1359.

Gleason, B. H., Suchomel, T. J., Brewer, C., McMahon, E. L., Lis, R. P., and Stone, M. H. (2024). Defining the sport scientist. *Strength & Conditioning Journal*, *46*(1), 2–17.

Haff, G. G., and Triplett, N. T. (Eds.). (2016). *Essentials of Strength Training and Conditioning* (4th ed.). Champaign, IL: Human Kinetics.

Hargens, T. A., Richardson, L. A., Brawner, C. A., Perry, D., Verrill, D. E., Porcari, J., and Kerrigan, D. J. (2022). CEPA 2020 Clinical Exercise Physiology Practice Survey. *Journal of Clinical Exercise Physiology*, *11*(1), 2–11.

Herrmann, S. D., Willis, E. A., Ainsworth, B. E., Barreira, T. V., Hastert, M., Kracht, C. L., Schuna, J. M., Jr., Cai, Z., Quan, M., Tudor-Locke, C., Whitt-Glover, M. C., and Jacobs, D. R., Jr. (2024). 2024 Adult Compendium of Physical Activities: A third update of the energy costs of human activities. *Journal of Sport and Health Science*, *13*(1), 6–12.

Kilpatrick, M., Newsome, A. N., Foster, C., Robertson, R., and Green, M. (2020). Scientific rationale for RPE use in fitness assessment and exercise participation. *ACSM's Health & Fitness Journal*, *24*(4), 24–30.

Kraemer, W. J., and Ratamess, N. A. (2004). Fundamentals of resistance training: progression and exercise prescription. *Medicine & Science in Sports & Exercise*, *36*(4), 674–688.

Liguori, G., Feito, Y., Fountaine, C., and Roy, B. A. (Eds.). (2021). *ACSM's Guidelines for Exercise Testing and Prescription* (11th ed.). Philadelphia, PA: Lippincott Williams & Wilkins.

Moore, G. R. (2014). The role of exercise prescription in chronic disease. *British Journal of Sports Medicine*, *38*(1), 6–7.

Murray, N., Salvatore, A., Powell, D., and Reed-Jones, R. (2014). Reliability and validity evidence of multiple balance assessments in athletes with a concussion. *Journal of Athletic Training*, *49*(4), 540–549.

Newsome, A. N. M., Reed, R., Sansone, J., Batrakoulis, A., McAvoy, C., and W. Parrott, M. (2024). 2024 ACSM worldwide fitness trends: future directions of the health and fitness industry. *ACSM's Health & Fitness Journal*, *28*(1), 14–26.

Nuzzo, J. L., Pinto, M. D., Nosaka, K., and Steele, J. (2024). Maximal number of repetitions at percentages of the one repetition maximum: a meta-regression and moderator analysis of sex, age, training status, and exercise. *Sports Medicine*, *54*(2), 303–321.

Overstreet, B., Ward-Ritacco, C., Neric, F., Brawner, C. A., Thompson, B., Hargens, T., and Thompson, W. (2023). Technical requirements for clinical exercise physiologists as qualified health professionals. *ACSM's Health & Fitness Journal*, *27*(2), 20–26.

Ozemek, C. (2023). Creating the first professional doctor of clinical exercise physiology program and a call to expand the model. *Journal of Clinical Exercise Physiology*, *12*(1), 1–2.

Ozemek, C., Kaminsky, L. A., Brubaker, P. H., Lavie, C. J., and Arena, R. (2019). Time to elevate the education of clinical exercise physiologists: a professional doctorate model. *Translational Journal of the American College of Sports Medicine*, *4*(18), 185–191.

PAR-Q+. (n.d.). The Physical Activity Readiness Questionnaire for Everyone: Print Versions. Available at: https://eparmedx.com/?page_id=79

Pojednic, R., O'Neill, D. P., Flanagan, M. G., Bartlett, A., Carter, B. L., and Kennedy, M. A. (2024). Exercise professional education, qualifications, and certifications: a content analysis of job postings in the United States. *Front Sports Act Living*, *6*, 1338658.

Powers, S. K., Howley, E. T., and Quindry, J. C. (Eds.). (2024). *Exercise Physiology: Theory and Application to Fitness and Performance* (12th ed.). McGraw-Hill.

Rapport, M. J. K., Stelzner, D., and Rodriguez, J. (2007). The Doctor of Physical Therapy degree: a new curriculum for a new degree. *Physical Disabilities: Education and Related Services*, *26*(1), 308–318.

Riebe, D., Franklin, B. A., Thompson, P. D., Garber, C. E., Whitfield, G. P., Magal, M., and Pescatello, L. S. (2015). Updating ACSM's recommendations for exercise preparticipation health screening. *Medicine & Science in Sports & Exercise*, *47*(11), 2473–2479.

Schoenfeld, B., and Dawes, J. (2009). High-intensity interval training: applications for general fitness training. *Strength & Conditioning Journal*, *31*(6), 44–46.

Schoenfeld, B. J., and Snarr, R. L. (Eds.). (2022). *NSCA's Essentials of Personal Training* (3rd ed.). Human Kinetics.

Scifers, J. R. (2020). The role of the DAT in the future of athletic training education. *Athletic Training and Sports Health Care*, *12*(1), 3–5.

Shurley, J. P., Todd, J. S., and Todd, T. C. (2017). The science of strength: reflections on the National Strength and Conditioning Association and the emergence of research-based strength and conditioning. *Journal of Strength & Conditioning Research*, *31*(2), 517–530.

Thompson, W. R., Sallis, R., Joy, E., Jaworski, C. A., Stuhr, R. M., and Trilk, J. L. (2020). Exercise is medicine. *American Journal of Lifestyle Medicine*, *14*(5), 511–523.

Tipton, C. M. (Ed.). (2014). *History of Exercise Physiology*. Human Kinetics.

Todd, J. S., Shurley, J. P., and Todd, T. C. (2012). Thomas L. DeLorme and the science of progressive resistance exercise. *Journal of Strength and Conditioning Research*, *26*(11), 2913–2923.

US Bureau of Labor Statistics. (2025a). Fitness Trainers and Instructors. *Occupational Outlook Handbook*. Available at: https://www.bls.gov/ooh/personal-care-and-service/fitness-trainers-and-instructors.htm

US Bureau of Labor Statistics. (2025b). Athletic Trainers. *Occupational Outlook Handbook*. Available at: https://www.bls.gov/ooh/healthcare/athletic-trainers.htm

US Bureau of Labor Statistics. (2025c). Physical Therapists. *Occupational Outlook Handbook*. Available at: https://www.bls.gov/ooh/healthcare/physical-therapists.htm

Wagner, D. R. (2023). Making sense of accreditation, certification, and licensure for careers in exercise science. *ACSM's Health & Fitness Journal*, *27*(2), 27–32.

Warburton, D., Jamnik, V., Bredin, S., Shephard, R., and Gledhill, N. (2022). The 2022 Physical Activity Readiness Questionnaire for Everyone (PAR-Q+) and electronic Physical Activity Readiness Medical Examination (ePARmed-X+): 2022 PAR-Q+. *The Health & Fitness Journal of Canada*, *15*(1), 54–57.

Westcott, W. L. (2012). Resistance training is medicine: effects of strength training on health. *Current Sports Medicine Reports*, *11*(4), 209–216.

Zhu, W., Geng, W., Huang, L., Qin, X., Chen, Z., and Yan, H. (2024). Who could and should give exercise prescription: physicians, exercise and health scientists, fitness trainers, or ChatGPT? *J Sport Health Sci*, *13*(3), 368–372.

7 Biomechanics

Tyler M. Wiles, Aaron D. Likens, and Nikolaos Stergiou

LEARNING OBJECTIVES

After studying this chapter, the student will be able to:

- define biomechanics, including its etymology and interdisciplinary nature, and understand how it integrates concepts from anatomy, engineering, and physics
- outline the fundamental principles of movement analysis, including statics, dynamics, kinematics, kinetics, and temporal analysis, and how these principles are used to evaluate human motion
- understand the diverse applications of biomechanics
- obtain further resources for advancing an education or career in biomechanics

INTRODUCTION

"Biomechanics" is a Greek word that arises from the synthesis of two words: "bio" and "mechanics." Therefore, a simple etymological definition of biomechanics is the study of the mechanics of living organisms. Stergiou (2020) defines **biomechanics** as the study of the forces that act on the body and the effects they produce. Winter (2009) defines biomechanics as an interdisciplinary field that describes and analyzes the mechanics and biophysics required to achieve any movement skill. Knudson (2007) defines biomechanics as the study of motion and its causes in living things. Although there are varying definitions of biomechanics, each describes the essential relationship between humans and mechanics found in biomechanics.

Science is a field of study that focuses on comprehending, forecasting, and elucidating phenomena in a particular subject area. Biomechanists study movement to gain a better understanding of the fundamental mechanisms governing movement as well as the development and control of skill. But rather than coming from a unique body of knowledge, biomechanics as a field of study emerges from the unique set of questions posed to comprehend human movement (Bates, 1991). Biomechanists apply strategies and techniques from other scientific fields, like engineering and physics, and relate them to human movement (Uchida, Delp, and Delp, 2021). In biomechanics, biological interpretations are always used to supplement mechanical evaluations (Higgins, 1977). Thus, biomechanics is a science and a key area of study.

The study of movement involves explaining and understanding the structural and functional mechanisms underlying human performance, in all its presentations, from fundamental motor skills to demanding exercise. Higgins (1977) proposed that skill is a

DOI: 10.4324/9781032697185-7

movement that allows the organism to respond or act effectively within the environment and to integrate past and present. To become skillful requires mastery of the redundant degrees of freedom (Bernstein, 1967). These degrees of freedom, or constraints, are morphological (having to do with the body's structure), biomechanical, environmental, and task-specific (Bartlett, 2007). The study of these constraints is required to explain and understand the underlying mechanisms of movement. Thus, movement must be approached from an interdisciplinary perspective. Movement, as a very broad phenomenon, appears in many different forms, such as play, dance, sport, work, and activities of daily living. This is why a biomechanist cannot study meaningful questions without adequate preparation in areas such as anatomy, motor control, physics, exercise physiology, and engineering.

HISTORICAL PERSPECTIVES

The history of biomechanics can be traced back to the ancient Greeks (Exhibit 7.1). According to Nigg and Herzog (2007), the contribution to biomechanics during the period 650 BC to 200 AD included the distinction between facts and fiction in the discipline, development of mechanical and mathematical models, development of anatomical models, and the first attempt to examine the human body biomechanically. Aristotle (384–322 BCE) was the first to examine and write about complex movements such as running and walking, and Archimedes (287–212 BCE) was the first to examine floating bodies and their movements in water.

Hippocrates (460–377 BCE), the Father of Western Medicine, advocated that humans should base observations on, and draw conclusions from, only what was perceived through the senses. Galen (131–201 CE) was the physician of the gladiators and developed anatomical descriptions and the present-day terminology used in many biological fields and, during the Renaissance, Leonardo da Vinci (1452–1519) examined the structure and function of the human body in a variety of movements. In fact, the contribution of the Renaissance period from 1450 to 1527 was particularly important to science since that is when the foundation of modern anatomy and physiology, and an early examination of movement and muscle action, began (Nigg and Herzog, 2007). In the centuries that followed, another group of scientists, including Galileo Galilei (1564–1642), Giovanni Alfonso Borelli (1608–1679), and Sir Isaac Newton (1643–1727) contributed to the growth of biomechanics. For example, Galileo studied the action of falling bodies and laid the basis for the mechanical analysis of movement.

Borelli, a student of Benedetto Castelli who studied under Galileo, examined muscular movement and mechanical principles. His work *De Motu Animalium* is considered the first biomechanical "textbook," in which he combined the sciences of mathematics, physics, and anatomy. Sir Isaac Newton developed his famous mechanical laws and was the founder of calculus, statics, and dynamics. Contributions to biomechanics during this time period included Newtonian mechanics, which provided a theory for mechanical analysis, as well as an improvement in science through development of the process of theory and experimentation (Nigg and Herzog, 2007).

During the 19th century, contributions to biomechanics included the foundation of electromyography, the development of measuring techniques to examine the kinematics and kinetics of movement, and the beginning of the use of engineering principles in biomechanical analysis (Nigg and Herzog, 2007). Around 1836, the Weber brothers investigated the influence of gravity on limb movements in walking and running and were the first to study the path of the center of gravity during movement. Eadweard Muybridge (1830–1894) was the first to develop cinematographical serial pictures to study animals (horses) and humans. Étienne Jules Marey (1830–1904) used various photographic methods to examine movement. These early examples of photographic techniques would develop into the motion capture used in modern cinema and biomechanics.

During the 20th century, biomechanics became an academic discipline and biomechanical research influenced applications in industrial, medical, and other practical areas, and evolved as a necessary discipline-based method in the study of human and animal movement (Nigg and Herzog, 2007). During this time, Jules Amar (1879–1935) summarized the physical and physiological aspects related to industrial work. His book *The Human Motor* was translated into English in 1920 and set the standards for human engineering in the United States and Europe. Nicholas Bernstein (1896–1966) examined walking, running, and jumping and his work laid the foundation for the study of motor control and coordination. A. V. Hill (1886–1977) investigated efficiency and energy cost in human movement, and in 1931, W. O. Fenn published one of the first biomechanical works in the exercise and sport science literature, a cinematographical analysis of sprint running (Fenn, 1931).

In the 1960s, the term "biomechanics" began appearing more frequently in the literature, and became a graduate specialization, first at Pennsylvania State University and then at the University of Indiana. Richard Nelson developed a laboratory for biomechanical research at Penn State in 1966, and it was the first that was identified with the term biomechanics (Atwater, 1980). His initial graduates were Charles Dillman and Doris Miller, and Dillman went on to establish a biomechanics program at the University of Illinois. Around this same time, in 1967, John Cooper developed a biomechanics laboratory at the University of Indiana. The first graduate was Barry Bates, who later developed the biomechanics program at the University of Oregon. From these pioneer laboratories, programs, and their graduates, many more programs were developed around the country. Others who made tremendous contributions to the development of biomechanics programs around the nation were James Hay (University of Iowa), Stanley Plagenhoef (University of Massachusetts), and Carol Widule (Purdue University).

The period from 1966 to the present has been an era of great growth in biomechanics. It includes the development of a number of new societies, journals, and professional meetings, such as the First International Seminar on Biomechanics, which was held in Zurich, Switzerland, in 1967, and the origination of the *Journal of Biomechanics* in 1968 (Wilkerson, 1997). In 1973, the Fourth International Seminar on Biomechanics was held at Penn State University ("The Fourth International Seminar on Biomechanics," 1974), and resulted in the founding of the International Society of Biomechanics (ISB) that promotes the study of biomechanics at the international level and includes members from several disciplines including anatomy, engineering, physiology, and rehabilitation science. In 1975, at the Fifth International Seminar on Biomechanics in Jyvaskyla, Finland, the American Society of Biomechanics (ASB) was first conceptualized. The following year in Chicago, Illinois, it was officially founded. The ASB includes members from physical education, medicine, ergonomics, biology, and engineering and seeks to advance the field of biomechanics and its application to benefit society (Wilkerson, 1997).

Another important meeting held in 1977 at the University of Illinois, was the first national conference on teaching kinesiology. At this conference, the differences between the terms biomechanics and kinesiology were discussed at length. Kinesiology was found to vary from the name of a course to the title of a college department (Dillman and Sears, 1977). It was also found that, in the United States, the use of mathematical and mechanical principles to study human movement was initially called kinesiology, whereas in Europe it was called biomechanics (Nelson, 1980). At this meeting, it was decided that kinesiology be defined as the parent discipline of biomechanics and, generally, as the science that investigates movement, and that biomechanics be defined as a subdiscipline of the study of forces that act on the body and the effects they produce.

In 1982, the International Society of Biomechanics in Sport (ISBS) was founded in San Diego, California. In the late 1980s, an international electronic mail communication list with the name BIOMCH-L (Biomechanics-List) was established at the University of Calgary, Canada, to help biomechanists from all over the world exchange ideas, problems, information, and the like (Van Den Bogert, Gielo-Perczak, and Woltring, 1992). Finally, in 1989, the Academy of Physical Education was renamed the Academy of Kinesiology and Physical Education, because kinesiology was defined as the overall science of human movement (Charles, 1994).

In 2016, the Department of Biomechanics at the University of Nebraska at Omaha was founded by Nick Stergiou, a previous doctoral student of Barry Bates, and became the first academic department of its kind to both conduct biomechanics research and offer undergraduate (BS) and graduate degree programs (MS and PhD) in biomechanics. The department is housed in the Biomechanics Research Building, established in 2013, and was the first building in the world dedicated exclusively to research in biomechanics.

Exhibit 7.1 Important dates in biomechanics

Date	*Event*
384–322 BCE	Aristotle examined and wrote about complex movements such as running and walking.
1501–1576	Girolamo Cardan opened the consideration of 3-D joint angles.
1452–1519	Leonardo da Vinci examined the function of the human body.
1564–1642	Galileo Galilei and the modern scientific method.
1596–1650	Rene Descartes' cartesian coordinates.
1608–1679	Alfonso Borelli wrote the first biomechanical text, *De Motu Animalium*.
1642–1727	Sir Isaac Newton developed calculus and his mechanical laws.
1668–1738	Hermann Boerhaave's application of Newtonian mechanics to the human body.
1707–1783	Leonhard Euler's theory on 3-D joint angles.
1783–1855	François Magendie and the physiology of walking.
1804–1871	Willhelm Eduard Weber and Eduard Friedrich Weber's anatomy and mechanics of walking.
1806–1875	The founder of electrophysiology, Guillaume Duchenne, and the Duchenne gait pattern.
1830–1894	Eadweard Muybridge developed cinematographical serial pictures to study animals and humans.

(*Continued*)

Exhibit 7.1 (Continued)

Date	*Event*
1831–1917	First 3-D gait analysis by Willhelm Braune and Otto Fischer.
1844–1924	Freidrich Trendelenberg's gait pattern.
1896–1966	Nikolai Bernstein's development of motor control theories.
1918–2013	Jacquelin Perry's influential work on clinical electromyography and observational gait analysis.
1920	Jules Amar's book, *The Human Motor*, was translated into English.
1923–2006	David Sutherland's digitization of data from cine film and development of walking in children.
1925–1984	Pat Murray's instrumented walking studies of normal men and women.
1926–2000	Jurg Baumann integrates cinematography and electromyography.
1931	W. O. Fenn published about the cinematographical analysis of sprint running.
unknown	Herbert Elftman's kinetics of walking
1965	The beginning of MATLAB
1966	Richard Nelson developed the first laboratory for biomechanical research at Penn State.
1967	First International Seminar on Biomechanics, Zurich, Switzerland.
1968	Origination of the *Journal of Biomechanics*.
1969	The first publicly available piezoelectric force plate by KISTLER
1973	Founding of the International Society of Biomechanics.
1976	Founding of the American Society of Biomechanics. The first publicly available strain gauge force plate by AMTI.
1982	Founding of the International Society of Biomechanics in Sports.
1984	Tom Brown receives the first American Society of Biomechanics Borelli Award
1995	Motion capture used to create visual effects in the movie Titanic and its development becomes tied to the entertainment industry.
1997	C-Motion is born from Move3D rehabilitation technology developed at the National Institutes of Health in the USA.
2013	The Biomechanics Research Building is completed at the University of Nebraska at Omaha, the first building dedicated to biomechanics research.
2016	The first academic department offering degrees at all levels in biomechanics is founded at the University of Nebraska at Omaha.

FUNDAMENTAL CONCEPTS

Biomechanics can be divided into the study of the mechanical and anatomical aspects of human movement and, therefore, requires an understanding of anatomy (discussed in Chapter 3), as well as the fundamental principles that govern human movement and the mechanical interactions in the body. The mechanical aspects can be further subdivided into statics and dynamics. **Statics** investigates bodies, masses, and forces at rest or in equilibrium. **Dynamics** investigates bodies, masses, and forces in motion and consists of temporal analysis, kinematics, and kinetics. **Temporal analysis** uses time as the sole basis for analysis, **kinematics** investigates motion without reference to masses or forces, and **kinetics** investigates the actions of forces in producing or changing the motion of masses. Understanding foundational principles in biomechanics sets the groundwork for more advanced study and practical applications in fields such as sports science, rehabilitation, and ergonomics. The following provides a brief introduction to the fundamental concepts mentioned above.

Statics

Statics in biomechanics focuses on analyzing conditions where the body or an object remains in a state of equilibrium, meaning it is either at rest or moving at a constant velocity without acceleration. For an object or body to be in static equilibrium, it must satisfy two key conditions: there must be no net force acting on it, and there must be no net torque. This means that the sum of all forces acting on the body must equal zero, preventing translational movement, and the sum of all torques around any axis must also equal zero, preventing rotational movement. These principles are crucial for understanding how the body maintains stability and balance during various activities, such as standing still, maintaining posture, or performing controlled movements.

In the context of statics, the concepts of the center of mass and center of gravity are pivotal in understanding balance and stability. The center of mass is the point within a body where its mass is evenly distributed in all directions, essentially acting as the balance point. The center of gravity, on the other hand, is the point at which the gravitational force can be considered to act. In most practical scenarios, especially near the Earth's surface, the center of mass and center of gravity are considered the same. The position of these centers affects how stable a body is: the lower the center of mass, the more stable the body, and vice versa. Proper alignment of the center of gravity over the base of support is crucial for maintaining balance. For instance, when standing upright, the human body continually makes slight adjustments to keep the center of gravity over the feet, ensuring stability (Horak, Diener, and Nashner, 1989). Understanding these principles of statics is essential for designing safe and efficient postures, improving athletic performance, and developing ergonomic solutions to prevent injuries.

Dynamics

Dynamics in biomechanics involves the study of how forces produce motion and how energy is transferred and utilized within the body. **Work, energy, and power** are fundamental concepts that help us understand these processes. **Work** is defined as the force applied to an object multiplied by the distance over which it is applied, and it represents the transfer of energy from one system to another. In the human body, work is performed when muscles exert force to move body parts or overcome resistance. **Energy**, on the other hand, is the capacity to perform work, and it exists in various forms, such as kinetic energy (associated with motion) and potential energy (stored energy due to position). Understanding how energy is converted between these forms is crucial for analyzing movements. **Power** is the rate at which work is done or energy is transferred, and it is a key factor in activities that require quick bursts of effort, such as sprinting or lifting weights. High power output indicates the body's ability to perform work rapidly, which is often associated with athletic performance and muscular strength (Suchomel, Nimphius, and Stone, 2016).

Another important aspect of dynamics is **mechanical advantage and efficiency**, which describe how body structures and movements optimize performance and reduce energy expenditure. **Mechanical advantage** refers to the leverage obtained by using a lever system, such as bones and joints, to perform work more effectively. This advantage allows for the amplification of force or speed, making movements more efficient. For example, the long bones in the human limbs act as levers that increase the range of motion and reduce the effort required to move the body. **Efficiency** in biomechanics is the ratio of useful work performed to the total energy expended, and it is a measure of how effectively the body converts metabolic energy into mechanical work. An efficient movement minimizes energy wastage and maximizes output, which is essential for endurance activities and daily tasks. By analyzing these principles, biomechanics helps in understanding how to optimize human motion, improve athletic performance, and develop rehabilitation strategies that enhance mechanical efficiency and reduce the risk of injury (Gaesser, Poole, and Angadi, 2022).

Temporal Analysis

Temporal analysis in biomechanics examines the timing aspects of human movement, focusing on how different phases and events unfold over time during an activity. This analysis is essential for understanding coordination, efficiency, and the rhythm of movements. By breaking down movements into distinct phases, such as the stance and swing phases in gait analysis, temporal analysis provides insight into the sequence and duration of actions, which can reveal how effectively different body segments work together. Key components of temporal analysis include measuring the time spent in various movement phases, calculating cadence (steps per minute) in activities like walking or running, and analyzing symmetry between limbs to identify potential imbalances or coordination issues. This approach is widely applied in sports science to optimize athletic performance by identifying ideal timing patterns and refining techniques. In clinical biomechanics, it assists in diagnosing gait abnormalities, monitoring rehabilitation progress, and evaluating balance and stability in patients with neurological or musculoskeletal conditions. For instance, analyzing a runner's gait might involve assessing how long each foot is in contact with the ground and the duration of the swing phase, helping identify inefficiencies like over-striding. Overall, temporal analysis is crucial for improving performance, minimizing injury risk, and developing targeted interventions by providing a detailed understanding of the timing and coordination of human movement (Harrison and Earhart, 2023; Stergiou, Kent, and McGrath, 2016; Wilson and Likens, 2023).

Kinematics

Kinematics in biomechanics is the study of motion without regard to the forces that cause it. It involves understanding basic concepts such as **position**, **velocity**, and **acceleration**, which are essential for describing how objects or body segments move in space over time. **Position** refers to the location of an object or body part relative to a reference point, providing a basis for tracking changes in movement. **Velocity** is the rate at which position changes, indicating how fast something is moving and in what direction. **Acceleration** is the rate of change of velocity, describing how quickly an object speeds up, slows down, or changes direction. By analyzing these parameters, kinematics provides a detailed picture of movement dynamics, helping to interpret the effectiveness and efficiency of human motion.

Kinematics can be further divided into **linear and angular kinematics**, which focus on different types of motion. **Linear kinematics** studies motion along a straight or curved path, involving parameters such as displacement (change in position), speed (magnitude of velocity), velocity (speed with a direction), and acceleration (change in velocity over time). For example, the linear kinematics of running examines how an athlete's stride length and frequency contribute to overall speed. In contrast, **angular kinematics** deals with rotational motion around an axis, characterized by angular displacement (change in angular position), angular velocity (rate of change of angular displacement), and angular acceleration (rate of change of angular velocity). Angular kinematics are crucial for analyzing movements such as joint rotations during walking or throwing a ball, where understanding the angles and speeds of limb segments can reveal insights into technique, performance, or injury (Ide et al., 2024). By studying both linear and angular aspects, kinematics provides a comprehensive framework for analyzing and optimizing human movement across a variety of contexts.

Kinetics

Kinetics in biomechanics is the study of the forces and torques that cause or result from motion. This involves examining both internal forces, such as muscle forces, and external forces, including gravity and friction. Internal forces are generated by muscles, tendons, and ligaments within the body, allowing for movement and stabilization of joints, while external forces act upon the body from the environment, influencing movement patterns and performance. Understanding these forces is crucial for analyzing human movement and identifying factors that can affect efficiency and injury risk.

A fundamental aspect of kinetics is the application of Newton's Laws of Motion to human movement. **Newton's First Law**, often called the law of inertia, states that an object will remain at rest or continue to move at a constant velocity unless acted upon by an external force. This principle helps explain why certain muscular actions are necessary to initiate or stop motion. **Newton's Second Law** focuses on the relationship between force, mass, and acceleration, expressed by the equation $F=ma$. This law is particularly important in biomechanics as it provides the basis for calculating the forces needed to produce specific movements or accelerate a body part. **Newton's Third Law** states that for every action, there is an equal and opposite reaction, which is observed when the body interacts with surfaces, such as the ground during walking or running, where ground reaction forces play a significant role.

Another key concept in kinetics is the relationship between impulse and momentum, which describes how forces affect changes in motion. Impulse is defined as the product of force and the time over which it acts, and it is directly related to the change in momentum of an object. In biomechanics, understanding impulse can help determine how forceful and prolonged an action needs to be to achieve a desired change in velocity or direction.

For instance, increasing the impulse can enhance performance in activities like jumping or sprinting, where rapid acceleration is crucial. Overall, kinetics provides essential insights into the mechanical aspects of human movement, enabling the optimization of performance, injury prevention, and rehabilitation strategies.

APPLICATIONS TO EXERCISE SCIENCE

As demonstrated above, biomechanics is integral to exercise science because it provides the tools and knowledge to understand and enhance human movement, optimize performance, prevent injuries, and tailor training programs to individual needs. By applying biomechanical principles, exercise scientists can ensure that athletes and individuals engage in safe, effective, and efficient physical activity, ultimately leading to improved health, performance, and well-being. For example, biomechanical analysis of a sprinter's stride can reveal inefficiencies that, when corrected, improve speed and performance. Additionally, biomechanics plays a crucial role in injury prevention by identifying movement patterns that may lead to injury, such as improper foot placement in running, and guides the development of training programs that enhance joint stability and reduce injury risks. Furthermore, biomechanics helps in understanding energy expenditure and mechanical efficiency, which is essential for designing exercises that maximize output while minimizing energy loss. This is particularly important in endurance sports where efficiency is key. Wearable technology and protective gear design also benefit from biomechanics, as they are developed to monitor movement patterns and absorb impact, respectively. These are just a few examples of how biomechanics applies to exercise science; however, given the diverse nature of the discipline, biomechanics has profound applications that extend to all aspects of life. The next section focuses upon other common applications in health related and clinical contexts, as well as within the context of sports and exercise performance.

HEALTH/CLINICAL ASPECTS

Developmental Biomechanics

Biomechanical research in human development focuses on evaluating essential movement patterns across the human life span. Individuals of different ages are examined while performing a variety of daily-living motor skills. The activities can then be quantified, described, and analyzed. Biomechanical analysis is specifically important in quantifying developmental motor skills and movement patterns related to walking, kicking, jumping, throwing, and catching. This research resulted in the characterization of typical activity patterns for each age group. These patterns can then be compared to an individual's performance to determine his or her level of ability at any age. This type of analysis has been performed for a variety of daily living activities across the human life span, including ascending and descending stairs, raising and lowering to a different level (such as a chair or bed), lifting and carrying objects, pushing and pulling objects, and working with short- and long-handled implements. Again, evaluations and quantifications of each type of activity at a variety of ages allow comparisons to be made between ages and the possibility to evaluate an individual's skill or ability in a specific activity at a particular age. For example, biomechanics experts use high-speed camera systems and force platforms to capture and analyze slight movement changes in young children. Based on this information, biomechanists objectively examine movements such as body sway during sitting and standing, and/or the range of motion at the joints during walking. These results are then shared with pediatricians and pediatric physical therapists to accurately evaluate developmental motor milestones during infancy and childhood. Such objective biomechanical measurements are used to evaluate therapies for children with developmental movement disorders (e.g., global developmental delay, cerebral palsy, and Down syndrome).

Another example of developmental biomechanical research focuses on the aging process. Through the developmental process, aging is the ultimate and inevitable stage. Activity levels and working capacity are diminished in older adults. Physiological and motor performance, such as reaction time, movement time, muscle strength, and flexibility, are also diminished with age. Biomechanical analysis is commonly used to assess movement changes in older adults to identify the causes of slips, trips, and falls that the elderly population experiences. In addition, biomechanists strive to develop biomedical devices that can improve the quality of life for older populations, prevent injury, and quantify the best treatment approaches for restoring diminished balance and other motor abilities.

Rehabilitative Biomechanics

Biomechanical research also involves studying the movement patterns of injured and disabled people. Biomechanists commonly analyze abnormal movement changes after injury. This information is crucial for clinicians, especially physical therapists and athletic trainers, when developing an appropriate rehabilitation protocol for individuals to re-learn motor skills (Odanye et al., 2023).

Biomechanical research in rehabilitative biomechanics has led to the development of sound exercises and exercise equipment to train injured individuals back to pre-injury functioning; the development of assistive devices such as canes, crutches, walkers, and orthotics; and the development of rehabilitative devices such as prostheses and wheelchairs. By using objective biomechanical measurements obtained through equipment such as goniometers, hand-held dynamometers, and force transducers, biomechanists can determine the effectiveness of those devices and provide professional opinions to help physicians and therapists improve their usage.

An example of rehabilitative biomechanics is the study of the effects of peripheral artery disease (PAD) on gait patterns (Bapat et al., 2023; Huisinga et al., 2010; Myers et al., 2015). PAD is a progressive disease that limits ambulation due to intermittent pain in the leg muscles and cramping pain induced by movement (i.e., walking). Rehabilitative biomechanists can identify specific abnormalities in a PAD patient's leg movement patterns. They can then evaluate the effects of pharmacotherapy, conservative treatment, and surgical interventions by biomechanically monitoring these abnormalities. Multiple sclerosis patients are another population that can benefit from rehabilitative biomechanics. Patients with multiple sclerosis can also benefit from rehabilitative biomechanics. This progressive neurological disorder, which often causes significant gait disturbances, can be studied using biomechanical techniques to identify specific gait impairments. These insights help develop targeted rehabilitation interventions to address the identified issues (Wurdeman et al., 2011, 2013).

Occupational Biomechanics

Biomechanical research often focuses on providing a safer and more efficient environment for the worker. The development of better safety equipment (e.g., helmets, shin guards, and footwear) for protecting the body from the impacts of falling or colliding with other objects is an important area of biomechanical research. In addition, the development of safer or more mechanically efficient tools, improvement in the design of transportation modules (e.g., airplanes, trains, boats, automobiles, and motorcycles), and decreased occupational injury are major contributions by biomechanists to various work environments.

To reduce the incidence of occupational injury, biomechanists objectively evaluate working performance and develop optimal environments. For example, biomechanists have created personalized robotic exoskeletons to make walking easier with less energy (Slade et al., 2022) and can identify overuse injuries that occur when making simple gestures on devices with a touchscreen (Asakawa et al., 2019). Today, biomechanists also have the technology to simulate realistic environments, even those that resemble the pitch and roll of a ship, to better understand fall risk in dynamic environments (Choi et al., 2024). Biomechanists have also investigated environmental factors, such as noise and distractions in the operating room (Siu et al., 2010; Suh et al., 2010), as well as robotic assistive surgical performance, muscle effort, and fatigue. These biomechanical studies have contributed to the development of an advanced surgical training program that optimizes surgeon performance and minimizes tissue injury during surgery (Suh et al., 2011).

Forensic Biomechanics

Another application for biomechanics research is related to questions that arise in legal situations. Forensic biomechanists are invited to analyze evidence, clarify some of the most important issues, and facilitate the decisions of the jury. In most cases, biomechanists provide forensic investigations, technical reports, and expert testimony for a broad range of human performance-related incidents involving personal injury. The work of an expert witness always involves a human element or component interacting with various aspects of the environment. Most accidents typically involve an initial perceptual component, some form of expectation, and an action, which typically results in a biomechanical consequence. Also, there is often a need to match the resulting injuries with the actions. For example, an analysis and evaluation may be run to determine the potential effects of lap belt and shoulder harness restraint systems on the injuries suffered by a passenger in an auto accident. Various forces on the spine could be calculated to demonstrate the differential effects of the restraint systems and body positions. Such case evaluations typically use a computer simulation program that estimates movement and forces of the head and neck.

Other legal disputes that a biomechanist may be called for, such as product liability, are a combination of occupational and forensic biomechanics in legal cases involving industrial design and safety. For example, a biomechanist may be asked to determine the factors that contribute to nail-gun accidents. The issues assessed could include the adequacy of the design relative to human performance capabilities, expected use patterns, and the use and effect of warnings. The adequacy of machine design relative to safety, when cleaning and operating the nail-gun, may be found to be of concern. Site and product examination, coupled with an analysis of human perceptions and expectations, may suggest that the design was unsafe and a contributing cause of an accident.

SPORTS/PERFORMANCE RELATED ASPECTS

Biomechanical research in exercise and sport has focused on postures and movement patterns that minimize the risk of injury during physical activity and improve performance. Among the contributions of biomechanics are the development of exercise machines for improving strength, endurance, flexibility, and speed; the development of new exercise modes, such as plyometrics and isokinetics to advance performance; the design of exercise and sports equipment to minimize injuries; and the development of exercise and sport techniques to optimize performance.

The design of sport footwear is an example of how biomechanics is used to improve performance and reduce injury. Until the beginning of the 1970s, changes in the design of sport shoes were based on the subjective observations of athletes and coaches. Because the movements of the lower extremities were too fast to be evaluated with the naked eye or even standard film cameras, a new technology needed to be developed. A groundbreaking invention that enabled biomechanists to analyze fast movements was high-speed cinematography. Sixteen-millimeter film taken at high speed could be displayed at normal speed or evaluated frame by frame for a detailed examination of the movement of the foot and leg during contact with the ground while walking or running. Today, advanced digital video camera systems are used to capture movements in sports that are extremely fast, such as the golf swing and baseball pitch (Ide et al., 2024).

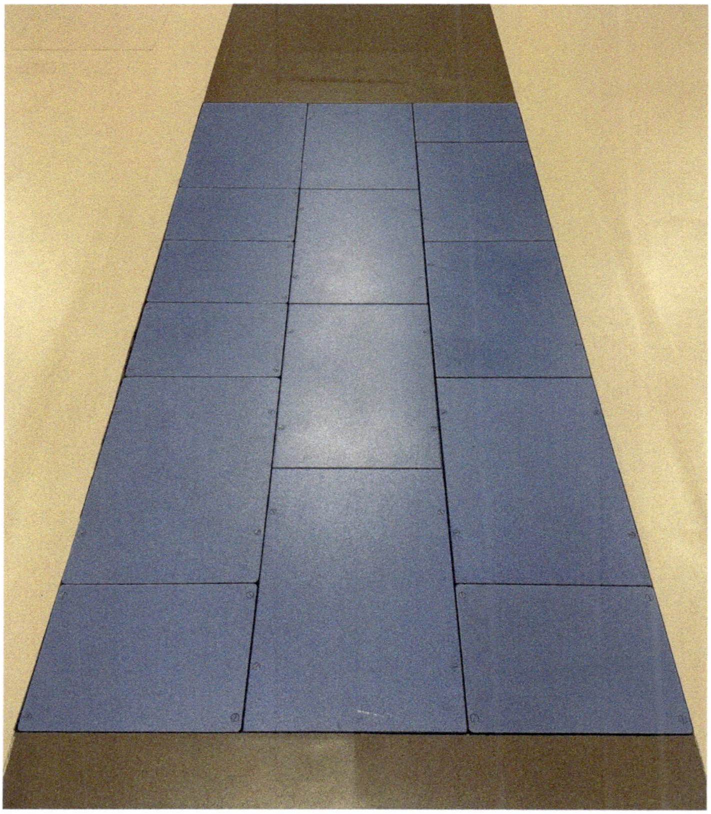

Exhibit 7.2 A force platform suite

The amount of force that is applied to a surface or an individual during a sport activity is also important to the biomechanist. To determine this force, biomechanists developed special scales, known as **force platforms** (Exhibit 7.2), that can measure the impact forces between the shoe and the ground. By measuring these forces, we know today that the foot and the shoe must absorb two to three times the body's weight with each running step.

Another device used by biomechanists is an instrumented insole (Exhibit 7.3) that can be worn within a shoe under the foot, where it measures the pressure between the shoe and the foot. With this device, biomechanists can determine the extent that each part of the foot plays in a specific activity. This information can then be used to determine which areas of the foot will sustain most of the load while the foot is in contact with the ground. Knowing the amount of force that each area receives allows the shoe manufacturer to adjust the amount of support and cushion in the shoe to best support the foot and reduce the chance of injury.

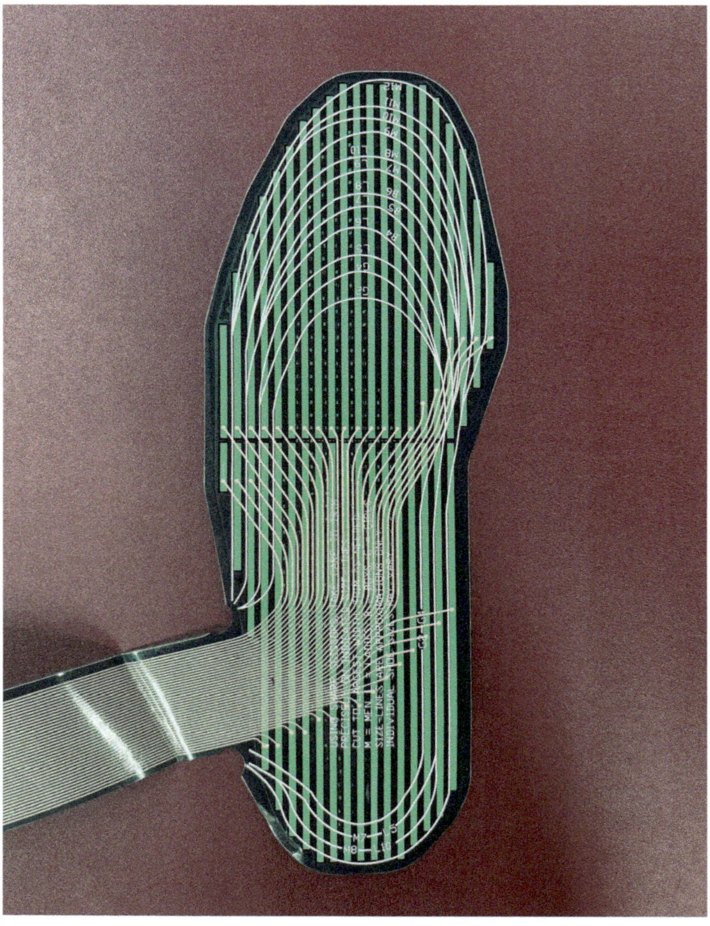

Exhibit 7.3 A pressure insole

Currently, most of the biomechanical shoe research is directed toward the cushioning and stability of the sport shoe. Some other important considerations in shoe design are the flexibility and density of the sole as well as the weight, performance, durability, and breathability of the upper part of the shoe. Using the techniques previously described, biomechanists analyze the demands of a specific sport (e.g., basketball or volleyball) in relation to the shoes that are designed for that sport. This research has dramatically improved the design of all sports shoes.

Biomechanists also contribute significantly to the design of exercise equipment for improving strength and endurance, as seen in the development of stair-stepping machines and exercise bicycles. They evaluate posture, force production, and injury risk to optimize user safety and performance on these devices. As a result, stair-steppers and exercise bikes have evolved to offer greater comfort and improved usability, while providing safe and effective resistance for improving strength and endurance.

Biomechanists also play an important role in the development and testing of protective devices (e.g., eye guards, football helmets, and pads) and in the development and testing of sports equipment (e.g., golf clubs, ice skates, and wetsuits). These devices help athletes prevent athletic injuries and improve performance. Some companies, like Nike, have also created dedicated facilities focused on athlete performance and the integration of apparel and performance. Examples of academic and industry pairings to develop sports or occupational equipment through biomechanical analysis are common, and have been useful to determine if a new product should continue to develop, or be discontinued (Wiles et al., 2022).

An example of the use of biomechanics to improve sport performance can be found in golf-swing analysis. With a high-speed video camera and speed-measuring device, the golf instructor can determine a player's position and movement throughout the golf swing. The speed and path of the golf club head, as well as the speed and path of the ball after contact, can also be determined. This data provides the instructor with the information necessary to describe the player's actions that result in the path of the golf ball. By adjusting the player's actions, the instructor can alter the path of the ball and perhaps improve performance. This type of analysis can be helpful to the beginner as well as the highly skilled player. More recently, many sports teams have begun to recognize the importance of creating a dedicated biomechanist position. Those who work as a biomechanist for a professional sports team (e.g., baseball, basketball, soccer) gain access to motion capture cameras installed in stadiums to analyze the movement of all players, for every play, during live games!

TECHNOLOGY AND RESEARCH TOOLS

Biomechanists use a variety of instruments to measure and record time, motion, and forces. These devices are often highly technical, but are essential for collecting data and analyzing human movement (Robertson et al., 2014).

To record time and motion, timing devices (e.g., watches and digital clocks) and motion image recording methods and devices (e.g., cinematography, videography, digital imaging, brain imaging, and goniometers) are used to provide temporal and kinematic data. Temporal and kinematic data can also be combined with force measurements quantified by force platforms, pressure insoles, accelerometers, inertial measurement units, and electromyography to obtain kinetic data such as joint movements and powers. Furthermore, this information can be integrated with modeling and simulation techniques to predict performance.

When body movement is captured by the motion recording device, the recorded images of reflective skin markers are converted into spatial coordinates (Exhibit 7.4 left). From the coordinates of the digitized markers, the displacements, velocities, and accelerations of each recorded moving body segment can be calculated (Exhibit 7.4 right).

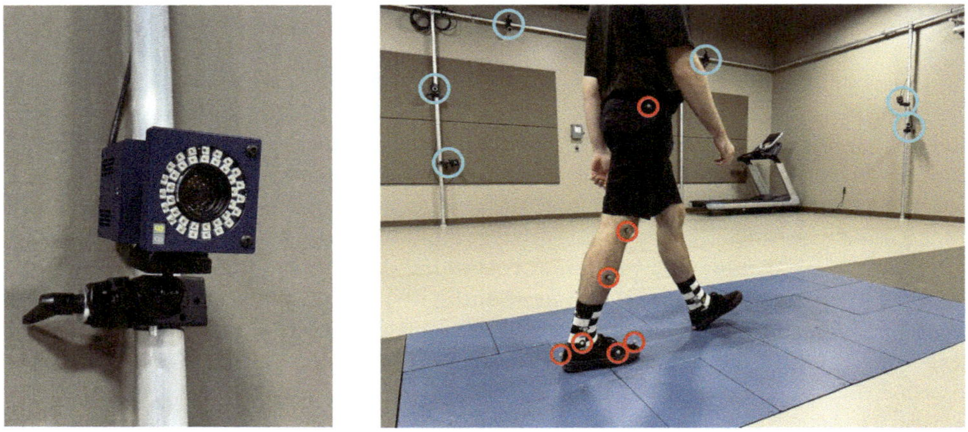

Exhibit 7.4 Measuring movement with passive motion capture

Motion recording devices use optical lenses to capture body motion and provide permanent recorded images of movement that can be evaluated with more precision than perception with the naked eye alone (Exhibit 7.4 left). Therefore, many activities, such as the contact of the foot with the ground while running, as described earlier, happen so quickly that they must be analyzed by specialized equipment that can capture the activity in many more frames per second. In this way, a biomechanist can more precisely analyze events like foot injuries that may occur while running.

Cinematography provides a sequence of images that can be displayed as a motion picture or be viewed one by one. Filming can be done at nearly any speed, from less than one frame per second to more than five million frames per second. Filming at high frame rates allows motion that is too fast to see with the naked eye to be captured and viewed in slow motion or as individual images. Although rarely used today, 16 mm film cameras used in cinematography, with variable focal length lenses and adjustable shutter speeds and apertures, are capable of adjustable frame rates of up to 500 frames per second. Videography also provides a sequence of images that can be displayed as a motion picture or viewed individually.

Videography has most of the features of cinematography, with the convenience of instant viewing and the ability to reuse the recording. The most common video cameras and recorders capture images at 60 frames per second using variable focal length lenses and adjustable shutter speeds and apertures. Today, video cameras have evolved into high-speed digital optoelectronic systems that directly capture the digital images of movement described by the trajectories of skin markers (Exhibits 7.4 and 7.5). The digital trajectories of the markers are then directly stored on a computer hard drive.

Videotapes are no longer needed in a digital optoelectronic motion capture system. Current motion capture systems are mostly of two types: passive and active systems. Passive motion capture systems use markers coated with a reflective material to reflect light

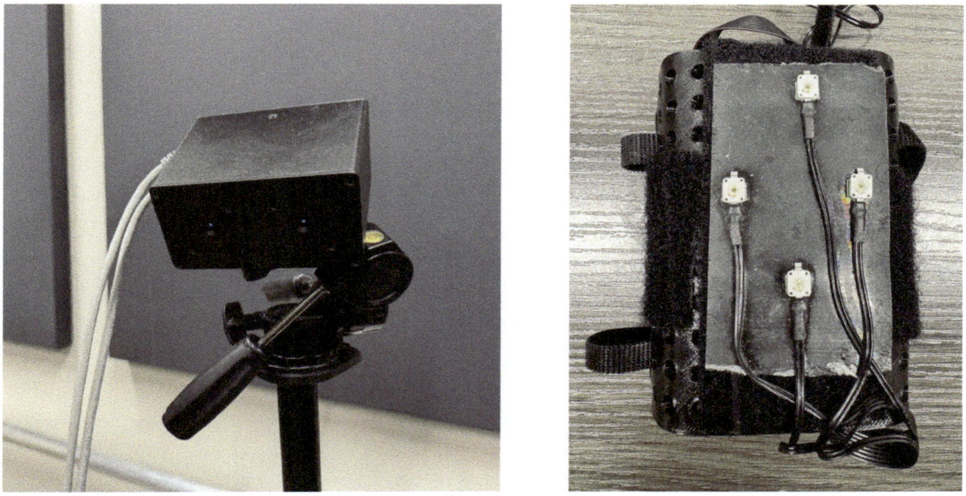

Exhibit 7.5 Measuring movement with active motion capture

from the cameras (Exhibit 7.4). Active motion capture systems use active markers with light-emitting diodes (LEDs); rather than reflecting light back to the camera, the active makers are powered to emit their own light and their relative positions are tracked by illuminating the LEDs (Exhibit 7.5).

For a more comprehensive biomechanics analysis, a motion capture system can be used with other equipment, such as an instrumented treadmill, to evaluate both kinematics and kinetics during walking. Motion of the leg can be captured by either an active or a passive marker of a motion capture system, while forces from the ground can be measured and captured by the force plate embedded in an instrumented treadmill or walkway. By combining the kinematic data from the motion capture system with kinetic data from the instrumented treadmill, the neuromuscular responses and their contributions, in the form of joint moments and their powers, can be evaluated during walking.

Dynamography provides kinetic or force data. An example of a dynamographic device is a force platform with built-in force transducers that provide electrical signals proportional to the components of force acting on it. A transducer is a measuring device that converts one form of energy into another. An electrical displacement transducer, for example, converts kinetic energy from movement into electrical energy. Force transducers used in a force platform can be strain gauges, which change their electrical resistance with strain, or piezoelectric elements, which generate a charge when stressed. The electrical energy can then be measured and recorded as an indication of the amount of force. The most common use of a force platform is to measure the three orthogonal components of ground reaction forces (GRFs) in vertical (Fz), anterior–posterior (Fy), and medial–lateral (Fx) directions, between the foot and the floor, during locomotor activities (refer to Exhibit 7.2). Force platforms can be used to assess the forces generated during contact with the ground in a variety of activities such as running, walking, jumping, landing, hopping, and stair climbing.

Instrumented treadmills have force platforms embedded below the belt. Multiple designs have been developed, including the split-belt instrumented treadmill, which has two force platforms under its dual belt design (Exhibit 7.6, c and d), and the tandem instrumented treadmill, which is divided between independent front and back belts (Exhibit 7.6, b). An additional unique feature of this device is its split-belt design, which can provide a different speed for each belt or even two different directions. It creates a more challenging environment for studying human locomotion. The most challenging environments can be created with the Computer Assisted Rehabilitation Environment (CAREN) and its associated instrumented treadmill (Exhibit 7.6, d). This split-belt treadmill can move in all axes, while a subject is immersed in a 180° virtual environment. In addition to the forces from the treadmill, the CAREN is also equipped with a large array of motion capture cameras. Instrumented treadmills allow biomechanists to conduct sophisticated biomechanical research studies, such as locomotion perturbations, for example asymmetrical walking, and even slip and trip assessments.

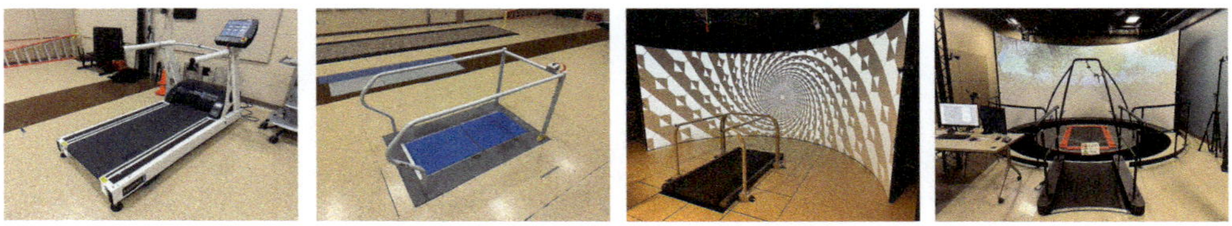

(a) (b) (c) (d)

Exhibit 7.6 Instrumented treadmill systems

Instrumented staircases are typically equipped with multiple force platforms. For example, in Exhibit 7.7, a force platform is embedded under the first three steps, and an additional force platform is connected to the handrail structure. An instrumented staircase can accurately measure the amount of force applied on each step during stair ascent and descent and can detect the usage of handrails during stair negotiation. Combining the force (kinetic) data, from the instrumented staircase, with the kinematic data, from motion recording devices, the neuromuscular responses and their contributions to power and joint movements can be estimated. In this fashion, biomechanists can fully understand the mechanism of human stair negotiation and help physicians and therapists to develop strategies for patients to regain their ability to climb stairs.

Computerized dynamic posturography, such as Bertec's Computerized Dynamic Posturography system (Exhibit 7.8), is used to measure body sway in a standing position. This sophisticated instrument provides different research protocols that allow biomechanists to study the contribution of different sensory systems (visual, vestibular, and somatosensory) in maintaining postural stability. The embedded force platform with rotation and translation capabilities provides either a stable or unstable support surface and measures the amount of force exerted by the participant. The movable visual surround provides additional complexity and challenge for participants attempting to maintain their postural stability in a static or dynamic visual environment.

Another example of a dynamographic device is a **pressure insole.** The pressure insole consists of a matrix of small-force transducers (Exhibit 7.3). When the area of each element is known, the pressure can be estimated. Because this device measures a pressure distribution it allows the force acting on individual anatomical foot regions to be measured, rather than just the resultant force on the entire foot generated by a force plate. This information is especially important in shoe design, diabetic foot evaluation, and

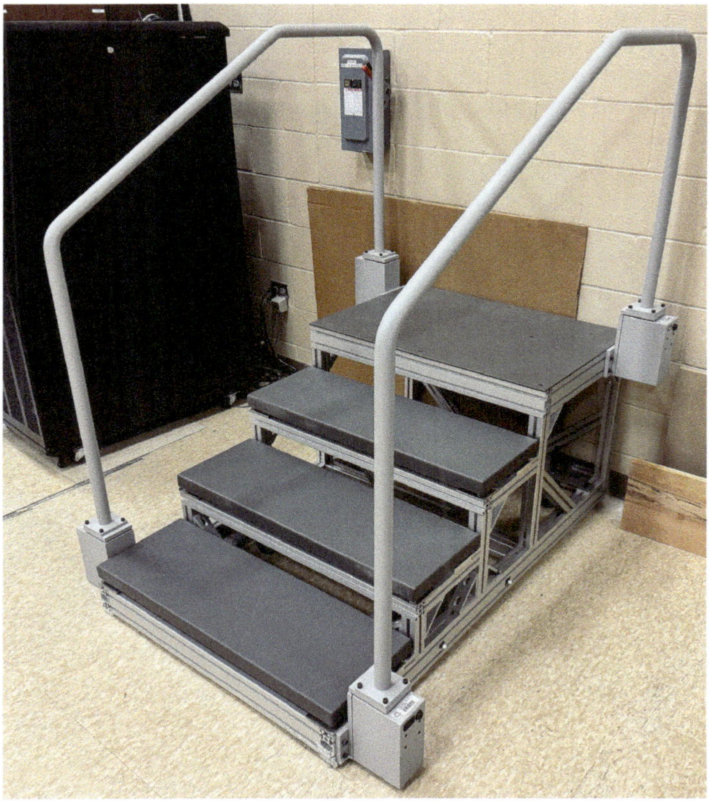

Exhibit 7.7 A custom instrumented staircase

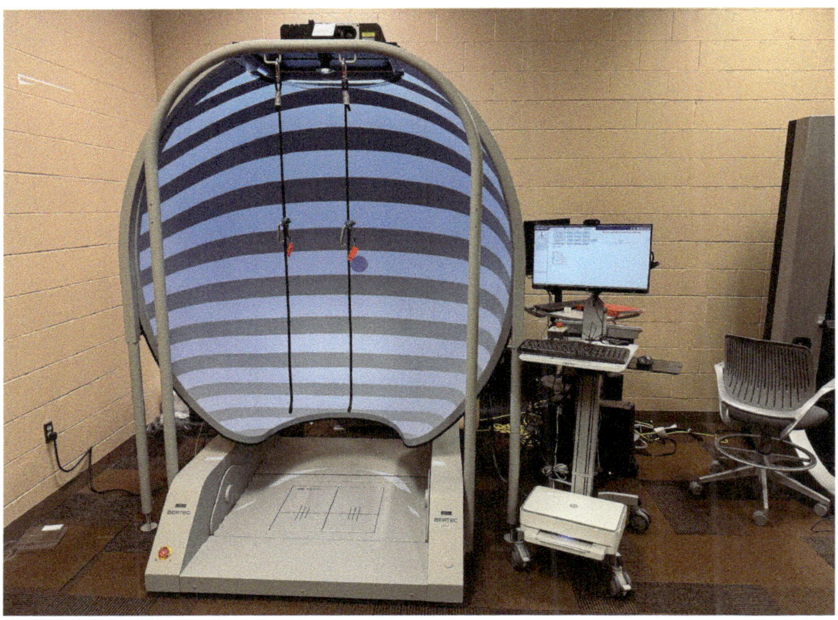

Exhibit 7.8 A system for testing vestibular, proprioceptive, and visual components to balance

pathological gait. Similar pressure technologies can be incorporated into seats, mats, or even treadmills (Exhibit 7.6, a), which allows measurement of more diverse activities including sitting, lying down, walking, and running. These systems can be used to evaluate risk for bedsore development or seat and back pressures, or to detail more information about foot contact during gait.

Computerized dynamic posturography can be combined with **eye tracking systems** specifically designed to capture data on eye movement, focus of vision, head position and rotation, eyelid aperture, lip and eyebrow movement, and pupil size (Exhibit 7.9, right). Software that accompanies these devices provides visual analysis tools that generate heat-maps and advanced eye-gaze analytics over video, still images, webpages, and interfaces. Such information is commonly used to investigate the coordination between eye and body movement, or to study how visual information influences movements, and postural sway (Haworth and Stergiou, 2018). Other applications for eye tracking include determining the points of gaze when someone is picking up an object, such as a cup, or planning future steps on an unstable surface. Additionally, eye tracking data can provide valuable insights into athletes' decision-making processes during their routines.

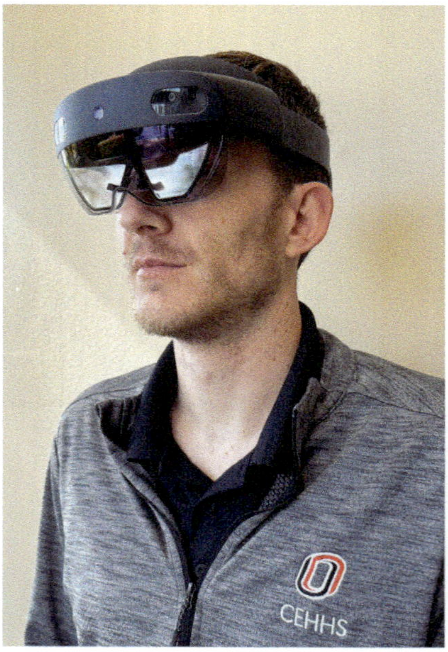

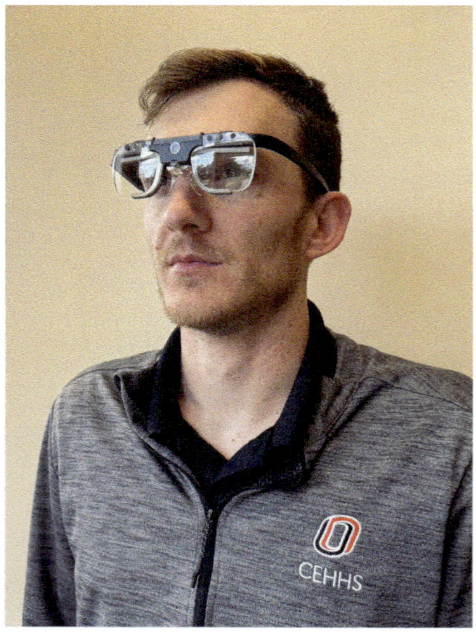

Exhibit 7.9 Head mounted displays that track the orientation of the eyes and head

Virtual reality systems can be incorporated with other biomechanics equipment to study the influence of visual flow or virtual environments on various aspects of movement. Virtual reality systems are commonly implemented using multiple projectors and screens that create a 180° (or greater) immersive view (Exhibit 7.6, c and d). Portable virtual reality or augmented reality systems also create an immersive virtual environment shown through a head-mounted display (Exhibit 7.9). Virtual reality systems create entirely new environments by displaying virtual images on a screen, like playing a video game. Augmented reality systems differ from virtual reality systems in that they overlay digital information onto the real world rather than creating an entirely new environment. For instance, smartphone apps allow users to place virtual furniture in their homes. Both types of systems utilize sophisticated software to create 3D virtual environments and can be used for rehabilitation, among many other applications. For example, virtual environments can be used to improve the feasibility of remote-therapy and tele-rehabilitation in stroke survivors (Dodakian et al., 2017; Parker et al., 2022). In addition, virtual environments can be incredibly useful for promoting increased daily activity, safely practicing surgical procedures, realistic occupational training for commercial pilots, or educational tools at all levels of academia.

Brain imaging, using **functional near-infrared spectroscopy (fNIRS), electroencephalography (EEG),** and **magnetic resonance imaging (MRI),** is becoming more common because recent systems permit measuring brain activity during movement. fNIRS sends near-infrared light through the scalp and brain to measure changes in oxygenated and deoxygenated hemoglobin to help determine the activity levels of neurons during mentally intensive tasks (Exhibit 7.10). For example, trying to synchronize finger tapping with more complex and difficult to follow auditory metronomes increases brain activity that mimics the metronome itself (Harrison et al., 2018). EEG is like fNIRS and records the tiny electrical signals produced by neurons in the brain through electrodes placed on the scalp or surface of the brain. Electrical activity occurs at all times, and EEG is useful for investigating how the behavior of electrical activity influences sleep patterns and seizures, or identifying brain regions that are more or less active when walking over uneven terrain (Liu et al., 2024). MRI utilizes strong magnetic fields and radio waves to provide a computer-generated two-dimensional image of a body part's soft tissue, such as muscles, ligaments, tendons, and internal organs. After the two-dimensional image is acquired, it is manipulated so that it can be viewed on a video monitor and reconstructed into a three-dimensional image. MRI

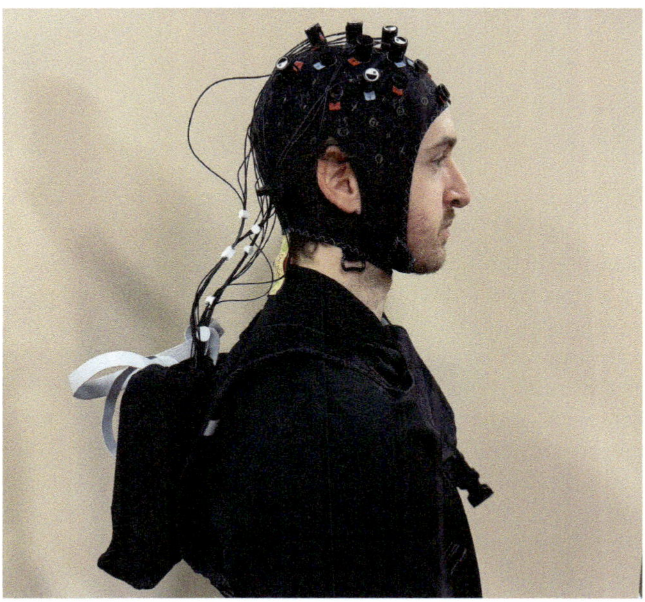

Exhibit 7.10 fNIRS setup that sends near-infrared light through the scalp and brain to measure blood flow and activity

provides a noninvasive means of viewing the structures under the skin, which allows for a more extensive evaluation of an injury or a muscle adaptation to training.

The **inertial measurement unit** is a very useful portable electronic device because it combines triaxial **accelerometers, gyroscopes, and magnetometers** into one small piece of equipment placed on the body (Exhibit 7.11). An **accelerometer** is an electronic device that measures acceleration forces. It usually consists of an inertial mass that exerts a force against an element, such as a beam, and the resulting strain is then measured. Because we know that force is the product of mass and acceleration, when mass is a constant and the acceleration is known, we can estimate forces. The **gyroscope** is the part of the inertial measurement unit that measures the rotation and direction of the sensor. The **magnetometer** is the part of the inertial measurement unit that can estimate direction and measures local magnetic fields, which can be used to determine if the sensor is deployed in an appropriate environment without many electronics. By utilizing one inertial measurement unit, accelerations and orientations can be estimated. If two or more inertial measurement units are synchronized and located on adjacent joints, it is possible to determine joint angles. A group of inertial measurement units serves as a portable version of a motion capture camera, which is typically restricted to a dedicated lab space. The portability of these synced devices gives researchers the freedom to collect data in many environments. For example, we can now collect high quality data when walking around an indoor track, along hiking trails, during sporting events, or underwater (Wiles et al., 2023). See Exhibit 7.13 for an example of a research study that used inertial measurements to collect kinematic data.

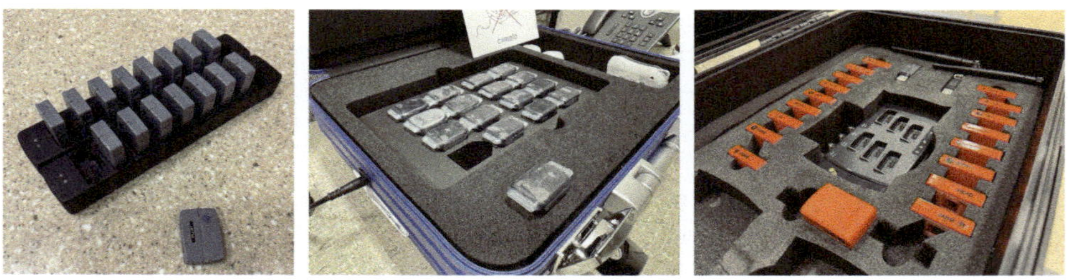

Exhibit 7.11 Inertial measurement units containing an accelerometer, gyroscope, and magnetometer

Like inertial measurement units, **goniometers** provide kinematic data on joint positioning. They are used to measure static positions of limb segments with respect to a joint axis. An electro-goniometer is a goniometer with a potentiometer (variable resistor) at its axis of rotation. The electrogoniometer provides an indication of joint position during movement and can be calibrated to determine speed of movement. The device is most often attached to the body with the axis of the potentiometer aligned with the long axis of segments. The electro-goniometer provides an output voltage, proportional to the joint angle, which can be measured, scaled, and recorded. This information can be used to assess flexibility for diagnosis, rehabilitation, and exercise prescription. When kinematic data of movement are measured, they can be combined with data from force platforms, pressure insoles, accelerometers, and electromyography to provide even more detail regarding body motion.

Electromyography provides data on muscle activity (Exhibit 7.12). An electromyograph records electrical changes that occur in a muscle before, during, or after contraction. This electrical activity can be captured, amplified, filtered, and recorded as an indication of muscle activity or fatigue during a performance. Recent advances have combined EMG and inertial measurement units into a single system. Such a combination allows researchers to directly monitor muscle activity and how those electrical signals drive movement in real-time. Waterproof alternatives also exist to evaluate underwater activities in swimming or with underwater treadmills (Exhibit 7.12 right).

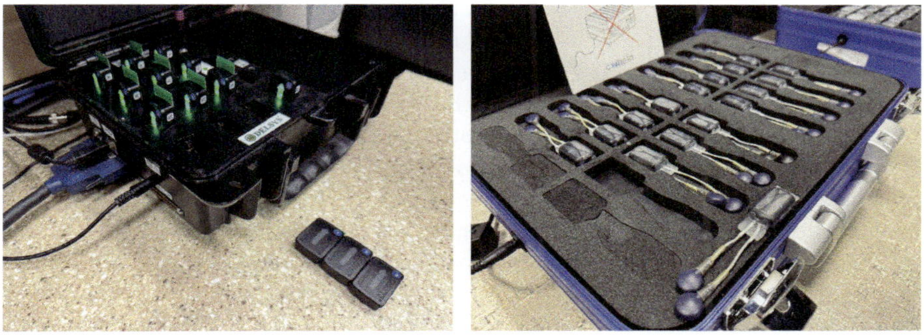

Exhibit 7.12 Electromyography sensors

For all pieces of equipment, **hardware**, **software**, and **coding** experience is becoming increasingly necessary as the sophistication and amount of data increases. With current technology, biomechanists can easily combine data from multiple pieces of equipment to form a comprehensive understanding of how and why the body moves in particular ways. Before these advancements in technology, biomechanists had the daunting task of hand calculating joint angles from individual images from a camera recording many images per second. Similar to the way the microscope changed the world and led to groundbreaking discoveries in fields such as biology, pathology, and genetics, biomechanists now have available to them the "microscope" of movement. Today, biomechanists can capture movements for hours or even days at very high sampling rates, using different systems, then store the data, and process it quite fast to solve complex problems. It is a great time to be a biomechanist as our "microscope" is finally fully available and our capabilities to analyze movement are amazing!

CAREER AND EMPLOYMENT OPPORTUNITIES

Employment opportunities in biomechanics are wide ranging because of the great variety of applications related to biomechanics discussed earlier in this chapter. The majority of employment opportunities fall under academic and research, and industry and government related positions. To gain a better understanding of the type and number of positions available, search the BIOMCH-L website (BIOMCH-L, n.d.). Social media is also a useful source to search for employment, especially in academia. Creating media accounts separate from your personal accounts can function as a virtual resume to reach out to future advisors, build connections, or advertise your skills and expertise.

EDUCATION REQUIREMENTS

Because of the diversity of the areas related to the field of biomechanics, a broad range of knowledge is required to be successful. For example, requirements for a doctoral degree in biomechanics typically require courses in mathematics, computer science, engineering, physics, and motor control and learning. Undergraduate programs accept students directly from high school and usually require coursework in physics, chemistry, mathematics, anatomy and physiology, programming, and biomechanics.

Although the general course requirements for a master's or doctoral degree in biomechanics are similar from one university to another, differences do exist between programs depending upon the research focus of the faculty in the program. Because biomechanics is a broad and diverse field, ideally, there should be variety in the academic training of the faculty. For example, the training for someone working in rehabilitative biomechanics will be distinctly different from that of someone working in sport biomechanics or industrial biomechanics. Therefore, depending upon your area of interest in biomechanics, it is important to determine if the school you wish to apply to has a faculty with the expertise and academic background to help you achieve your goals.

Graduate degree (i.e., doctoral and master's) programs typically fall under an engineering, kinesiology, or exercise science department, although there are programs under varied areas including ophthalmology and physical therapy. New areas of study in computational biomechanics and bio-mechatronics are emerging, with a focus on merging biology and mechatronics to create assistive and implantable devices, prosthetics, and robots. This convergence is being driven by recent technological advances in computers and manufacturing. A list of available graduate programs in biomechanics can be found on the website of the American Society of Biomechanics (n.d.).

If you are an interested in pursuing an advanced degree in biomechanics, there are some key skills that separate good and great students, as well as good and great scientists (Stergiou, 2020). For example, the ability to succinctly, and clearly, communicate a biomechanical issue through writing or oral presentation is a very important skill. Biomechanists often spread into overlapping fields, and it is important to convey critical information that can be easily digestible between professions (i.e., clinicians, executives, material designers, etc.). Although much of biomechanics does not explicitly rely heavily on mathematics, a sufficient level of knowledge and confidence will help young researchers tackle more computationally focused research questions. Finally, biomechanics lends itself to large, and sometimes confusing datasets that cannot be handled by memory alone, therefore, working knowledge in hardware, software, as well as coding experience in languages such as MATLAB, R, and Python are recommended. Certainly not all students meet these requirements when beginning graduate school or joining the work force. Playing to your strengths, developing your weaknesses, and staying curious, will help you become a successful biomechanist. After all, it is never too late to learn a new skill!

PROFESSIONAL ORGANIZATIONS

Several professional associations in the field of biomechanics allow biomechanists to meet and discuss specific topical areas. For more information about these organizations, you can visit their respective websites. The **American Society of Biomechanics (ASB)** was founded in 1977 and has nearly 1,000 members today. The purpose of ASB is to provide a forum for the exchange of information and ideas among researchers. The society is affiliated with the *Journal of Biomechanics*. Meetings are held on an annual basis throughout the United States. (See American Society of Biomechanics, n.d.).

The Canadian Society of Biomechanics (CSB) was founded in 1973. Its purpose is similar to the ASB's; however, the CSB has successfully expanded internationally, as evidenced by the large participation of international scientists. The meetings are held biannually (CSB, n.d.). CSB and ASB put on a joint conference titled the North American Congress on Biomechanics.

The European Society of Biomechanics (ESB) was founded in 1976 at a meeting in Brussels. The goal of the ESB is to encourage research, disseminate knowledge, and promote progress in Biomechanics. It is now the largest Biomechanics society in Europe with over 1,500 members. The ESB congress is held annually (ESB, n.d.).

The International Society of Biomechanics (ISB) was founded in 1973 and has about 1,000 members today. The purpose of the ISB is to promote the study of all areas of biomechanics at the international level, although special emphasis is given to the biomechanics of human movement. The ISB meetings are held on a biannual basis (ISB, n.d.).

The International Society of Biomechanics in Sports (ISBS) was set up to provide a forum for the exchange of ideas between sport biomechanics researchers, coaches, and teachers; to bridge the gap between researchers and practitioners; and to gather and disseminate information and materials on biomechanics in sports. The first meeting took place in 1982, and a constitution was developed by 1983. Meetings are held on an annual basis (ISBS, n.d.).

JOURNALS

Because of the breadth of scientific inquiry in the field of biomechanics, several journals publish articles related to the field.

Primary Journals

Clinical Biomechanics
Journal of Applied Biomechanics
Journal of Biomechanics
Sports Biomechanics

Related Publications in Engineering and Modeling

Biomechanics and Modeling in Mechanobiology
Computer Methods in Biomechanics and Biomedical Engineering
Journal of Biomechanical Engineering

Muscle and Bone

BMC Musculoskeletal Disorders
Foot and Ankle International
Footwear Science
Journal of Bone and Joint Surgery
Journal of Electromyography and Kinesiology
Journal of Orthopaedic Research
Journal of the American Podiatric Medical Association

Movement Science and Rehabilitation

Ergonomics
Gait & Posture

Human Factors
Human Movement Science
Journal of Human Movement Studies
Journal of Orthopaedic and Sports Physical Therapy
Physical Therapy & Rehabilitation Journal

Sports Medicine

American Journal of Sports Medicine
British Journal of Sports Medicine
International Journal of Sports Medicine
Journal of Sports Medicine and Physical Fitness
Journal of Strength and Conditioning Research
Medicine & Science in Sports & Exercise
Research Quarterly for Exercise and Sport

The BIOMCH-L newsgroup is a discussion group for biomechanics and human and animal movement science. To subscribe, and for more information on the resources available on BIOMCH-L, visit their site (BIOMCH-L, n.d.).

Exhibit 7.13 Example of a typical abstract presented at The American Society of Biomechanics Scientific Conference

What can 400 miles of overground walking tell us about the individuality of gait?
Tyler M. Wiles[1], Seung Kyeom Kim[1], Nick Stergiou[1,2], Aaron D. Likens[1]
[1]Department of Biomechanics, University of Nebraska at Omaha
[2]Department of Physical Education & Sports Science, Aristotle University, Thessaloniki

Introduction: Picture yourself in a crowded concert venue. You spot someone you think you recognize. At a distance, their facial features are obscured by the darkness and flashing stage lights, but the way they walk gives you a clue. You walk closer. Finally, you recognize what was once only the outline of your roommate who joined you for the concert. What makes it possible for you to recognize your friend from only a distant, shadowy figure? In this paper, we investigate what has been termed a *gaitprint*, a set of gait features observable when walking that uniquely identify someone, similar in fashion to a fingerprint [1]. In previous work, we showed that a curated set of biomechanically meaningful gait features could reliably identify a person with >98% accuracy [1]. Presently, we expand that work by asking: Can people be identified from a few seconds of walking using just a handful of gait features?

Methods: 25 (12 female, 24.5 ± 2.1 years old, 174.4 ± 7.2 cm tall, weighing 72.9 ± 15.7 kg), 31 middle (24 female, 46.5 ± 6.0 years old, 171.4 ± 8.2 cm tall, weighing 82.1 ± 15.1 kg), and 35 older adults (16 female, 64.3 ± 5.9 years old, 172.3 ± 9.1 cm tall, weighing 81.4 ± 15.6 kg) were sampled from the NONAN GaitPrint datasets. Participants completed 18, four-minute overground walking bouts, evenly split into two days. Only participants that returned one week following their first session were used. Lower body kinematic data was collected using inertial measurement units recording at 200Hz from approximately 400 miles (n = 1,638 trials) walked at a preferred pace. Next, we calculated the 14 most important gait features for the entire four-minute duration, as well as for the final two minutes, one minute, 30 seconds, 15 seconds, and five seconds of data. Then, a random forest, support vector machine, multilayer perceptron, and ADA Boost algorithm were initiated across a range of parameters while trained on a random 70% of the data (70/30), trials from day one (Day 1), or the first trial (Trial 1).

Results and Discussion: We iterated through 1,296 support vector machines with differing parameters and achieved our best accuracy of 99.39% in identifying participants. This accuracy was achieved twice when training our models on 70% of the data from one minute of walking—once with 13 features and once with 14 features. Surprisingly, identification accuracy did not consistently decrease with walking duration. Four minutes of walking was not always the most accurate, nor was five seconds always the least accurate. The range of maximum accuracies only spanned by 3.25% (70/30), 10.99% (Day 1), and 15.71% (Trial 1). This inconsistent trend suggests a small degree of stochasticity in either our data or models. We observed two expected trends: accuracy decreased as training size decreased (70/30 > Day 1 > Trial 1) and increased with the number of features. Notably, we achieved 87.19% accuracy using only the five most important features (four-minutes). Remarkably, just seven features measured over five seconds were enough to achieve 80.28% accuracy, suggesting that unique gait characteristics emerge within roughly five strides using only a handful of features.

Significance: We supplement previous research by demonstrating the uniqueness of human walking, a person's gaitprint. Our results also demonstrate that even brief walking durations and a limited set of gait features are sufficient to capture the unique signatures of an individual's movement. Furthermore, because unique movement can be characterized within only a few strides, the identification of clinical groups with mobility deficits becomes more feasible.

Acknowledgements: NSF 212491, NIH P20GM109090, P20GM152301, University of Nebraska Collaboration Initiative, the Center for Research in Human Movement Variability at the University of Nebraska at Omaha, NASA EPSCoR, IARPA.

FUTURE DIRECTIONS

In the future, biomechanics will be applied across many professional domains to understand fundamental movement in sports, exercise, medicine, robotics, biology, gaming, and occupational science. Applications of biomechanical analysis, utilizing various measurements and tools, will examine human movement from infants to the elderly and from healthy to pathological populations. In recent years, new and innovative analyses in biomechanics—for example, nonlinear analysis for human movement variability (Stergiou,

2004, 2016)—have been developed to study human performance. By using advanced mathematical algorithms, biomechanists can understand human movement variability in a novel fashion. Such approaches will expand the current understanding of human movement in many biomechanical applications, especially in clinical areas. Furthermore, human movement will be studied to a greater extent using virtual and augmented reality. The use of such technologies takes biomechanical research beyond the laboratory settings to simulate actual environments from which natural human movement responses can be detected. Examples are the VENLab at Brown University (Brown University, n.d.), the Medical Virtual Reality Center at the University of Pittsburgh (University of Pittsburgh, n.d.), and the laboratories of the Biomechanics Research Building at the University of Nebraska at Omaha (Exhibit 7.14) (University of Nebraska Omaha, n.d.).

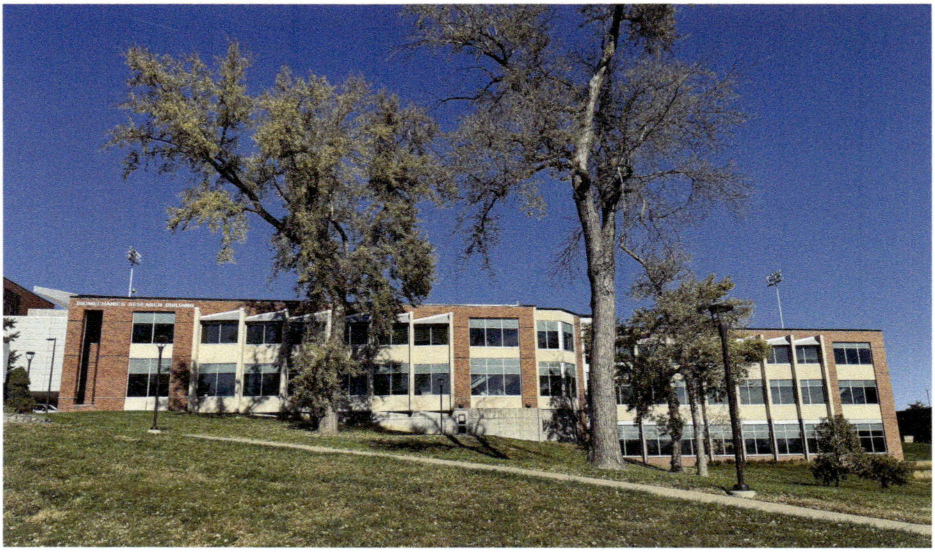

Exhibit 7.14 The Biomechanics Research Building, University of Nebraska at Omaha

In sports and exercise research, an increasing emphasis is being placed on obtaining accurate measures to determine the outcomes of various training protocols. Computer modeling, simulation, and machine learning can be used to evaluate a training protocol that is designed to enhance athletic performance. Such advanced biomechanical methodologies can optimize performance and further improve the design of training programs. In the future, successful training in sports and exercise will rely on both computer technology and various biomechanical measurements of movement.

In clinical settings, biomechanical approaches and methods will commonly be used by physicians, physical therapists, and other specialists. The goals will be to examine pathological human movement and develop more effective treatments for patients to regain their quality of life by using motion analysis and gait evaluations that can be conducted away from the laboratory with inexpensive wireless technology. This technology will also be incorporated into standard clinical examinations in hospitals to increase the precision of the clinical diagnoses.

In occupational science, biomechanically designed environments will be the norm. Currently, the focus is on the engineering of the workplace; however, it is slowly being realized that the interface between the human and the machine is equally important. Thus, biomechanists are needed to work with engineers to design more biologically sound workplace layouts that are safe and will improve productivity.

As the scientific and clinical professions using biomechanical analysis of human movement expand further, the development of new training protocols for athletes and an exploration of new treatments and rehabilitation procedures for patients will follow. Advanced biomechanical technology, such as exoskeletons or exosuits or 3D printed prosthetics, will become essential in the future.

SUMMARY

Biomechanics is a discipline that utilizes a wide variety of instruments, techniques, and technologies to study movement. Biomechanists work in several areas including developmental biomechanics, biomechanics of exercise and sport, rehabilitative biomechanics, occupational biomechanics, and forensic biomechanics. Because of this diversity, a broad range of knowledge is required and many students of biomechanics pursue advanced expertise in master's and doctoral programs. As a result of the variety of applications related to biomechanics, employment opportunities are extremely varied. These opportunities include positions in academia as well as industry and government.

STUDY QUESTIONS

1. Explain the focus of developmental biomechanics.
2. The safety and mechanical efficiency of tools would most likely be evaluated by which type of biomechanist?
3. List and describe some optical recording devices.
4. Define biomechanics.
5. Is biomechanics a discipline? Explain.
6. Why do we need to study movement using an interdisciplinary approach?
7. What is the difference between biomechanics and kinesiology?
8. Define kinetics, kinematics, dynamics, and statics.
9. Identify the major areas of research in biomechanics.
10. Give five examples of biomechanical applications.
11. What is a force platform?
12. List the three sensors of an inertial measurement unit.
13. Name five journals where biomechanists publish their research.
14. Name two new and emerging areas of study in biomechanics.
15. Where can you find biomechanics programs in North America?

LEARNING ACTIVITIES

1. Go to either the International Society of Biomechanics in Sport website (ISBS, n.d.) or the Canadian Society of Biomechanics website (CBS, n.d.). Write a brief description of the website's contents.
2. Find two different professional journals that publish articles related to biomechanics. Retrieve one article from each. In your own words, write an abstract for each article.
3. Explore (using the Internet and/or written sources) the job market for biomechanics and write a brief report on one potential career opportunity.

4. The "Health" app on your phone likely records kinematic information about your gait such as walking speed and step length. Compare your gait kinematics to a friend that is taller or shorter than you.

SUGGESTED READING AND RELATED WEBSITES

American Society of Biomechanics. (n.d.). American Society of Biomechanics Website. Available at: https://asbweb.org/programs-and-labs/

BIOMCH-L. (n.d.) BIOMCH-L Forums. Available at: https://biomch-l.isbweb.org/

Brown University. (n.d.). VENLab: Virtual Environment Navigation Laboratory. Available at: https://sites.brown.edu/venlab/

Canadian Society of Biomechanics. (n.d.). Canadian Society of Biomechanics Website. Available at: www.csb-scb.com

European Society of Biomechanics (ESB). European Society of Biomechanics Website. Available at: www.esbiomech.org

Hall, S. J. (2022). *Basic Biomechanics*. Ninth edition. New York: McGraw Hill LLC.

International Society of Biomechanics (ISB). (n.d.). International Society of Biomechanics Website. Available at: www.isbweb.org/

McNeill Alexander, R. (1992). *The Human Machine*. New York: Columbia University Press.

McGinnis, P. M. (2020). *Biomechanics of Sport and Exercise*. Fourth edition. Champaign, IL: Human Kinetics.

Nordin, M., Frankel, V. H., Meere, P. A., Mullerpatan, R. P., Wilke, H.-J., and Leger, D., eds. (2022). *Basic Biomechanics of the Musculoskeletal System*. Fifth edition. Philadelphia, PA: Wolters Kluwer.

Stergiou, N. (2020). *Biomechanics and Gait Analysis*. San Diego, CA: Academic Press.

Stergiou, N., ed. (2016). *Nonlinear Analysis for Human Movement Variability*. Boca Raton, FL: Taylor & Francis.

Thomas, S. J., Zeni, J. A., and Winter, D. A. (2022). *Biomechanics and Motor Control of Human Movement*. Fifth edition. Hoboken, NJ: Wiley.

University of Pittsburgh. (n.d.). Medical Virtual Reality Center. Available at: www.mvrc.pitt.edu/index.html

University of Nebraska Omaha. (n.d.). Biomechanics Core Facility. Available at: http://biomech.unomaha.edu

REFERENCES

American Society of Biomechanics. (n.d.). American Society of Biomechanics Website. Available at: https://asbweb.org/programs-and-labs/

Asakawa, D. S., Becker, M. G., Asaro, J. M., and Hein, J. L. (2019). Shoulder, elbow, and wrist joint angle excursions vary by gesture during touchscreen interaction. *Journal of Electromyography and Kinesiology, November*, 102377–102377. https://doi.org/10.1016/j.jelekin.2019.102377

Atwater, A. E. (1980). Kinesiology/Biomechanics: perspectives and trends. *Research Quarterly for Exercise and Sport*, *51*(1), 193–218. https://doi.org/10.1080/02701367.1980.10609283

Bapat, G. M., Bashir, A. Z., Malcolm, P., Johanning, J. M., Pipinos, I. I., and Myers, S. A. (2023). A biomechanical perspective on walking in patients with peripheral artery disease. *Vascular Medicine*, *28*(1), 77–84. https://doi.org/10.1177/1358863X221146207

Bartlett, R. (2007). *Introduction to Sports Biomechanics: Analysing Human Movement Patterns* (2nd ed). London: Routledge.

Bates, B. T. (1991). The need for an interdisciplinary curriculum. In *Third National Symposium on Teaching Kinesiology and Biomechanics in Sports Proceedings* (pp. 163–166). Ames, IA: Iowa State University Press.

Bernstein, N. A. (1967). *The Coordination and Regulation of Movements*. Oxford: Pergamon Press.

BIOMCH-L. (n.d.) BIOMCH-L Forums. Available at: https://biomch-l.isbweb.org/

Brown University. (n.d.). VENLab: Virtual Environment Navigation Laboratory. Available at: https://sites.brown.edu/venlab/

Canadian Society of Biomechanics. (n.d.). Canadian Society of Biomechanics Website. Available at: www.csb-scb.com

Charles, J. M. (1994). *Contemporary Kinesiology: An Introduction to the Study of Human Movement in Higher Education*. London: Morton Pub. Co.

Choi, J., Knarr, B. A., Youn, J.-H., and Song, K. Y. (2024). Machine learning-based approach to identifying fall risk in seafarers using wearable sensors. *Journal of Marine Science and Engineering*, *12*(2), 356. https://doi.org/10.3390/jmse12020356

Dillman, C. J., and Sears, R. G. (Eds.). (1977). Kinesiology: a national conference on teaching. In *Kinesiology: A National Conference on Teaching*. Urbana-Champaign, IL: University of Illinois.

Dodakian, L., McKenzie, A. L., Le, V., See, J., Pearson-Fuhrhop, K., Burke Quinlan, E., Zhou, R. J., Augsberger, R., Tran, X. A., Friedman, N., Reinkensmeyer, D. J., and Cramer, S. C. (2017). A home-based telerehabilitation program for patients with stroke. *Neurorehabilitation and Neural Repair*, *31*(10–11), 923–933. https://doi.org/10.1177/1545968317733818

European Society of Biomechanics (ESB). European Society of Biomechanics Website. Available at: www.esbiomech.org

Fenn, W. O. (1931). A cinematographic study of sprinters. *The Scientific Monthly*, *32*(4), 346–354. JSTOR.

Gaesser, G. A., Poole, D. C., and Angadi, S. S. (2022). Quantifying the benefits of inefficient walking: Monty Python inspired laboratory based experimental study. *BMJ*, e072833. https://doi.org/10.1136/bmj-2022-072833

Harrison, E. C., and Earhart, G. M. (2023). The effect of auditory cues on gait variability in people with Parkinson's disease and older adults: a systematic review. *Neurodegenerative Disease Management*, nmt-2021–0050. https://doi.org/10.2217/nmt-2021-0050

Harrison, S. J., Hough, M., Schmid, K., Groff, B. R., and Stergiou, N. (2018). When coordinating finger tapping to a variable beat the variability scaling structure of the movement and the cortical BOLD signal are both entrained to the auditory stimuli. *Neuroscience*, *392*, 203–218. https://doi.org/10.1016/j.neuroscience.2018.06.025

Haworth, J., and Stergiou, N. (2018). Orderliness of visual stimulus motion mediates sensorimotor coordination. *Frontiers in Physiology*, *9*, 1441. https://doi.org/10.3389/fphys.2018.01441

Higgins, J. R. (1977). *Human Movement: An Integrated Approach*. Los Angeles, CA: Mosby.

Horak, F. B., Diener, H. C., and Nashner, L. M. (1989). Influence of central set on human postural responses. *Journal of Neurophysiology*, *62*(4), 841–853. https://doi.org/10.1152/jn.1989.62.4.841

Huisinga, J. M., Pipinos, I. I., Stergiou, N., and Johanning, J. M. (2010). Treatment with pharmacological agents in peripheral arterial disease patients does not result in biomechanical gait changes. *Journal of Applied Biomechanics*, *26*(3), 341–348. https://doi.org/10.1123/jab.26.3.341

Ide, T., Hamer, T. J., Rosen, A. B., Vogel, C., Haan, D., Knarr, B. A., and Wilkins, S. J. (2024). Limited total arc range of motion increases sheer stress in the shoulder while pitching in collegiate baseball pitchers. *Journal of Athletic Training*. https://doi.org/10.4085/1062-6050-0565.23

International Society of Biomechanics (ISB). (n.d.). International Society of Biomechanics Website. Available at: www.isbweb.org/

International Society of Biomechanics in Sports (ISBS). (n.d.) International Society of Biomechanics in Sports (ISBS) Website. Available at: www.isbs.org/

Knudson, D. V. (2007). *Fundamentals of Biomechanics* (2nd ed). Springer.

Liu, C., Downey, R. J., Salminen, J. S., Arvelo Rojas, S., Richer, N., Pliner, E. M., Hwang, J., Cruz-Almeida, Y., Manini, T. M., Hass, C. J., Seidler, R. D., Clark, D. J., and Ferris, D. P. (2024). Electrical brain activity during human walking with parametric variations in terrain unevenness and walking speed. *Imaging Neuroscience*, *2*, 1–33. https://doi.org/10.1162/imag_a_00097

Myers, S. A., Huben, N. B., Yentes, J. M., McCamley, J. D., Lyden, E. R., Pipinos, I. I., and Johanning, J. M. (2015). Spatiotemporal changes posttreatment in peripheral arterial disease. *Rehabilitation Research and Practice*, *2015*, 1–10. https://doi.org/10.1155/2015/124023

Nelson, R. C. (1980). Biomechanics: past and present. In J. M. Cooper and B. Haven (Eds.), *Proceedings of the Biomechanical Symposium* (pp. 4–13). Indiana State Board of Health.

Nigg, B. M., and Herzog, W. (Eds.). (2007). *Biomechanics of the Musculo-skeletal System* (3rd ed). John Wiley & Sons.

Odanye, O., Steffensen, E., Hinton, E., Bierner, S., Hsiao, H.-Y., and Knarr, B. (2023). Treadmill handrail-use increases the anteroposterior margin of stability in individuals' post-stroke. *Journal of Motor Behavior*, 1–10. https://doi.org/10.1080/00222895.2023.2285383

Parker, S. M., Andreasen, S. C., Ricks, B., Kaipust, M. S., Zuniga, J., and Knarr, B. A. (2022). Comparison of brain activation and functional outcomes between physical and virtual reality box and block test: a case study. *Disability and Rehabilitation: Assistive Technology*, *19*(2), 273–280. https://doi.org/10.1080/17483107.2022.2085334

Robertson, D. G. E., Caldwell, G. E., Hamill, J., Kamen, G., and Whittlesey, S. N. (2014). *Research Methods in Biomechanics* (2nd ed.). Champaign, IL: Human Kinetics.

Siu, K.-C., Suh, I. H., Mukherjee, M., Oleynikov, D., and Stergiou, N. (2010). The impact of environmental noise on robot-assisted laparoscopic surgical performance. *Surgery*, *147*(1), 107–113. https://doi.org/10.1016/j.surg.2009.08.010

Slade, P., Kochenderfer, M. J., Delp, S. L., and Collins, S. H. (2022). Personalizing exoskeleton assistance while walking in the real world. *Nature*, *610*(7931), 277–282. https://doi.org/10.1038/s41586-022-05191-1

Stergiou, N. (Ed.). (2004). *Innovative Analyses of Human Movement*. Champaign, IL: Human Kinetics.

Stergiou, N. (Ed.). (2016). *Nonlinear Analysis for Human Movement Variability*. Boca Raton, FL: Taylor & Francis.

Stergiou, N. (2020). *Advice for the Novice Investigator: Examples Taken from Movement Sciences*. Boca Raton, FL: CRC Press.

Stergiou, N., Kent, J. A., and McGrath, D. (2016). Human movement variability and aging. *Kinesiology Review*, *5*(1), 15–22.

Suchomel, T. J., Nimphius, S., and Stone, M. H. (2016). The importance of muscular strength in athletic performance. *Sports Medicine*, *46*(10), 1419–1449. https://doi.org/10.1007/s40279-016-0486-0

Suh, I. H., Chien, J., Mukherjee, M., Park, S., Oleynikov, D., and Siu, K. (2010). The negative effect of distraction on performance of robot-assisted surgical skills in medical students and residents. *The International Journal of Medical Robotics and Computer Assisted Surgery*, *6*(4), 377–381. https://doi.org/10.1002/rcs.338

Suh, I. H., Mukherjee, M., Schrack, R., Park, S.-H., Chien, J.-H., Oleynikov, D., and Siu, K.-C. (2011). Electromyographic correlates of learning during robotic surgical training in virtual reality. *Studies in Health Technology and Informatics*, *163*, 630–634.

The Fourth International Seminar on Biomechanics. (1974). *The Fourth International Seminar on Biomechanics*, *45*, 69–70.

Uchida, T. K., Delp, S., and Delp, D. B. (2021). *Biomechanics of Movement: The Science of Sports, Robotics, and Rehabilitation*. Cambridge, MA: MIT Press.

University of Nebraska Omaha. (n.d.). Biomechanics Core Facility. Available at: http://biomech.unomaha.edu

University of Pittsburgh. (n.d.). Medical Virtual Reality Center. Available at: www.mvrc.pitt.edu/index.html

Van Den Bogert, T., Gielo-Perczak, K., and Woltring, H. J. (1992). BIOMCH-L: An electronic mail discussion forum for biomechanics and movement science. *Journal of Biomechanics*, *25*(11), 1367. https://doi.org/10.1016/0021-9290(92)90293-A

Wiles, T. M., Mangalam, M., Sommerfeld, J. H., Kim, S. K., Brink, K. J., Charles, A. E., Grunkemeyer, A., Kalaitzi Manifrenti, M., Mastorakis, S., Stergiou, N., and Likens, A. D. (2023). NONAN GaitPrint: an IMU gait database of healthy young adults. *Scientific Data*, *10*(1), 867. https://doi.org/10.1038/s41597-023-02704-z

Wiles, T., Simmons, M., Gomez, D., Schubert, M. M., Newcomer, S. C., and Nessler, J. A. (2022). Foamed neoprene versus thermoplastic elastomer as a wetsuit material: a comparison of skin temperature, biomechanical, and physiological variables. *Sports Engineering*, *25*(1), 6. https://doi.org/10.1007/s12283-022-00370-9

Wilkerson, J. D. (1997). Biomechanics. In J. D. Massengale and National Association for Physical Education in Higher Education (Eds.), *The History of Exercise and Sport Science* (pp. 321–366). Champaign, IL: Human Kinetics.

Wilson, T. J., and Likens, A. D. (2023). Running gait produces long range correlations: a systematic review. *Gait & Posture*, *102*, 171–179. https://doi.org/10.1016/j.gaitpost.2023.04.001

Winter, D. A. (2009). *Biomechanics and Motor Control of Human Movement* (4th ed). Wiley.

Wurdeman, S. R., Huisinga, J. M., Filipi, M., and Stergiou, N. (2011). Multiple sclerosis affects the frequency content in the vertical ground reaction forces during walking. *Clinical Biomechanics*, *26*(2), 207–212. https://doi.org/10.1016/j.clinbiomech.2010.09.021

Wurdeman, S. R., Huisinga, J. M., Filipi, M., and Stergiou, N. (2013). Multiple sclerosis alters the mechanical work performed on the body's center of mass during gait. *Journal of Applied Biomechanics*, *29*(4), 435–442. https://doi.org/10.1123/jab.29.4.435

8 Motor Behavior

David I. Anderson and Anthony M. Mayo

LEARNING OBJECTIVES

After studying this chapter, the student will be able to:

- discuss the importance of studying motor behavior
- distinguish between motor control, motor learning, and motor development
- identify some of the important issues researchers study in motor behavior
- describe what tools researchers use to study these issues
- discuss how motor behavior relates to other sub-disciplines within kinesiology/exercise science
- describe how practitioners can use their knowledge of motor behavior to improve health and performance

INTRODUCTION

Have you ever wondered how you coordinate your incredibly complicated body to perform seemingly simple tasks like sitting, standing, walking, and pointing? Have you ever considered how a hapless newborn transforms into a willing toddler, an adventurous child, a rebellious adolescent, and a skilled adult capable of controlling the wide diversity of actions needed to work, play, and make it through the day? Have you ever marveled at how a professional athlete, a circus performer, an experienced surgeon, or an accomplished musician makes a seemingly impossible feat seem easy? If so, you will enjoy learning more about the field of motor behavior, which studies these intriguing issues and many more.

Kinesiology is traditionally defined as the study of physical activity. However, kinesiology really focuses on the study of *skillful* physical activity. Can you think of anything of importance to humans that does not require the capacity to control actions with some degree of skill? Humans enter the world with a capacity to move but must learn to move skillfully to survive and flourish. Skill is thus a biological, social, and cultural necessity; without a minimum level of it, we would perish. We need it to escape from predators, to secure food, to find or build shelter, and to procreate. Life becomes unimaginable without a minimum level of skillfulness, as anyone who has lost the capacity to control their movements through accident, injury, or disease will quickly tell you.

The study of motor behavior is vitally important because skilled activity is fundamental to human life. It is the food of life. How humans become skillful represents the essence of becoming human. It is the core of what we study in motor behavior and so the study of motor behavior makes a vital contribution to our understanding of the human experience.

DOI: 10.4324/9781032697185-8

HISTORICAL PERSPECTIVES

Three sub-disciplines comprise the discipline of **motor behavior**: motor control, motor learning, and motor development, and each will be formally defined later in this chapter. Researchers generally study these areas from either a behavioral or a neurophysiological perspective, though some take both perspectives. Consequently, the history of motor behavior intertwines with the histories of biology, medicine, and psychology.

Role of Skill in Human Evolution and Ancient Cultures

Skillful physical activity has played a significant role in human evolution and has sculpted not only our physical capacities but also our mental capacities. The Nobel Laureate English neuroscientist Charles Sherrington (1857–1952) argued that humans developed a brain and mind far superior to those of other species because of our evolutionary ancestors' needs to acquire control over increasingly sophisticated patterns of muscular coordination to survive the environments they lived in. Skill played a significant role in the lives of early humans and those who lived in ancient times. Early humans observed other animals closely and mimicked their movements in their dances (Sörgel, 2015). They relied heavily on the learning and teaching of skills like hunting, fishing, and gathering. The Egyptians engaged enthusiastically in dance, acrobatics, swimming, wrestling, ball games, and bullfighting. The Chinese developed kung fu and the feudal Japanese developed jujitsu for combat and self-defense and they used martial arts to promote physical fitness, self-discipline, and mastery of the body.

Yoga, which involves mastery of thinking, breathing, and physical postures, emerged as a spiritual and philosophical practice in India. The Greeks integrated dance into military training to improve unity of mind and body, muscle strength, and discipline, and the Romans used various physical activities for military training. The Roman physician of Greek origin, Galen (c. 129–216 AD), who served as the emperors' physician, stressed the importance of physical skill and fitness.

Evolution of the Scientific Knowledge Bases in Motor Behavior

Historians credit Galen as the first person to distinguish between motor and sensory nerves and agonist and antagonist muscles (Inglis, 1965). He also advanced one of the first models of muscle contraction, wherein the flow of a vital force or fluid referred to as "animal spirits" down the nerves caused the muscles to inflate. This model continued to influence thinking for centuries and well into the Renaissance period, as evidenced by a model proposed by René Descartes (1596–1650), in which a sensory signal caused the heart and arteries to release animal spirits into the muscles. Descartes's model persisted into the latter part of the Enlightenment period (the late 1700s), until scientists discovered bioelectricity after witnessing the ability of some animals, like eels, to produce electric shocks.

The Neuromuscular Control of Movement

Jan Swammerdam (1637–1680), a Dutch biologist and anatomist, conducted some of the earliest experiments dispelling the notion that animal spirits caused human movement. He performed detailed dissections of muscles and nerves, mapping out their structure and connections, and observed that muscles contained fibers that could contract and relax. The work of Luigi Galvani (1737–1798) finally put the animal spirits theory to rest. He observed that an electric current applied to a frog's muscle caused it to contract, and then, working with his cousin Giovanni Aldini (1762–1834), showed that touching a frog's muscle with a nerve from another frog could also cause the muscle to contract (Sabbatini, 1998).

Following adoption of the bioelectric model of muscle contraction, scientists made a number of breakthroughs in their understanding of how the brain and nervous system-controlled movement. Scientists had accepted the notion of *cerebral localization* of function well before neurosurgical techniques confirmed it, after noting relations between unusual talents and unique facial and cranial features. Marie-Jean-Pierre Flourens (1794–1867) introduced a neurosurgical technique to study localization when he uncovered the brains of pigeons, removed a specific part of the brain, and recorded the effects on the pigeon's behavior (Wozniak, 1992).

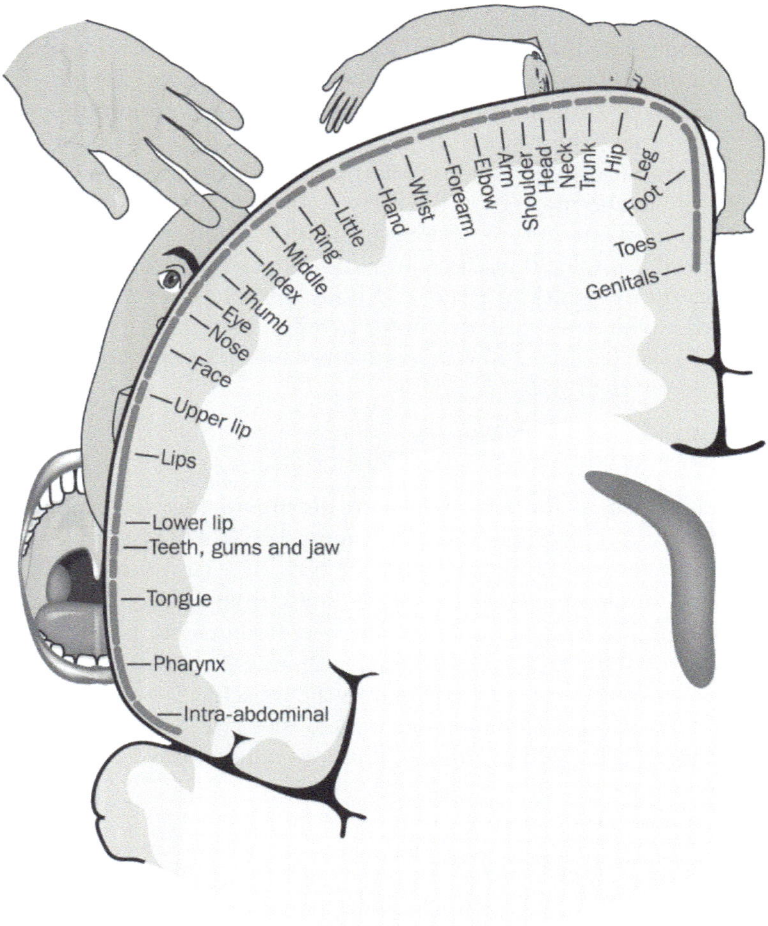

Exhibit 8.1 A drawing of Penfield's homunculus showing body parts mapped to areas of the cerebral cortex

Scientists later studied cerebral localization by electrically stimulating areas of the cortex and observing an animal's behavior. This ultimately led to a series of classic experiments by Wilder Penfield (1891–1976) and his colleagues showing that the motor cortex and the somatosensory cortex represent movements and sensory information from different body parts in a *somatotopic* configuration (see Exhibit 8.1). In other words, specific points on the body correspond to specific points on the cortex (Penfield and Rasmussen, 1950). This model persisted for many decades until Evan Gordon and colleagues (Gordon et al., 2023) recently updated it with their integrate-isolate model of motor control, which suggests that the motor cortex plays a much greater role in postural regulation, gross motor control of axial muscles, and movement coordination than previously thought.

Several other notable scientific contributions and scientists during the 18th and 19th centuries warrant mention. These include the discovery of the *reflex arc* by the English physician and physiologist Marshall Hall (1790–1857), the discovery of how action potentials travel along the axons of nerves by the French anatomist and physiologist Louis Ranvier (1835–1922), and the discovery of how brain disorders influence movement control by the English neurologist John Hughlings Jackson (1835–1911).

The rate of knowledge acquisition related to the role of the neuromuscular system in motor behavior expanded exponentially during the 20th century. Santiago Ramon y Cajal (1852–1934) deepened our understanding of the structure of the nervous system, as did Charles Sherrington, who also introduced the concept of *reciprocal inhibition*, whereby the nervous system inhibits the activity of antagonist muscles as it stimulates agonist muscles to contract. Willem Einthoven (1860–1927) pioneered the use of electromyography to study muscle activity and others refined the techniques for recording and analyzing muscle electrical activity, ultimately leading to their widespread adoption in research and clinical practice.

Behavioral Research in Motor Behavior

At the behavioral level of analysis, a number of "baby biographers," including Friedrich Tiedemann (1781–1861), William Preyer (1841–1897), and Milicent Shinn (1858–1940) pioneered the methodology used to document changes in children's behavior as they developed (Clark and Whitall, 1989). Scientists also made notable contributions to our understanding of the processes that underlie changes in behavior. Charles Darwin's (1809–1882) insights into how the environment and adaptation to the environment shape behavior, as well as his insights into continuities within and across species, continues to shape theorizing about the developmental process. Francis Galton (1822–1911) introduced the study of twins as a way to unravel the contribution of heredity and the environment to development. In the area of motor control and learning, Franciscus Donders (1818–1889) developed a method to study the speed of mental processes, and Wilhelm Wundt (1832–1920) and William James (1842–1910) provided insight into the psychological processes that underlie behavior. Robert Woodworth (1869–1962) spurred our understanding of how we use vision to control movement and how we regulate the speed and accuracy of our movements, and Bryan and Harter (1897, 1899) conducted classic experiments on the acquisition of telegraphy skills that drew attention to plateaus during motor learning.

Eric von Holst (1908–1962) conducted many studies on movement coordination in animals and humans and he introduced the *reafference principle*, which proposes that animals compare self-generated (reafferent) sensory information with externally generated (exafferent) sensory information to distinguish their own movements from movements imposed on them. Nicolai Bernstein (1897–1966) highlighted that a good theory of motor control needed to explain how the motor system solves the *degrees of freedom problem* and deals with *context-conditioned variability*. In other words, how does the motor system manage to assemble its multitude of moveable components into a manageable organization, and how does it deal with the enormous variation in the environment and the body from one movement to the next? He also introduced the concept of *muscle synergies*, wherein the muscles work together as functional groups.

John Watson (1878–1958) introduced the principles of *behaviorism*, which focuses on the analysis of observable behavior, and which used Ivan Pavlov's (1849–1936) concepts of conditioned and unconditioned reflexes to argue that learning occurred by associating stimuli with responses. Edward Thorndike introduced a way to conceptualize transfer of learning, and his *law of effect* (Thorndike, 1927) inspired a large volume of work on the role of augmented feedback in motor learning, which continues today. Clark Hull drew on Watson's and Thorndike's ideas to propose *drive theory* (Hull, 1943), which inspired considerable research in motor learning.

Notable scientists working in the motor development area in the first half of the 20th century included Arnold Gesell, Myrtle McGraw, Mary Shirley, Henry Halverson, and Nancy Bayley. Whereas behaviorism focused heavily on the role the environment played in shaping behavior, Gesell (1928) and McGraw (1935) explored how biological maturation influenced changes in motor behavior. They did so by carefully mapping detailed descriptions of changes in infants' behavior to presumed underlying changes in the nervous system. Shirley (1933) chronicled the mental and motor development of 25 babies over a 2-year period, Halverson (1931) published an important study on the development of reaching and grasping, and Bayley (1936) developed a normative scale of motor development, still in use today, based on her observations of children's behavior over the first three years of life.

World War II had a major influence on the research conducted in motor behavior from the middle of the 20th century onward. Motor learning researchers during the first half of the century had focused on characterizing learning curves and studying the effects of augmented feedback and the distribution of practice on motor learning (Adams, 1987). They also had an interest in transfer of training, the retention of motor learning, and the influence of individual differences on learning and performance. Observational learning emerged as a topic of interest toward the latter part of the first half of the century (McCullagh, 1993). During and immediately following the war, research shifted heavily toward the study of individual differences. The military had a major interest in predicting flying ability, among other military skills, from perceptual, motor, and intellectual abilities, and Edmund Fleishman had a major influence on the research conducted in this area (e.g., Fleishman, 1972).

Emergence of the Contemporary Field of Motor Behavior

The 1960s represented a crucial period in the history of the field of motor behavior. The modern discipline emerged during this time which, ironically, coincided with a decline in experimental psychologists' interest in motor learning, and an increase in interest by physical educators. Prominent physical educators working on issues of motor learning and control during this period included Franklin Henry, Alfred Hubbard, and Arthur Slater-Hammel, while Jack Adams represents one of the major psychologists who made significant contributions during this time. Much of the work during the 1960s and 1970s focused on motor control, thanks to the newly dominant *information processing* approach in experimental psychology, which researchers like Kenneth Craik (1947/1948) had introduced a couple of decades earlier as a counter to behaviorism. Prominent physical educators leading up to and during the 1960s in the motor development area included Anna Espenschade, Helen Eckert, Ruth Glassow, and G. Lawrence Rarick. Their descriptive work kept the field of motor development alive and set the stage for a surge of experimental work and theorizing in the decades that followed.

Although the information processing framework dominated much of the research in motor behavior from the 1960s through the 1980s, led by Jack Adams' students Richard Schmidt, George Stelmach, and Ronald Marteniuk, the theorizing of the American psychologist James Gibson and the Russian neurophysiologist Nicolai Bernstein spurred the development of the *dynamical systems* perspective as a counter perspective in motor behavior. Gibson introduced an *ecological approach* to the study of perception and action (e.g., Gibson, 1966), whereas Bernstein, whose work did not receive attention in the West until the 1960s (Bernstein, 1967), highlighted the contribution of non-neural factors to coordination dynamics. Their ideas inspired Peter Kugler, Scott Kelso, and Michael Turvey to write two seminal chapters introducing the dynamical systems perspective to the broader motor behavior audience (Kugler, Kelso, and Turvey, 1980, 1982) which, in turn, inspired an enormous amount of research and theorizing for the next couple of decades. Esther Thelen and her colleagues spearheaded the research in motor development conducted from a dynamical systems perspective and Karen Adolph and her colleagues led a more specific research agenda inspired by Gibson's ecological approach to perception and action.

Since the start of the new millennium, research in motor behavior has expanded at a rapid pace. The information processing and dynamical systems perspectives continue to inspire researchers; however, models and frameworks developed within the neurosciences, coupled with a growing interest in public health issues, have had a much greater influence (Whitall et al., 2020a, 2020b). The global obesity epidemic, for example, has encouraged researchers to examine how the development of motor competence influences physical activity patterns, physical fitness, weight status, and longer-term health outcomes (e.g., Stodden et al., 2008). Researchers have also examined how motor development contributes to psychological development (e.g., Anderson et al., 2013). Technological innovations within the neurosciences have encouraged much more sophisticated explorations of how the brain controls movement and how the brain changes as we acquire new skills. At the same time, we have seen much greater application of the principles of motor control and learning to the rehabilitation of function following accidents, injuries, and disease, as well as to the prevention of the declines associated with aging. In many respects, motor behavior is entering a golden age because the knowledge bases, skillsets, and technologies that characterize the field have such relevance to so many of the big challenges that confront contemporary society.

FUNDAMENTAL CONCEPTS

As noted earlier, the term motor behavior is used to describe the work conducted in motor control, learning, and development. Magill and Anderson (2024) and Schmidt and colleagues (Schmidt et al., 2019) define **motor control** as a field focused on *the study of the neural, physical, and behavioral processes underlying the performance of a motor skill*. They define **motor learning** as *the study of the processes associated with practice or experience that lead to relatively permanent changes in the capacity to perform motor skills*. The practice or experience component of the definition distinguishes learning-related changes in behavior from changes that might result from processes like growth and maturation. The reference to relatively permanent changes highlights the need to differentiate learning from short-term changes in behavior that might result from temporary changes in motivation or some similar variable, and the reference to the capacity to perform skills highlights that we cannot observe learning directly but must infer it from changes in behavior.

Clark and Whitall (1989) define **motor development** as the study of *the changes in motor behavior over the lifespan and the process(es) which underlie these changes*. Development represents a broader process than learning because it encompasses changes associated with growth and maturation in addition to learning. We can also tie motor control to learning and development because many would argue that motor learning and development represent changes in motor control over the lifespan and the processes underlying these changes. Students of motor behavior need to recognize that considerable overlap exists in the issues examined in the field and the issues studied within a number of other sub-disciplines within kinesiology and exercise science, including biomechanics, sport and exercise psychology, and physical education and sport pedagogy.

The field of motor behavior is very broad thanks to its focus on control, learning, and development. In the next paragraphs, we highlight some of the key questions and findings in each area within motor behavior.

Motor Control

When someone touches their nose, what events occur in the neuromuscular system between the intention to touch the nose and the finger landing on the nose? What structures play a role in supporting these events and how does injury or disease influence these structures and their function? These represent some of the most basic questions motor control researchers ask, although we can layer a myriad of other questions on top of these. We have a very good understanding of the structures that participate in motor control, but our understanding of the processes that underlie the organization of these structures continues to develop.

Let us start with the most basic component of the nervous system, the nerve cell, or *neuron* (see Exhibit 8.2). The human nervous system contains tens of billions of neurons that we classify into three basic types. These include *sensory neurons* (also called afferent neurons), which send neural impulses to the central nervous system (CNS) from the periphery, *motor neurons* (also called efferent neurons), which send neural impulses to skeletal muscle fibers, and *interneurons*, which lie within the brain and spinal cord and connect motor and sensory neurons as well as other interneurons together. The *central nervous system*, which includes the brain and spinal cord, serves as the "command center" for human behavior. The brain areas most directly involved in motor control include the *cerebrum*, the *diencephalon*, the *cerebellum*, and the *brainstem*.

The Brain

The cerebrum has two halves, the left and the right *cerebral hemispheres*, and each hemisphere has four lobes: the *frontal lobe*, the *parietal lobe*, the *temporal lobe*, and the *occipital* lobe (see Exhibit 8.3). A thin layer of nerve cell bodies, called the gray matter, covers the surface of the cerebrum. The frontal lobe plays a key role in the planning, initiation, and execution of voluntary movement. Key structures within the frontal lobe include the *motor cortex*, which directly controls voluntary contractions of skeletal muscles, the

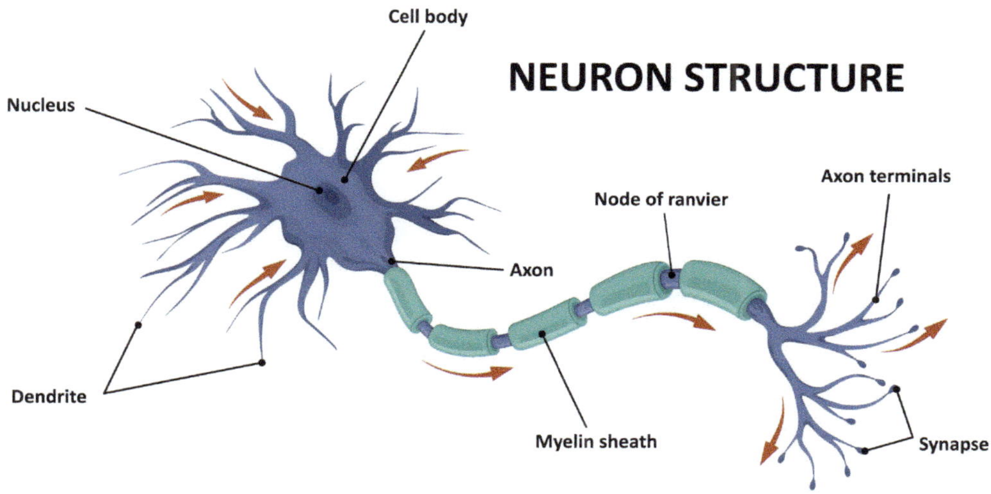

Exhibit 8.2 A diagram of the structure of a neuron

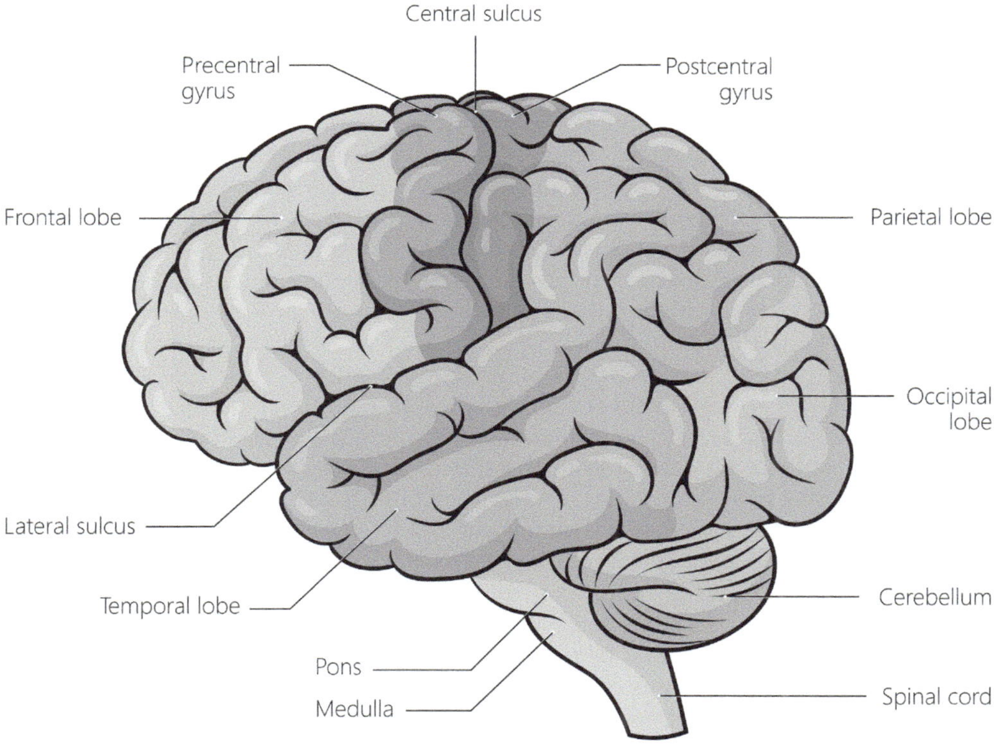

Exhibit 8.3 A drawing of the human brain

premotor area, which plays a role in the planning and preparation of movements, and the *supplementary motor area* (SMA), which also plays a role in the planning of movements, particularly those involving movement sequencing and bimanual coordination.

The parietal lobe integrates sensory information from various modalities like touch, proprioception, vision, and audition to create a spatial representation of the body and the surrounding environment. This spatial awareness makes a key contribution to accurate motor planning and execution. The *sensory cortex* (also known as the somatosensory cortex) represents an important area within the parietal lobe because it receives sensory input from the body and plays a role in sensorimotor integration. Because the sensory cortex sits just behind the motor cortex, they are often referred to together as the *sensorimotor cortex*. These two cortical areas run as a strip of cortical tissue across the middle of the brain, roughly from one ear to the other. As noted earlier in the historical section, the sensorimotor cortex represents movements and sensory information from different body parts in a somatotopic configuration (see Exhibit 8.1) (Gordon et al., 2023; Penfield and Rasmussen, 1950).

The temporal lobe plays a role in the coordination of complex movements and the integration of sensory information with motor planning. Specific areas within the lobe, like the superior temporal gyrus, contribute to the processing of auditory and visual information relevant to movement control. The occipital lobe contains the primary visual cortex, which processes visual information that enables humans to monitor the environment and guide their movements.

The *diencephalon* lies between the cerebrum and the brainstem and contains two important structures, the *thalamus* and the *hypothalamus*. The thalamus serves as a relay station, receiving and integrating most of the sensory inputs from the spinal cord and brain stem and steering them through to the cortex. The cerebellum sits behind the cerebral hemispheres and attaches to the brainstem. Like the cerebrum, it has two hemispheres and a cortex, under which lie the deep cerebellar nuclei: the *red nucleus* and the *oculomotor nucleus*. The cerebellum receives sensory input from the spinal cord, the brainstem, and the cerebral cortex and sends motor output to the spinal cord and the cortex via a neural highway known as the *cerebello-thalamo-cortico pathway*. Detecting and correcting errors represent two key functions of the cerebellum and so it makes a major contribution to the execution of smooth and accurate movements. It also plays an important role in motor learning.

Bridging the cerebral hemispheres and the spinal cord, the brainstem contains three areas significantly involved in motor control. The *pons*, at the top of the brainstem, plays a role in chewing, swallowing, salivating, and breathing, and may play a role in balance control. The *medulla*, an extension of the spinal cord, plays a vital role in regulating physiological processes like respiration and heartrate. It also represents the site where motor tracts from the cortex to the spinal cord and the sensory tracts from the spinal cord to the brain cross over and merge. The *reticular formation* represents the third area of the brainstem involved in motor control. It primarily functions as an integrator of sensory and motor neural impulses.

Lying deep within the cerebral hemispheres, the *basal ganglia* represent the final brain structures that play a significant role in motor control. They consist of four large nuclei: the *caudate nucleus*, the *putamen*, the *substantia nigra*, and the *globus pallidus*. They receive neural input from various cortical and subcortical regions and send it to multiple brain regions, including the thalamus, brainstem, and cerebral cortex. The basal ganglia play critical roles in the planning and initiation of movement, the coordination of agonist and antagonist muscles, and the control of force. Much of what we know about the basal ganglia comes from research involving people with Parkinson's disease and cerebral palsy (CP), both of which involve the basal ganglia. People with Parkinson's disease lose neurons in the substantia nigra that produce dopamine, an important regulator of various functions within the nervous system. An injury to the basal ganglia is the cause of motor problems in a specific type of CP.

The Spinal Cord and the Motor Unit

Researchers once viewed the spinal cord (see Exhibit 8.4) as a simple telephone cable that relays messages, but they recognize it now as a complex system that interacts with a variety of other systems and plays a critical role in motor control. The *gray matter* and the *white matter* represent the two major portions of the spinal cord. The butterfly-shaped gray matter occupies the central portion of the cord. It consists of cell bodies and axons that lie within the cord. Two pairs of "horns" protrude from the gray matter: the *dorsal horns* on the posterior side of the cord, which contain cells involved in transmitting sensory information, and the *ventral horns* on the anterior side, which contain the cell bodies of the alpha motor neurons that transmit signals from the CNS to the skeletal muscles. The gray matter also contains the cell bodies of interneurons, referred to as Renshaw cells. The white matter in the spinal cord (and in the brain) is composed of bundles of axons coated with a mixture of proteins and lipids known as myelin. The myelin speeds the conduction of nerve signals and helps to protect the axons.

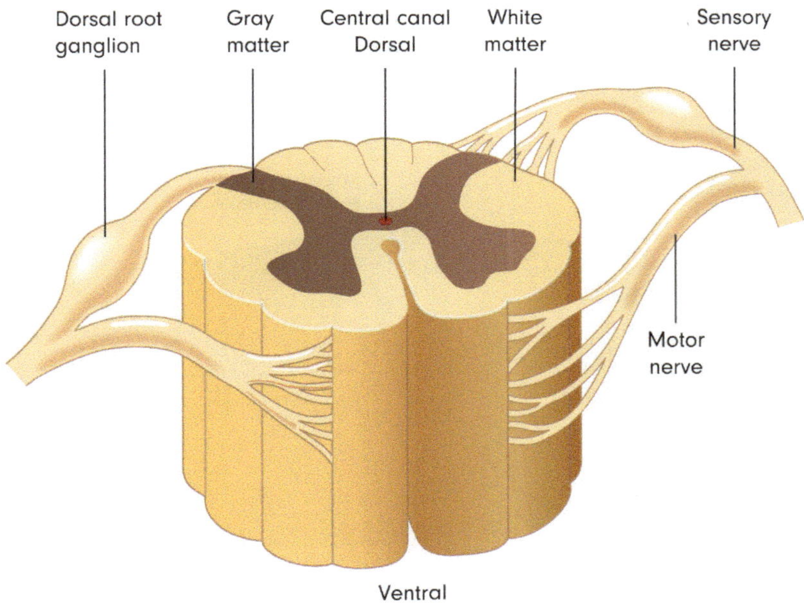

Exhibit 8.4 A diagram of a cross-section through the spinal cord

The spinal cord contains sensory neural pathways, called *ascending tracts*, which connect with various sensory areas within the cortex and cerebellum, and motor neural pathways, called *descending tracts*, which connect neurons in the cortex and brainstem with neurons whose axons terminate on skeletal muscles. The *dorsal column* and the *anterolateral system* represent two important ascending tracts that transmit sensory information relevant for motor control to the sensory cortex. The *spinocerebellar tracts* transmit sensory information to the cerebellum. The *pyramidal* and *extrapyramidal tracts* represent the two primary sets of descending tracts. The pyramidal tract (also known as the *corticospinal tract*) originates in various parts of the cerebral cortex, though primarily the motor cortex. Most of the fibers in the tract cross the midline at the medulla, such that each cerebral hemisphere controls muscles on the opposite side of the body. The pyramidal tract functions primarily in the control of fine motor skills. The extrapyramidal tracts originate in the brainstem and most of these fibers do not cross to the opposite side of the body. These tracts play a central role in the control of posture and in the facilitation and inhibition of muscles involved in finger and hand flexion and extension.

The *motor unit* (see Exhibit 8.5) represents the final target of the descending motor neural outflow. Comprised of an alpha motor neuron and the muscle fibers it innervates, the motor unit represents the smallest functional unit of motor control. The alpha motor neuron connects to the skeletal muscle fibers at the neuromuscular junction, a special type of synapse that allows the transmission of neural information from nerve cells to muscle cells.

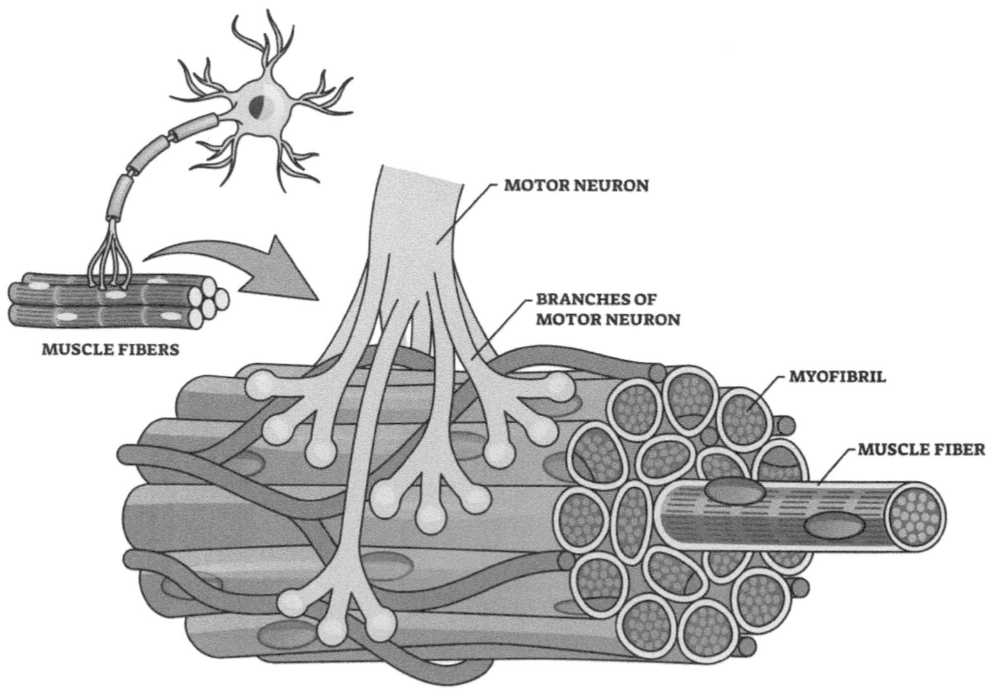

Exhibit 8.5 A drawing of a motor unit

Theories of Motor Control

As noted earlier, Bernstein (1967) highlighted that a good theory of motor control needed to explain the degrees of freedom problem and context conditioned variability. Theorists have generally addressed these issues by positing central control structures within the brain or by stressing how the field of external forces generated by the interaction between the body and the environment simplifies the nervous system's role in controlling movements. Control structure theorists have taken their lead from the open and closed loop control systems studied by mechanical engineers, computer scientists, and information processing theorists. *Open loop systems* (see Exhibit 8.6) send commands from an executive control structure to the device(s) it controls (the effectors). In human motor control, the effectors refer to muscles and the joints they move. *Closed loop systems* (see Exhibit 8.7) operate in the same way but they also compare feedback from the effectors with a reference mechanism, which allows modification of the commands to ensure the control system achieves its goal.

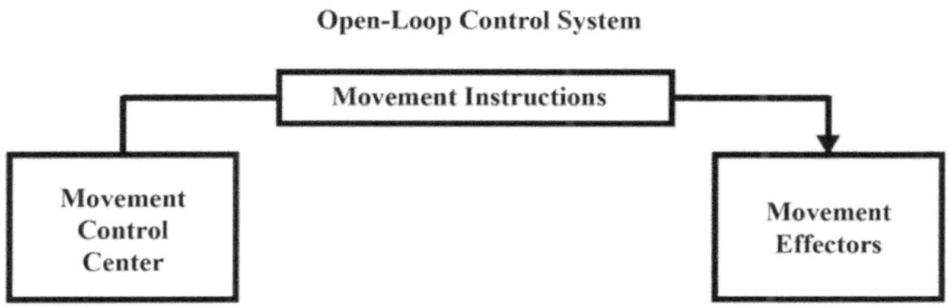

Exhibit 8.6 Open-loop control system

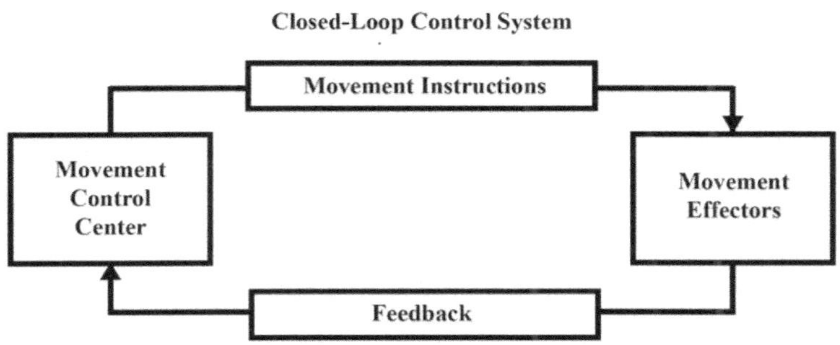

Exhibit 8.7 Closed-loop control system

The *motor program* represents the core structure in central control-oriented theories of motor control. Karl Lashley (1917) was the first person to use the term motor program, although the concept dates back to the Greek philosophers. Schmidt's *schema theory* represents the most influential motor program-based theory of motor control (Schmidt, 1975). Schema theory proposes that a generalized motor program, which can operate in an open or closed loop manner, controls the invariant features of a class of actions (e.g., throwing). The performer retrieves the program from memory and updates it with movement-specific parameters suitable to the current context via a recall schema. A recognition schema serves as a reference of correctness that allows comparison between actual sensory feedback and expected sensory feedback and updating of movement parameters if necessary. According to schema theory, motor learning occurs as we acquire new motor programs, as well as recall and recognition schemas, and we refine them through practice and experience.

Dynamical systems theory (DST) represents the most influential non-central-control-structure theory. It takes its inspiration from Bernstein's (1967) ideas about motor control, Gibson's (1966, 1979) ideas about ecological realism, and specific tenets from physics, physical biology, and thermodynamics. The theory argues that movement control emerges in response to a broad collection of constraints associated with the person, the task, and the environment (Newell, 1986). Non-specific CNS output harnesses the dynamical field of external forces to simplify the control processes by taking advantage of the self-organizing tendencies inherent to physical systems. DST stresses the tight and reciprocal coupling between perception and action, arguing that we perceive the environment in terms of opportunities for action, also known as *affordances* (Stoffregen, 2003). *Coordinative structures*—groups of muscles constrained to act as a functional unit—represent a key construct within the theory. They reduce the number of degrees of freedom the CNS has to organize and their "soft" and flexible assembly in response to contextual constraints heightens their responsiveness to contextual variability. The softly assembled coordinative structure serves as a counterpoint to the "hard wiring" we tend to associate with a motor program. DST views motor learning as increasing attunement to and exploitation of information specifying the constraints surrounding action.

Motor Learning

We noted earlier in the history section that motor learning researchers have studied a variety of topics ranging from the shape of learning curves to the appropriate way to schedule practice and provide augmented feedback to the way in which individual differences influence learning. Researchers have also devoted considerable attention to characterizing the stages that learners progress through as they acquire new skills. Although the interest in these topics has waxed and waned over the last 125 years and researchers have studied them unsystematically, they continue to receive attention. Schmidt's (1975) schema theory inspired considerable research on practice variability following its prediction that practicing multiple task variations rather than a single task variation strengthened the development of recall and recognition schemas. A landmark study by Shea and Morgan (1979) subsequently inspired numerous studies on the appropriate way to schedule the practice of multiple task variations. They showed that a blocked schedule, wherein the learner completes practice on one task variation before beginning practice on the next variation and so on, enhanced performance during practice but degraded learning as measured by retention and transfer tests, compared to a random switching between tasks during practice. Researchers referred to the paradoxical effects of task switching on performance and learning as the *contextual interference effect*.

Some years after Shea and Morgan's contextual interference study, Salmoni, Schmidt, and Walter (1984) published a review paper showing that the scheduling of knowledge of results, or KR (a type of augmented feedback), also had paradoxical effects on performance and learning. When researchers presented KR too frequently or in a way that made it too easy to use, learners became dependent on it. They performed well in practice but poorly on retention and transfer tests when the researchers removed KR. The explanation for the poor retention and transfer performance became known as the *guidance hypothesis*. The contextual interference effect and the guidance hypothesis reinforced the need for researchers to separate out a variable's temporary effects on performance from its more permanent effects on learning in any study of motor learning. The distinction between *performance* and *learning* represents a key construct in motor learning.

Three other important review papers and one experimental paper have had an outsized influence on the research conducted within motor learning over the last 40 years. Newell's (1986) "constraints" chapter dramatically increased the reach of the dynamical systems perspective by explaining how constraints associated with the task, the environment, and the performer influenced the organization of movement patterns (see Exhibit 8.8) and encouraged researchers to study the range of different ways in which manipulating constraints influenced performance and learning. Newell and colleagues also popularized Bernstein's description of the acquisition of a new coordination pattern as a process of *freezing and freeing degrees of freedom* (Vereijken et al., 1992).

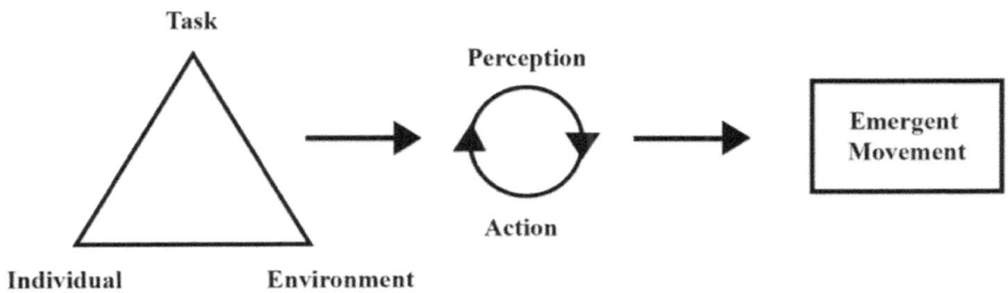

Exhibit 8.8 Newell's Constraints Model

Ericsson, Krampe, and Tesch-Romer (1993) published an influential paper that described the development of expertise in musicians. After collecting the practice histories of the musicians, who varied considerably in their level of expertise, they concluded that with sufficient amounts of the right kind of practice, what they referred to as *deliberate practice*, almost anyone could become an expert musician. Researchers have conducted numerous studies testing whether the deliberate practice notion applies to the development of expertise in sport. Reviews of this work suggest that it makes a significant contribution, but perhaps not as great of a contribution as Ericsson and colleagues had argued (Hambrick et al., 2020).

In the second influential review paper, Guadagnoli and Lee (2004) published their *challenge point framework*, bringing some needed organization to the literature on contextual interference and augmented feedback, which had produced some inconsistent and contradictory findings. They posited that the inconsistencies arose because researchers had not considered the variations that occurred because of the interaction between the learners' skill and the difficulty of the tasks they had to learn. They argued that learning is optimized when the combination of task difficulty and skill level presents the learner with an optimal challenge.

In the third influential review paper, Wulf and Lewthwaite (2016) argued that previous theorizing in motor learning had focused heavily on how certain practice conditions affected learning by encouraging, or discouraging, certain types and levels of task-related information processing. They developed their *OPTIMAL* (optimizing performance through intrinsic motivation and attention for learning) theory to highlight the significant body of evidence demonstrating motivational and attentional effects on performance and learning and to challenge assumptions about the most effective ways to facilitate them (see Exhibit 8.9). Specifically, they highlighted research demonstrating the benefits of enhancing the performer's or learner's expectancies about future performance,

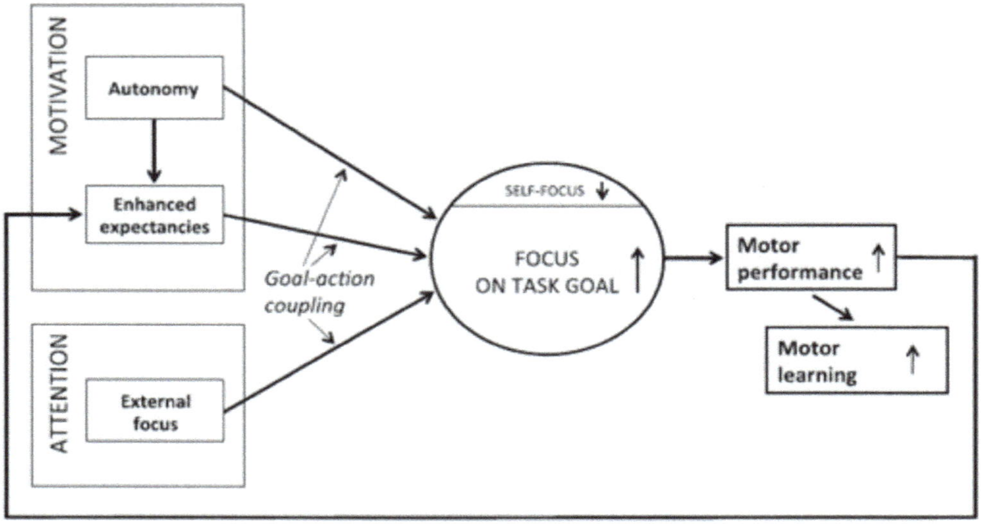

Exhibit 8.9 Wulf and Lewthwaite's (2016) OPTIMAL Theory

providing autonomy during practice, and encouraging an external focus of attention on the intended effect of a movement rather than on the movement itself.

Motor Development

A quick scan of any contemporary textbook on motor development reveals that the table of contents reads like a mini curriculum in kinesiology or exercise science. Researchers have studied with children nearly every issue they have studied with adults. Nevertheless, few researchers take a truly developmental perspective in which they study how change occurs over developmental time scales of months, years, and decades. True developmentalists seek to understand what behavior looks like now and why it looks that way, what it looked like earlier and why, and what it will look like in the future and why.

Clark and Whitall's (1989) definition of motor development provides a useful approach for understanding the questions that have attracted the attention of scholars of motor development. Much of the work in the field in the late 19th and 20th centuries focused on describing the changes that occur in motor behavior over time. This started with detailed descriptions of the motor milestones infants acquired over the first two years of life and moved on to the fundamental motor skills (like running, hopping, skipping, jumping, throwing, catching, and striking) they acquired in early childhood (see Exhibit 8.10). That work continues today, though with much greater focus on the causes underlying these changes and ways to promote these changes, particularly in children at risk of developmental delays.

At the process level, the nature vs. nurture debate dominated scholarly discussion in motor development during the first half of the 20th century, with biological maturation receiving a privileged position as the major cause of developmental change for much of that time. That began to change when systems theories began to infiltrate the broader field of developmental science and when researchers introduced dynamical systems

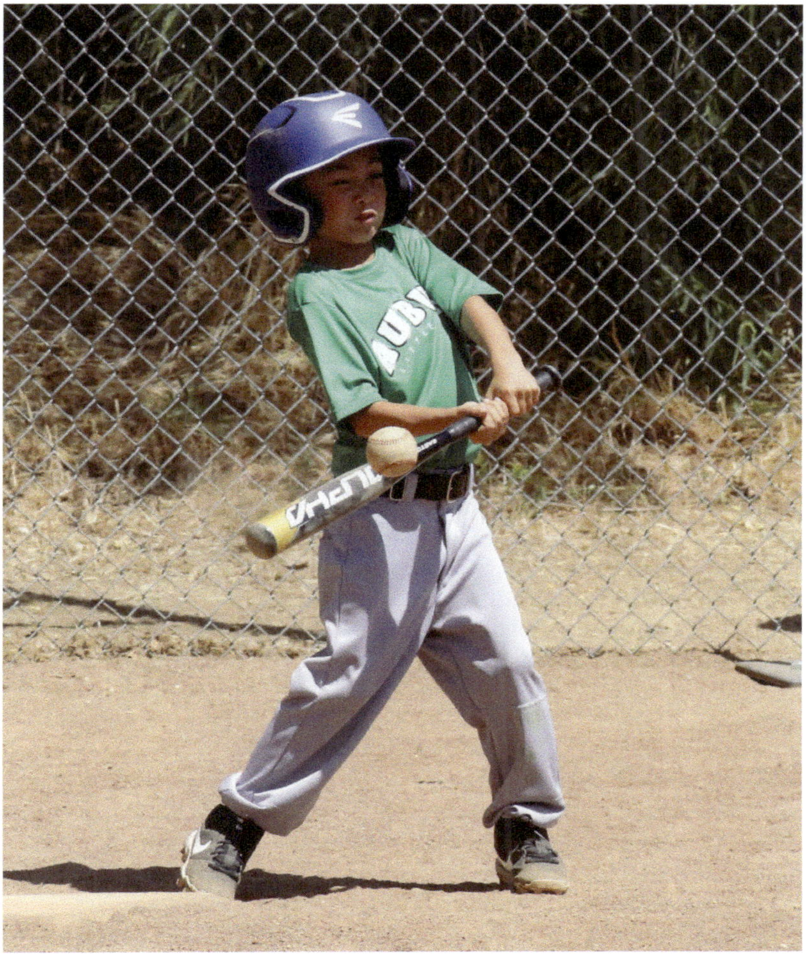

Exhibit 8.10 A child displaying the fundamental motor skill of striking while playing baseball

Note: Photo courtesy of Anthony Mayo

theory to motor behavior. Of course, we now realize the absurdity of attempting to ascribe developmental change to either hereditary or environmental factors or to attempt to parse out what contribution each makes. The critical question is how hereditary and environmental factors work together to induce and facilitate developmental change. The field of *epigenetics* has made important strides towards understanding how these factors co-act during development.

Consistent with the centrality of movement in human life, much of the contemporary work in motor development has focused on the consequences of developing movement competence for other domains of functioning, most notably those concerned with physical and mental health and psychological performance (Anderson, 2018). Considerable research has attempted to predict motor competence, health, academic performance, brain development, and psychological functioning from early measures of motor behavior and physical fitness. Research that includes a product and process focus has replaced research that focused on one or the other. Researchers have documented remarkable capabilities in the newborn and young infant to coordinate perception and action control, particularly when the context is optimal (Forma et al., 2019; Thelen and Ulrich, 1991). They have described the reorganization and refinement in neural circuitry that occurs during and after the acquisition of new skills (Corbetta, Friedman, and Bell, 2014) and documented the massive amounts of experience and practice infants and young children accrue when they develop species-specific skills (i.e., *phylogenetic* vs. *ontogenetic* skills) like upright walking (Adolph et al., 2012), and when they learn to perceive new capabilities. At the other end of the lifespan, researchers have documented age-related declines in perception and performance and developed interventions to promote motor competence in older adults and preserve a high level of brain functioning and independence (Rose, 2010).

APPLICATIONS TO EXERCISE SCIENCE

Because skilled behavior relates to every aspect of human life in every context in which it occurs, the study of motor behavior has almost limitless application to exercise science. The next sections briefly focus on some of the more common applications in health and clinical contexts and sports and performance contexts. Students should realize that the availability of research funding drives much of the research conducted in motor behavior. In the United States, much more funding exists to support health-related research than sport-related research and so researchers conduct more of the former than the latter. Most other countries provide more money than the United States to conduct sport-related research and so you see a better balance between health- and sport-related research in those countries.

HEALTH/CLINICAL ASPECTS

The study of developmental trajectories in infants at risk of developmental delay and the development of interventions and medical devices to facilitate motor, neurological, and psychological development represent two common applications of motor behavior to health and clinical contexts. Similarly, researchers and clinicians have a keen interest in developing statistical models to predict physical, motor, psychological, and academic outcomes from early measures of motor behavior. Researchers have also devoted considerable attention to the development of risk taking in young children and its implications for injury and mortality. The importance of this type of research becomes readily apparent when one realizes that accidents represent a major cause of injuries, long-term disability, and death in children (Peden et al., 2008).

Another line of application focuses on the development of interventions to help children with disabilities like CP, down syndrome, and developmental coordination disorders. Researchers have also shown considerable interest in uncovering the motor control deficits in children with various "non-motor" disorders like autism, attention deficit hyperactivity disorder (ADHD), and dyslexia. With reference to typically developing children and adolescents, a surge of research in recent years has focused on documenting the relationships among motor competence, physical activity, physical fitness, weight status, and health (Stodden et al., 2008) (see Exhibit 8.11). Studies showing declines in children's competence in performing fundamental motor skills, in parallel with decreases in time spent in physical activity and increases in rates of childhood obesity, have inspired much of this research (Barnett et al., 2022). Over 30 years ago, Jane Clark highlighted the importance of motor competence to physical health when she wrote: "To begin, I offer a reminder to those in the broad field of physical activity and physical education, in particular, that motor skillfulness is a critical component in achieving a nation of physically active people" (Clark, 1995, p. 173).

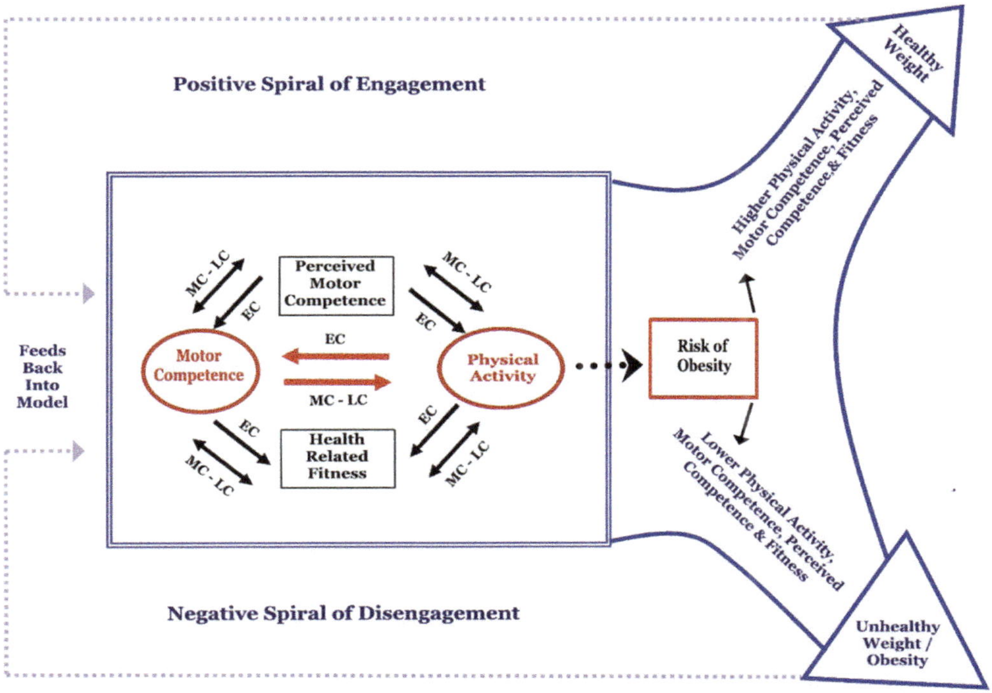

Exhibit 8.11 A diagram highlighting Stodden et al.'s (2008) model showing the relation between motor competence and physical activity (motor competence and PA are bi-directional)

Researchers and clinicians have also shown a keen interest in characterizing a variety of motor diseases like Parkinson's disease, Huntington's disease, dystonia, ataxia, and essential tremor. They have also devoted considerable time to developing and studying interventions to help people manage their diseases or to rehabilitate after accidents like strokes. A major line of research has focused on understanding and preventing falls in the elderly.

SPORTS/PERFORMANCE ASPECTS

Because theorists assume that acquiring fundamental motor skills is a prerequisite for developing sport-specific skills and leading an active lifestyle, considerable research has explored when and how children acquire these skills, as well as the factors that influence their development. The abstract below (see Exhibit 8.12) suggests that certain basketball skills improve more rapidly during specific stages of physical growth and maturation, particularly around the adolescent growth spurt. These findings highlight the importance of aligning skill development with biological maturity rather than chronological age to help coaches and practitioners better support athletes' progress.

Researchers have also studied how children and adolescents develop sport-related knowledge in parallel with sport-specific skills (French and Thomas, 1987). These lines of research highlight part of a broader agenda devoted to understanding youth sports participation. Researchers and practitioners who seek to understand competitive sport, particularly at the elite level, have shown an enduring interest in talent identification and development (Williams, Ford, and Drust, 2020). One question that has received considerable attention within this line of research concerns whether early specialization within a particular sport or early participation in a wide range of sports (referred to as diversification) is more likely to lead to long-term success in the sport (Anderson and Mayo, 2015).

Exhibit 8.12 Abstract of a research study on motor skill acquisition and development

Guimarães, E., Baxter-Jones, A. D. G., Williams, A. M., Anderson, D. I., Janeira, M. A., Garbeloto, F., Pereira, & Maia, J. (2024). Are there sensitive periods for skill development in male adolescent basketball players? *Medicine and Science in Sports and Exercise*, *56*(8), 1437–1445. DOI: 10.1249/mss.0000000000003439. PMID: 38598419.

Purpose: Although spurts in physical capacities during adolescence are well-known, little is known about the existence of such spurts in sport-specific skill development, especially during the period of rapid growth in stature. Our aims were to examine the timing, intensity, and sequence of basketball-specific skill spurts aligned with biological (years from peak height velocity [PHV]) rather than chronological age. We then defined putative sensitive periods (windows of optimal development) for each skill aligned to the adolescent growth spurt. **Methods:** Altogether, 160 adolescent male basketballers, aged 11–15 years, were tested bi-annually over three consecutive years. The years from attainment of PHV were estimated and six skill tests were aligned to each year from PHV in 3-month intervals. Skill velocities were estimated using a non-smooth polynomial model.

Results: Maximal gains in slalom dribbling occurred 12 months prior to PHV attainment (intensity = 0.18 $m \cdot s^{-1} \cdot year^{-1}$), whereas in speed shot shooting (intensity = 9.91 $pts \cdot year^{-1}$), passing (intensity = 19.13 $pts \cdot year^{-1}$), and slalom sprinting (intensity = 0.19 $m \cdot s^{-1} \cdot year^{-1}$) these skill spurts were attained 6 months prior to PHV attainment. The mean gains in control dribbling (intensity = 0.10 $m \cdot s^{-1} \cdot year^{-1}$) and defensive movement (intensity = 0.12 $m \cdot s^{-1} \cdot year^{-1}$) peaks coincided with attainment of PHV. We identified different sized windows for optimal development for each skill.

Conclusions: Peak spurts in skill development, for most basketball skills, were attained at the same time as PHV. The multiple peaks observed within the defined windows of optimal development suggest that there is room for skill improvement even if gains might be greater earlier rather than later in practice. Our findings highlight the need to make coaches aware of where their players are relative to the attainment of PHV since different skills appear to develop differently relative to PHV. Such knowledge may help in designing more relevant training regimes that incorporate the athlete's current growth status so that skill development can be maximized.

Moving beyond the prediction of long-term success in sport, motor behavior researchers and practitioners have worked alongside specialists from other sub-disciplines within kinesiology and exercise science to optimize sports performance. Much of the work in this area manipulates variables like practice, augmented feedback, and demonstration (modeling) known to enhance skill acquisition. Researchers and practitioners have combined our understanding of the principles that underlie the effective design of practice and instruction with advancements in technologies to measure brain activity, muscle activity, and movement kinematics and kinetics to enhance the skill acquisition process further (Williams and Hodges, 2023).

TECHNOLOGY AND RESEARCH TOOLS

Motor behavior researchers and practitioners use a variety of tools to understand and enhance motor performance and learning. The tools generally relate to the measurement of activity occurring at different levels of analysis within the motor system. Various motion capture (MOCAP) systems and devices exist to measure movement kinematics and kinetics at the behavioral level. At the most basic level, people use smartphones and video cameras to record movement patterns and use a variety of apps or pieces of software to conduct spatiotemporal and kinematic analyses of the patterns. Scientists have used machine learning and artificial intelligence technologies to automate many aspects of these analyses. A number of other devices exist to measure movement kinematics and kinetics, including accelerometers, goniometers, activity trackers, force plates, and force transducers.

Expensive MOCAP systems can automate the collection and analysis of human movement data by using banks of infrared cameras or clusters of electromagnetic or inertial sensors and custom algorithms to combine the data from the cameras or sensors. At the muscular level, scientists have used electromyography (EMG) recordings to study the activity of muscles since the 19th century and more recently have developed whole muscle mechanomyography (wMMG) and near-infrared spectroscopy (NIRS) as additional techniques. wMMG measures the displacement of a muscle belly following muscle stimulation via an electric current whereas NIRS determines the level of oxygenation in the muscle, as a proxy for work done by the muscle, by analyzing the absorption of different wavelengths of light.

Scientists also use NIRS, and the more recently developed functional near-infrared spectroscopy (fNIRS), to measure cerebral blood flow as a proxy for brain activity. More common tools for studying and analyzing brain activity include electroencephalography (EEG) (see Exhibit 8.13), positron emission topography (PET), functional magnetic resonance imaging (fMRI), magnetoencephalography (MEG), and transcranial magnetic stimulation (TMS). TMS is not strictly a neuroimaging technique like the others. It uses magnetic fields to induce changes in neural activity and so is also used to facilitate motor learning and as a therapeutic tool to treat various neurological conditions. Each neuroimaging tool uses a different technology and technique to detect brain activity, and each provides different degrees of spatial and temporal resolution. For example, EEG has excellent temporal resolution but poor spatial resolution whereas fMRI has excellent spatial resolution, but relatively poor temporal resolution and MEG has excellent spatial and temporal resolution.

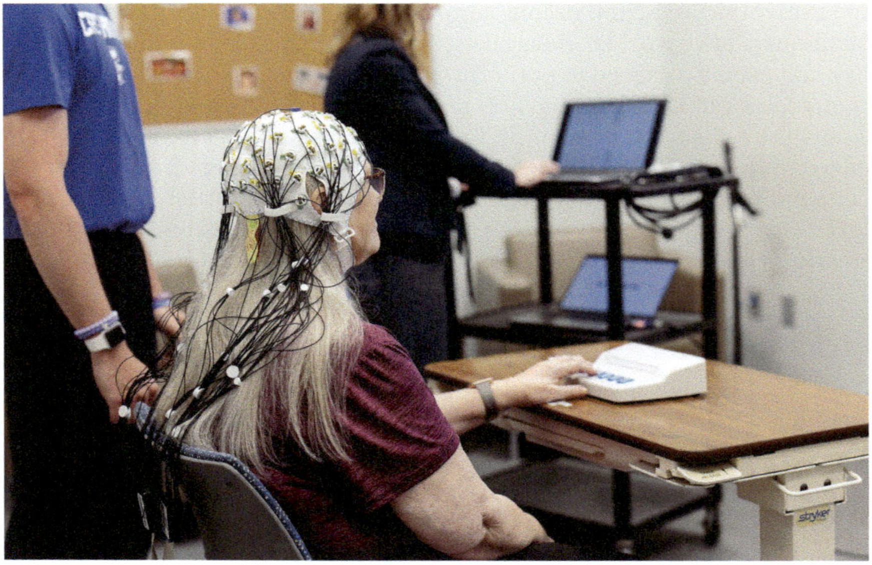

Exhibit 8.13 An individual participating in an experiment wearing an EEG cap
Source: Photo courtesy of Joan Eckerson

Simulators represent a research tool that has existed for decades. However, with improvements in technology this tool has become increasingly sophisticated and increasingly utilized by motor behavior researchers and practitioners. Simulators offer many advantages: people can practice difficult skills without concerns about the costs of accidents or performance errors, they can often practice for longer periods of time, especially when it is difficult to secure the time or equipment needed in the ultimate performance context, and they can often practice at higher levels of intensity. Virtual reality simulators have become an increasingly popular type of simulator (see Exhibit 8.14). Researchers have used them to train athletes, surgeons, pilots, military and police personnel, and to help rehabilitate people with specific diseases or after accidents or injuries.

CAREER AND EMPLOYMENT OPPORTUNITIES

Many of the career opportunities for those with an interest in motor behavior lie in teaching, coaching, and the allied health professions, including athletic training (AT), physical therapy (PT) and occupational therapy (OT). Motor behavior specialists also work in professional sports alongside video analysts, statisticians, and sport psychologists and most countries employ specialists at their Institutes of Sport and Olympic Training centers. Career opportunities also exist in human factors and ergonomics, related to optimizing work performance and preventing injuries, and in the video game industry, given the importance of perceptual-motor learning in game play. Motor behavior specialists also find work in military settings, training military personnel in the use of new technologies like remotely operated drones, for example. Given the importance of skill in everyday life, numerous opportunities exist for the entrepreneurial student to apply their understanding of motor behavior to enhancing performance and learning in many different personal and professional settings.

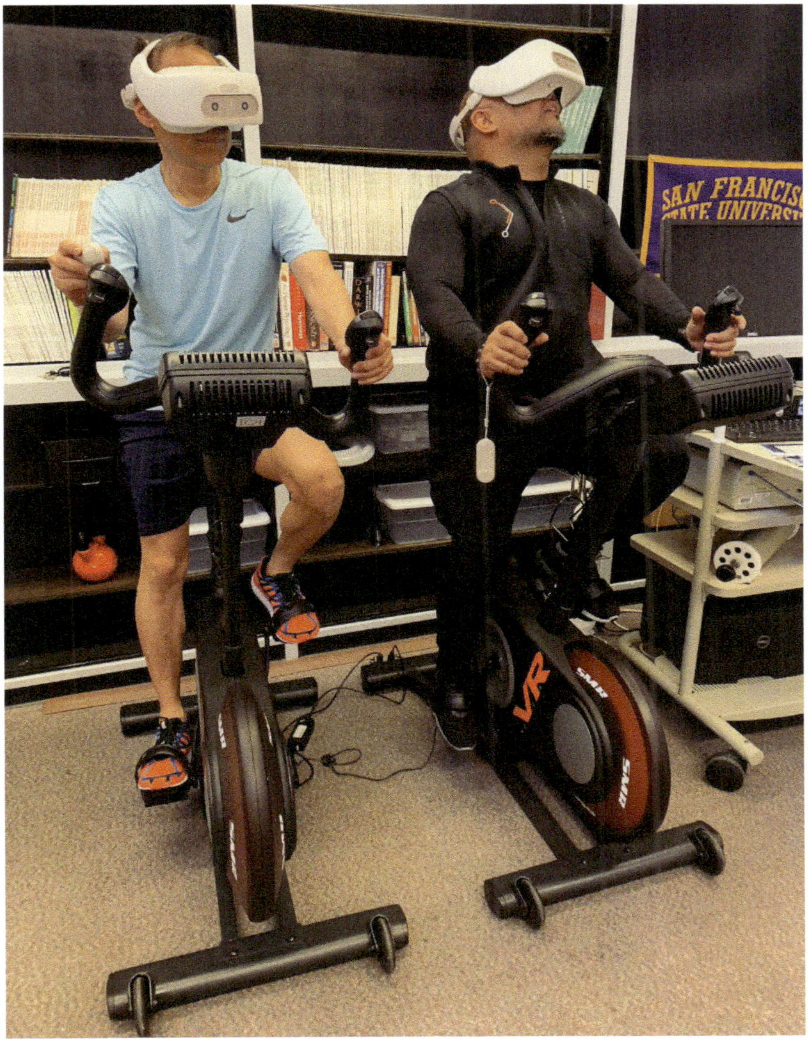

Exhibit 8.14 Two individuals participating in an active virtual reality game study

Source: Photo courtesy of Angelina Wong

EDUCATION REQUIREMENTS

A bachelor's degree in kinesiology or exercise science represents the minimum requirement for working in the field. It provides the credibility a person needs to secure an entry-level job or set up a personal business and it provides entry into graduate level professional programs like PT, OT, AT, and teaching physical education. Those who wish to teach in higher education require a minimum of a master's degree in kinesiology or exercise science, though a PhD represents the typical degree higher education faculty possess.

CERTIFICATIONS AND LICENSURE

People seeking to teach physical education will need a teaching credential and people seeking to coach could profit from obtaining a coaching certification or an academic minor in coaching. Individuals desiring to work in strength and conditioning and fitness industries could benefit from obtaining certifications related to those careers.

PROFESSIONAL ORGANIZATIONS

American College of Sports Medicine (ACSM)
Canadian Society for Psychomotor Learning and Sport Psychology (SCAPPS)
International Motor Development Research Consortium (IMDRC)
International Society for Ecological Psychology (ISEP)
International Society of Motor Control (ISMC)
International Society for Posture and Gait Research (ISPGR)
North American Society for the Psychology of Sport and Physical Activity (NASPSPA)
Society for Neuroscience
SHAPE America

JOURNALS

High Ability Studies
Human Movement Science
Journal of Experimental Psychology (Human Learning and Memory)
Journal of Experimental Psychology (Human Perception and Performance)
Journal of Motor Behavior
Journal of Motor Learning and Development
Journal of Sport and Exercise Psychology
Journal of Sports Sciences
Medicine & Science in Sports & Exercise
Motor Control
Perceptual and Motor Skills
Research in Developmental Disabilities
Research Quarterly for Exercise and Sport

FUTURE DIRECTIONS

Over the next two decades researchers will continue to pursue the questions and themes that have become prevalent over the first two and a half decades of the 21st century, albeit with new technologies, new paradigms, and in potentially new contexts, even though researchers have already studied skill acquisition in nearly every context in which human behavior occurs. These themes include (a) exploration of how the multitude of interacting constraints residing at different levels of analysis and changing at different time scales influence motor skill performance and learning; (b) exploration of how the acquisition of certain motor skills initiates developmental cascades in the motor and psychological domains; (c) mapping the relations between brain and behavior as individuals acquire new skills; (d) examination of changing relations among motor competence, physical activity, and health and the development of interventions to improve health by improving motor competence; (e) exploration of how motivational and attentional factors influence motor performance and learning; (f) examination of the role of practice in the development of motor expertise, particularly in sport, and application of motor learning principles to sports coaching; and (g) development of interventions to help prevent or manage diseases or the consequences of injuries/accidents that impair motor control.

Changing technology will play a major role in the work conducted in motor behavior. The COVID-19 pandemic accelerated a shift toward online data collection and the online delivery of interventions, and that shift will continue to accelerate. The nature of data collection has also changed considerably and will continue to change, given the ubiquity of web cameras and smartphones and their ability to collect multiple streams of data. The massive volumes of data we now collect has accelerated a trend toward analyzing "big data" and advances in machine learning and artificial intelligence have and will influence what we can extract from our data repositories. The nature of the skills we examine will also continue to shift. An increasing number of studies have examined the development of skill in online video gamers; a trend that will likely accelerate with the exponential increase in esports participation. Owing to the demands of modern warfare and our appetite for exploring worlds beyond our immediate reach, we will see an increasing amount of research devoted to optimizing performance and learning in tasks like operating a vehicle remotely. We will see much greater use of technologies like virtual reality to promote motor learning/re-learning, and a concomitant increase in research on the transfer of learning from the virtual environment to the "real" environment. Finally, we will see continued enhancement in neuroimaging and brain stimulation technologies and these technologies will deepen our understanding of the neural control of movement, and how to enhance it, considerably.

SUMMARY

The subfields of motor control, motor learning, and motor development comprise the broader field of motor behavior. The field studies how we acquire and control motor skills and how we can promote the development of skill. This represents a key endeavor because skilled activity has played a significant role in human evolution and development, and it is fundamental to human life. The history of motor behavior overlaps with the histories of biology, medicine, and psychology. The evolution of the scientific knowledge bases within motor behavior began with the Greeks and Romans, but the contemporary field of motor behavior did not emerge until the 1960s. Scientists who study motor behavior generally adopt either a behavioral or a neurophysiological perspective. Researchers in motor control, motor learning, and motor development address distinct issues; however considerable overlap exists among these subfields in terms of the questions asked, the tools used to answer them, and the application of the knowledge gained to health, clinical practice, and sports and performance settings. Motor behavior is entering a golden age because the knowledge bases, skillsets, and technologies that characterize the field have such relevance to so many of the big challenges that confront contemporary society.

STUDY QUESTIONS

1. Why is the study of skillful physical activity important?
2. What did Bernstein mean by the degrees of freedom problem and context-conditioned variability?

3. What issues did motor learning researchers study prior to World War II and how did that shift during and after the war?
4. What are the major brain areas involved in motor control and what are some of the important structures within each area?
5. What are the major neural tracts in the spinal cord?
6. What are the main differences between motor program-based theories of motor control and dynamical systems theory?
7. What do the contextual interference effect and guidance hypothesis reveal about the relation between performance and learning?
8. How do researchers now conceptualize the role of hereditary and environmental factors in motor development?
9. Provide some examples to highlight how research in motor behavior is applied in health-related, clinical, and sports settings.
10. Why do researchers and clinicians use a range of neuroimaging tools to study motor behavior?
11. In terms of future research directions, what issues interest you the most?

LEARNING ACTIVITIES

1. Search online for information about a specific disease or disorder that interferes with motor control. In a 300-word paper, describe the symptoms patients experience, the cause of the disease/disorder, and the brain structures and processes involved. Relevant examples include Parkinson's disease, Huntington's disease, cerebellar ataxia, multiple sclerosis (MS), amyotrophic lateral sclerosis (ALS), and dystonia.
2. Visit your local playground or search online for a picture of a playground apparatus. Post a picture of the apparatus into a document and generate a list of all of the actions the playground affords. In your own words, define the affordance concept and provide some examples of features of your apparatus that might afford different actions for a young child versus an adult.
3. Search online for the "stick test of coordination" and locate three "sticks" you could use to perform the task (unsharpened pencils work well). Practice the task for 10 minutes. Write a 300-word paper that describes your experience as a novice learner. Consider the following questions in your paper: did you improve? Did you set a specific goal and did the goal change? Did you try different strategies? What did you tell yourself during practice? What did you focus on and did it help? Did you experience frustration? Did you notice signs of unnecessary tension or effort and experience freezing of degrees of freedom? What might you do in future practice to speed up the learning of this task?
4. Find a piece of paper and a small waste paper basket. Scrunch up the paper into a ball and place the basket 10 to 15 feet away from you. Attempt to throw the ball into the basket multiple times and alternate what you attend to each time between the ball and its initial trajectory (external focus) and the movement of the wrist and elbow (internal focus). In a 300-word paper, describe your experience. Did you have more success with one focus of attention than the other? Why do you think this occurred?

SUGGESTED READING AND RELATED WEBSITES

American College of Sports Medicine (ACSM). (n.d.). American College of Sports Medicine website. Available at: https://www.acsm.org/

Anderson, D. I. (2023). Mastering motor skills: The contributions of motor learning and motor development to the growth and maturation of kinesiology. *Kinesiology Review*, *13*(1), 28–41.

Canadian Society for Psychomotor Learning and Sport Psychology (SCAPPS). (n.d.). Canadian Society for Psychomotor Learning and Sport Psychology website. Available at: https://www.scapps.org/

Clark, J. E., and Whitall, J. (2021). Motor development: A perspective on the past, the present, and the future. *Kinesiology Review*, *10*(3), 264–273.

International Motor Development Research Consortium (IMDRC). (n.d.). International Motor Development Research Consortium website. Available at: https://www.i-mdrc.com/

International Society for Ecological Psychology (ISEP). (n.d.). International Motor Development Research Consortium website. Available at: https://commons.trincoll.edu/isep/

International Society for Posture and Gait Research (ISPGR). (n.d.). International Society for Posture and Gait Research website. Available at: https://ispgr.org/

International Society of Motor Control (ISMC). (n.d.). International Society of Motor Control website. Available at: https://i-s-m-c.org/

Latash, M. L. (2021). Motor control: Creating a natural science of biological movement. *Kinesiology Review*, *10*(3), 257–263.

Lee, T. D., and Carnahan, H. (2021). Motor learning: Reflections on the past 40 years of research. *Kinesiology Review*, *10*(3), 274–282.

North American Society for the Psychology of Sport and Physical Activity (NASPSPA). (n.d.). North American Society for the Psychology of Sport and Physical Activity website. Available at: https://www.naspspa.com/

SHAPE America. (n.d.). SHAPE America website. Available at: https://www.shapeamerica.org/

Society for Neuroscience. (n.d.). Society for Neuroscience website. Available at: https://www.sfn.org/

REFERENCES

Adams, J. A. (1987). Historical review and appraisal of research on the learning, retention, and transfer of human motor skills. *Psychological Bulletin*, *101*, 41–74.

Adolph, K. E., Cole, W. G., Komati, M., Garciaguirre, J. S., Badaly, D., Lingeman, J. M., Chan, G. and Sotsky, R. B. (2012). How do you learn to walk? Thousands of steps and dozens of falls per day. *Psychological Science*, *23*(11), 1387–1394.

Anderson, D. I. (2018). Motor development is concerned with far more than the development of motor skills. *Kinesiology Review*, *7*(2), 99–114.

Anderson, D. I., Campos, J. J., Witherington, D. C., Dahl, A., Rivera, M., He, M., Uchiyama, I., and Barbu-Roth, M. (2013). The role of locomotion in psychological development. *Frontiers in Psychology*, *4*, 440.

Anderson, D. I., and Mayo, A. M. (2015). A skill acquisition perspective on early specialization in sport. *Kinesiology Review*, *4*, 230–247.

Barnett, L. M., Webster, E. K., Hulteen, R. M., De Meester, A., Valentini, N. C., Lenoir, M., Pesce, C., Getchell, N., Lopes, V. P., Robinson, L. E., Brian, A., and Rodrigues, L. P. (2022). Through the looking glass: A systematic review of longitudinal evidence, providing new insight for motor competence and health. *Sports Medicine*, *52*, 875–920.

Bayley, N. (1936). *The California Infant Scale of Motor Development.* University of California Press.

Bernstein, N. (1967). *The co-ordination and regulation of movement.* Pergamon Press.

Bryan, W. L., and Harter, N. (1897). Studies in the physiology and psychology of the telegraphic language. *Psychological Review*, *4*, 27–53.

Bryan, W. L., and Harter, N. (1899). Studies on the telegraphic language: The acquisition of a hierarchy of habits. *Psychological Review*, *6*, 345–375.

Clark, J. E. (1995). On becoming skillful: Patterns and constraints. *Research Quarterly for Exercise and Sport*, *66*(3), 173–183.

Clark, J. E., and Whitall, J. (1989). What is motor development? The lessons of history. *Quest*, *41*(3), 183–202.

Corbetta, D., Friedman, D. R., and Bell, M. A. (2014). Brain reorganization as a function of walking experience in 12-month-old infants: Implications for the development of manual laterality. *Frontiers in Psychology*, *5*.

Craik, K. J. W. (1947/1948). Theory of the human operator in control systems. I. The operator as an engineering system. *British Journal of Psychology*, *38*, 56–61.

Ericsson, K. A., Krampe, R. T., and Tesch-Romer, C. (1993). The role of deliberate practice in the acquisition of expert performance. *Psychological Review*, *100*, 363–406.

Fleishman, E. A. (1972). On the relationship between abilities, learning, and human performance. *American Psychologist*, *27*, 1017–1032.

Forma, V., Anderson, D. I., Provasi, J., Soyez, E., Martial, M., Huet, V., Granjon, L., Goffinet, F., and Barbu-Roth, M. (2019). What does prone skateboarding in the newborn tell us about the ontogeny of human locomotion? *Child Development*, *90*(4), 1286–1302.

French, K. E., and Thomas, J. R. (1987). The relation of knowledge development to children's basketball performance. *Journal of Sport Psychology*, *9*(1), 15–32.

Gesell, A. (1928). *Infancy and human growth*. The Macmillan Company.

Gibson, J. J. (1966). *The senses considered as perceptual systems*. Houghton Mifflin.

Gibson, J. J. (1979). *The ecological approach to visual perception*. Houghton Mifflin.

Gordon, E. M., Chauvin, R. J., Van, A. N., et al. (2023). A somato-cognitive action network alternates with effector regions in motor cortex. *Nature*, *617*, 351–359.

Guadagnoli, M. A., and Lee, T. D. (2004). Challenge point: A framework for conceptualizing the effects of various practice conditions in motor learning. *Journal of Motor Behavior*, *36*, 212–224.

Halverson, H. M. (1931). An experimental study of prehension in infants by means of systematic cinema records. *Genetic Psychology Monographs*, *10*(2–3), 107–286.

Hambrick, D. Z., Macnamara, B. N., and Oswald, F. L. (2020). Is the deliberate practice view defensible? A review of evidence and discussion of issues. *Frontiers in Psycholology*, *11*, 1134.

Hull, C. L. (1943). *Principles of behavior*. Appleton-Century-Crofts.

Inglis, B. (1965). *A history of medicine*. World.

Kugler, P. N., Kelso, J. A. S., and Turvey, M. T. (1980). On the concept of coordinative structures as dissipative structures: I. Theoretical lines of convergence. In G. E. Stelmach and J. Requin (Eds.), *Advances in psychology: Tutorials in motor behavior* (pp. 3–47). North-Holland.

Kugler, P. N., Kelso, J. A. S., and Turvey, M. T. (1982). On the control and coordination of naturally developing systems. In J. A. S. Kelso and J. E. Clark (Eds.), *The development of movement control and coordination* (pp. 2–78). John Wiley.

Lashley, K. S. (1917). The accuracy of movement in the absence of excitation from the moving organ. *American Journal of Physiology*, *43*, 169–194.

Magill, R. A., and Anderson, D. I. (2024). *Motor learning and control: Concepts and applications*. McGraw-Hill.

McCullagh, P. (1993). Modeling: Learning, development, and social psychological considerations. In R. N. Singer, M. Murphey, and L. K. Tenant (Eds.), *Handbook of research on sport psychology* (pp. 106–126). Macmillan.

McGraw, M. B. (1935). *Growth: A study of Johnny and Jimmy*. Appleton-Century-Crofts.

Newell, K. M. (1986). Constraints on the development of coordination. In M. G. Wade and H. T. A. Whiting (Eds.), *Motor development in children: Aspects of coordination and control* (pp. 341–360). Martinus Nijhoff.

Peden, M., Oyegbite, K., Ozanne-Smith, J., Hyder, A. A., Branche, C. Rahman, A. F., Rivara, F., and Bartolomeos, K. (2008). World report on child injury prevention. *World Health Organization*. Available at: https://www.who.int/publications/i/item/9789241563574

Penfield, W., and Rasmussen, T. (1950). *The cerebral cortex of man: A clinical study of localization of function*. Macmillan.

Rose, D. J. (2010). *Fallproof! A comprehensive balance and mobility training program.* Human Kinetics.

Sabbatini, R. M. E. (1998). The discovery of bioelectricity. *Brain and Mind*, *2*, 1–4.

Salmoni, A. W., Schmidt, R. A., and Walter, C. B. (1984). Knowledge of results and motor learning: A review and reappraisal. *Psychological Bulletin*, *95*, 355–386.

Schmidt, R. A. (1975). A schema theory of discrete motor skill learning. *Psychological Review*, *82*, 225–260.

Schmidt, R. A., Lee, T. D., Winstein, C. J., Wulf, G., and Zelaznik, H. N. (2019). *Motor control and learning: A behavioral emphasis* (6th ed.). Human Kinetics.

Shea, J. B., and Morgan, R. L. (1979). Contextual interference effects on the acquisition, retention, and transfer of a motor skill. *Journal of Experimental Psychology: Human Learning and Memory*, *5*, 179–187.

Sörgel, S. (2015). *Dance and the body in the western theatre: 1948 to the present.* Bloomsbury Publishing.

Shirley, M. M. (1933). *The first two years: A study of twenty-five babies.* Greenwood Press.

Stodden, D. F., Goodway, J. D., Langendorfer, S. J., Roberton, M. A., Rudisill, M. E., Garcia, C., and Garcia, L. E. (2008). A developmental perspective on the role of motor skill competence in physical activity: An emergent relationship. *Quest*, *60*(2), 290–306.

Stoffregen, T. A. (2003). Affordances as properties of the animal-environment system. *Ecological Psychology*, *15*(2), 115–134.

Thelen, E., and Ulrich, B.D. (1991). Hidden skills: A dynamic systems analysis of treadmill stepping during the first year. *Monographs of the Society for Research in Child Development*, *56*, i–103.

Thorndike, E. L. (1927). The law of effect. *American Journal of Psychology*, *39*, 212–222.

Vereijken, B., van Emmerik, R. E. A., Whiting, H. T. A., and Newell, K. M. (1992) Free(z)ing degrees of freedom in skill acquisition. *Journal of Motor Behavior*, *24*(1), 133–142.

Whitall, J., Bardid, F., Getchell, N., Pangelinan, M., Robinson, L. E., Schott, N., and Clark, J. E. (2020a). Motor development research: II. The first two decades of the 21st century shaping our future. *Journal of Motor Learning and Development*, *8*(2), 363–390.

Whitall, J., Schott, N., Robinson, L., Bardid, F., and Clark, J. E. (2020b). Motor development research: I. The lessons of history revisited (the 18th to the 20th century). *Journal of Motor Learning and Development*, *8*(2), 345–362.

Williams, A. M., Ford, P. R., and Drust, B. (2020). Talent identification and development in soccer since the millennium. *Journal of Sports Sciences*, *38*(11–12), 1199–1210.

Williams, A. M. and Hodges, N. J. (2023). Effective practice and instruction: A skill acquisition framework for excellence, *Journal of Sports Sciences*, *41*(9), 833–849, DOI: 10.1080/02640414.2023.2240630

Wozniak, R. H. (1992). *Mind and body: Rene Descartes to William James.* American Psychology Association. Available at: https://archive.org/details/9301710.nlm.nih.gov/page/n15/mode/2up

Wulf, G., and Lewthwaite, R. (2016). Optimizing performance through intrinsic motivation and attention for learning: The OPTIMAL theory of motor learning. *Psychonomic Bulletin and Review*, *23*, 1382–1414.

9 Exercise and Sport Psychology

Barbara B. Meyer and Carly A. Wahl

LEARNING OBJECTIVES

After studying this chapter, the student will be able to:

- describe exercise and sport psychology
- understand developments in the history of exercise and sport psychology
- comprehend health-related psychological aspects relevant to exercise and mental health, quality of life, cognitive function, adherence, and addiction to exercise
- comprehend sports-related psychological aspects relevant to stress, arousal, and anxiety; motivation; confidence and self-efficacy; team dynamics; and burnout and recovery
- recognize various types of technology used in research and practice
- describe educational requirements, career opportunities, and professional organizations relevant to exercise and sport psychology

INTRODUCTION

Exercise and sport psychology is the scientific study of behavior in exercise and sport environments in both individual and group contexts (Gill, Williams, and Reifsteck, 2017). Two primary objectives studied within the discipline are (1) to gain a better understanding of the relationships between psychological factors and physical activity, focusing on how these factors influence both the initiation and maintenance of exercise and sports participation, and (2) to examine the effects of exercise and sport participation on psychological well-being. Therefore, this chapter explores the dual objectives of the discipline by examining how various psychological elements, such as motivation, confidence, and stress and anxiety regulation, impact an individual's ability to adopt and adhere to exercise routines or excel in sports; and how regular participation in exercise and sports contributes to improved mental health, cognitive functioning, resilience, and overall quality of life.

HISTORICAL PERSPECTIVES

The foundation of exercise and sport psychology can be traced back to the late 19th century when Norman Triplett, a psychologist at the University of Indiana, published a paper in 1898 that examined the influence of social facilitation on cycling performance. His research, which showed that cyclists performed better when racing against others compared to when they raced alone, is often cited as one of the first studies in sport

DOI: 10.4324/9781032697185-9

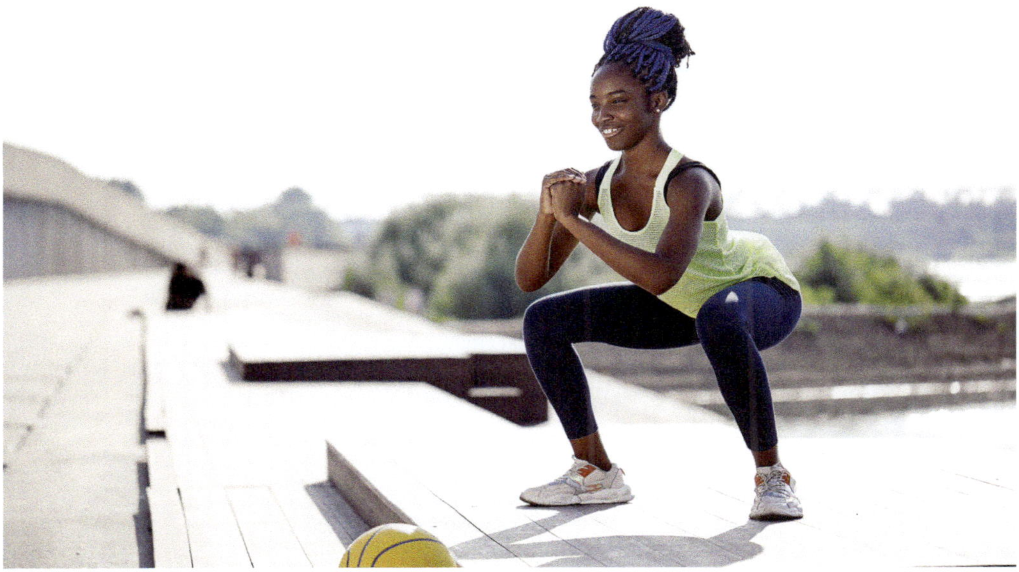

psychology. In the early 20th century, Coleman Griffith, who many consider the "father of American sport psychology," conducted extensive research on athletic performance and motivation, and established the first sport psychology laboratory at the University of Illinois in 1925. His work with professional athletes, including the Chicago Cubs baseball team, marked the beginning of applied sport psychology (Granito, 2017; Schmidt, 2018).

Interest in the psychological aspects of sport and exercise intensified in the mid-to-late 20th century, particularly in Europe and North America, and the field became more formalized with the establishment of professional organizations, such as the International Society of Sport Psychology (ISSP) in 1965, and, later, the Association for Applied Sports Psychology (AASP) in 1986. In the 1960s and 1970s, research expanded into areas including personality, motivation, and the psychological benefits of physical activity. Researchers also began to explore the mental aspects of performance, such as the role of anxiety and mental imagery, which laid the groundwork for modern techniques used in sport psychology today (Schmidt, 2018).

Since the 1980s, exercise and sport psychology has grown into a well-defined discipline with a strong emphasis on both research and applied practice and has diversified, addressing not only elite athletic performance but also the psychological benefits of physical activity for the general population. The American Psychological Association (APA) recognized sport psychology as a proficiency area in 2003, further solidifying its professional status. Advances in technology and neuroscience have also deepened the understanding of the mind-body connection, enabling more sophisticated approaches to improving performance and well-being through psychological interventions. Today, exercise and sport psychology is an interdisciplinary field that bridges psychology, exercise science, and health sciences, focusing on optimizing human potential across all levels of physical activity and sport. While a comprehensive review of the history of exercise and sport psychology can be found elsewhere (Granito, 2017; Schmidt, 2018), its key points are depicted in Exhibit 9.1.

1898	• Norman Triplett publishes the first experimental study in exercise psychology, examining the influence of social facilitation on cyclists' performance.
1920	• Carl Diem establishes the world's first sport psychology laboratory in Berlin, Germany.
1925	• Coleman Griffith, the Father of American Sport Psychology, is appointed director of the newly created Athletics research laboratory at the University of Illinois. A scientist practitioner, Griffith is known for teaching the first course and publishing the first textbook in sport and exercise psychology.
1965	• The International Society of Sport Psychology is founded.
1966	• Clinical psychologist Bruce Ogilvie is the catalyst to applied sport psychology as he begins to consult with athletes and teams.
1980	• The United States Olympic Committee develops the Sport Psychology Advisory Board.
1986	• The Association for Applied Sport Psychology (AASP) is established.
2020	• Certified Mental Performance Consultant (CMPC®) becomes the only nationally accredited certification for mental performance consultants in the world.

Exhibit 9.1 Key points in exercise and sport psychology history

FUNDAMENTAL CONCEPTS

Exercise psychology is described as the application of psychology to promote, maintain, and enhance exercise and physical activity (Lox et al., 2017). Applied research in exercise psychology addresses questions such as:

- Do individuals who participate in group exercise have higher rates of adherence than individuals who exercise alone?
- Do exercisers who monitor daily heart rate variability have improved confidence in their perceived recovery compared to exercisers who do not monitor daily heart rate variability?
- What is the relationship between an exercise physiologist's communication style and a heart attack survivor's adherence to cardiopulmonary rehabilitation?

Sport psychology is described as a multifaceted discipline, informed by principles of exercise science and psychology, and applied within a sport or performance context (Gill, Williams, and Reifsteck, 2017). Applied research in sport psychology addresses questions such as:

- Are athletes with lower levels of trait anxiety selected higher in the National Basketball Association draft than athletes with higher levels of trait anxiety?
- What is the relationship between psychological factors and knee injuries among Olympic level soccer players?
- How does engagement in a mindfulness practice influence the performance of military personnel in the field?

In the following sections, several key theories, principles, and practical applications are introduced within the contexts of exercise science, health and clinical related aspects, and sports that are essential for understanding how psychological factors contribute to promoting well-being, enhancing performance, and overcoming challenges across various physical activities.

APPLICATIONS TO EXERCISE SCIENCE

Historically, much emphasis in the field of exercise science has been placed on the **physical** aspects of health and performance. Yet, given recent advancements in research and practice it is prudent to place equal emphasis on the **psychological** aspects of health and performance (Hess and Meyer, 2021). Within a fitness or holistic health context, psychological strategies can be used as individuals strive to achieve the ideal mindset to pursue personal health goals. For example:

- setting weekly short-term goals might be used to increase a runner's motivation to complete marathon training
- utilizing positive self-talk might be used to improve a novice exerciser's self-esteem during strength training
- mindfulness might be used to help an individual slow down when eating or to choose more nutrient-dense food options

Within a sport or performance context, psychological strategies can be used as individuals strive to achieve the optimal mindset necessary for competition or other performance-related pursuits. For example:

- deep breathing might be used to reduce the heart rate of a biathlete, who is required to cross country ski between rifle shots at a target
- imagery might be used to improve confidence in proprioception as a gymnast learns a new floor routine
- implementing verbal and visual cues might be used to help a soldier improve the concentration required of them to scan the environment for relevant cues, block out distractions, and attend to the immediate tasks at hand

As the above examples indicate, psychological aspects of exercise and sport complement the foundational disciplines of exercise science (e.g., exercise physiology, biomechanics).

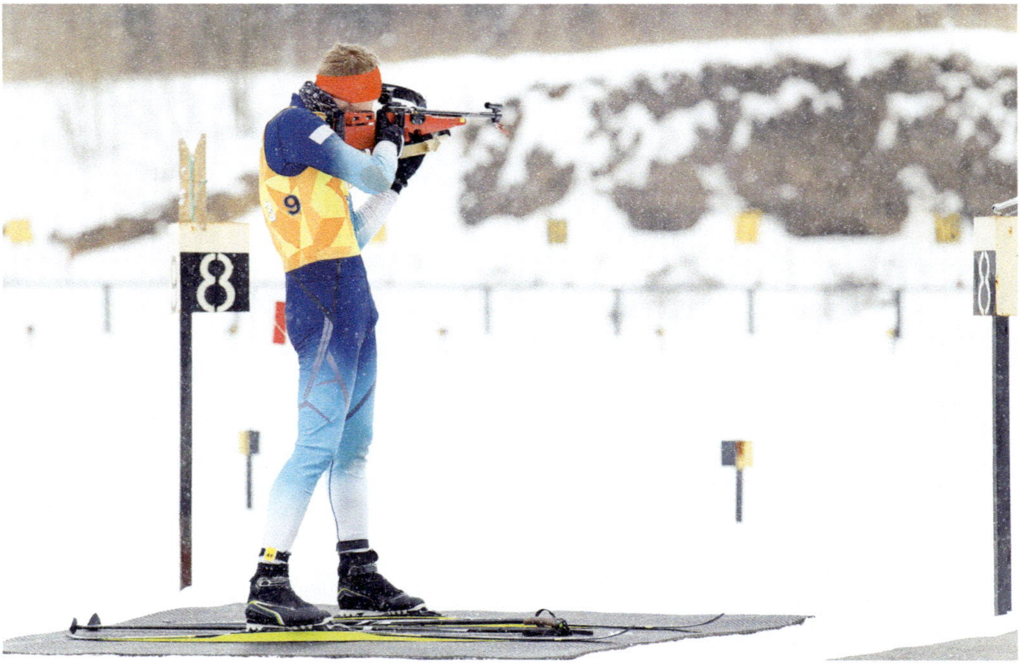

Moreover, psychological strategies can be used to improve the mind-body connection along with aerobic and anaerobic activities in both healthy and special populations.

HEALTH/CLINICAL ASPECTS

Exercise psychology pertains to several areas. A brief overview of five specific areas is provided next.

Exercise and Mental Health

One of the most researched areas in exercise psychology is the relationship between acute and chronic exercise and improvement of mental health. *Mental health* is used to characterize psychological function on a continuum from suboptimal to optimal (Henriksen et al., 2020). Suboptimal mental health is contemporarily referred to as a mental illness. Both acute and chronic exercise, as well as aerobic and anaerobic exercise, are known to reduce stress (Herbert et al., 2020), state anxiety (Ensari et al., 2015), and depression (Heissel et al., 2023), as well as to improve mood (Smith and Merwin, 2021) and self-esteem (Kim and Ahn, 2021). Several mechanisms have been hypothesized to explain the increases in positive affect following an acute bout of exercise including the **endorphin hypothesis**, which holds that an increase in circulating endorphins produces feelings of euphoria; and the **mastery hypothesis**, which holds that exercise may increase one's sense of self-mastery or accomplishment, thereby leading to improved affect (Brown, 1991; Ransford, 1982; Steinberg and Sykes, 1985).

Exercise and Quality of Life

Regular engagement in exercise improves various aspects of mental health, which in turn improves quality of life. **Quality of life** is characterized as the overall standard of living with regard to mental and physical health, social relationships, level of independence, personal beliefs and spirituality, and relationship to the environment (Felce and Perry, 1995). Research by Martin et al. (2009) reported a significant positive dose-response relationship between amount of exercise completed and physical and psychological quality of life measurements. Specifically, postmenopausal women who completed just 74 minutes per week of exercise reported improved quality of life (i.e., physical functioning, role limitations because of physical problems, bodily pain, general health perception, role limitations because of emotional problems, social functioning, vitality, and mental health) compared to individuals who did not exercise. Other researchers have identified the positive impact exercise participation has on improving quality of life in apparently healthy individuals (Berger and Tobar, 2011) as well as in special populations such as people with cancer (Knobf, Musanti, and Dorward, 2007) and stroke survivors (Chen and Rimmer, 2011).

Exercise and Cognitive Function

Regular engagement in exercise also improves **cognitive functioning**, the process by which individuals take in, use, and respond to information (Morley, 2018). Research supports the notion that aerobic exercise improves the speed, efficiency, and accuracy of cognitive functioning (Ferrer-Uris et al., 2022). Specifically, exercise facilitates cognitive functioning by improving attentional focus and concentration, storage and retrieval of information, and execution of motor skills. The combination of aging and a sedentary lifestyle reduces cognitive functioning (Anshel, 2011), yet both acute and chronic exercise have demonstrated short-term and long-term improvements in cognitive functioning.

Exercise Adherence

An area of concern among exercise professionals is the high rate of attrition commonly seen in exercise programs. **Exercise adherence** refers to the degree to which an individual follows the recommended frequency, intensity, and duration in any given program or activity. Research has shown that approximately 50 percent of those who begin exercise programs discontinue within the first 6 months (Biddle and Mutrie, 2008). Exercise psychology professionals are interested in learning more about the discrepancy between the desire to exercise and the ability to adhere to an exercise regimen.

To that end, researchers have identified a multitude of psychological, physiological, social, and program factors that affect exercise adherence. Psychological factors include aspects of personality such as self-motivation, attitudes toward exercise, and health knowledge and beliefs (Willis and Campbell, 1992). Physiological factors include body weight, body fat, angina pectoris, and left ventricular ejection fraction (Markland and Ingledew, 2007). Social factors include marital status, spousal and family social support, peer social support, and work demands (Willis and Campbell, 1992). Program factors include enjoyment, convenience, quality of the exercise facility and equipment, program social support, group versus individual programs, program leadership, and program intensity (Willis and Campbell, 1992).

Exercise Addiction

Exercise addiction refers to the psychological dependence on regularly scheduled exercise (Landolfi, 2013). An individual who is addicted to exercise will continue to exercise regardless of physical injury, personal inconvenience, or scheduling conflicts, and experiences a high degree of anxiety, depression, and discomfort if they miss an exercise session (Colledge et al., 2020). Addiction to exercise is considered positive when it occurs in an individual chasing a runner's high (i.e., a psychological phenomenon experienced by some runners whereby the runner has heightened euphoria and awareness; Sachs, 1984), and it is considered negative when it occurs in an individual who presents with symptoms of a clinical eating disorder or body dysmorphia. Practitioners working with exercisers should monitor exercise intensity, duration, and general affect with regard to exercising and make referrals to the appropriate medical and/or mental health professional if it is observed that the exerciser is experiencing tolerance, loss of control, persistence to exercise in the face of injury or illness, excessive time, and/or conflicts with occupational or social activities (Juwono, Tolnai, and Szabo, 2022).

SPORTS/PERFORMANCE ASPECTS

Sport psychology pertains to several areas. A brief overview of five specific areas is provided next.

Stress, Arousal, and Anxiety

Many individuals use the terms stress, arousal, and anxiety interchangeably, yet distinct differences exist. **Stress** is described by contemporary researchers within a sport context as a collection of demands that disturb the homeostasis of physiological and metabolic processes (Kellmann et al., 2018). Smith (1986) conceptualized a cognitive-affective model of stress, consisting of four interrelated stages, that helps to explain the relationship between stress and performance:

- stage 1: an objective demand is placed on the athlete (e.g., increased training load)
- stage 2: the athlete cognitively appraises the demand to determine if resources are available to meet the demand (e.g., increased rest and/or fuel)
- stage 3: cognitive appraisal of the demand results in a physiological response. In the case of a perceived inability to meet the demand, negative physiological responses that are deleterious to performance and/or health (e.g., elevated heart rate, increased anxiety, susceptibility to illness or injury) may occur
- stage 4: the athlete responds by trying to cope with the demand (e.g., increased rest and/or fuel) or by eliminating the demand altogether (e.g., withdrawing from the activity)

As indicated by Smith's model, the antecedents of stress might include event importance, uncertainty, history or past experiences, confidence, and/or trait anxiety. These sources of stress, in turn, generate a psychological and physiological response to the stressor which may subsequently impact performance. For example, a freshman collegiate swimmer who is navigating their first experience with course finals as well as the travel schedule might have a negative appraisal toward these demands. The swimmer does not perceive they have the resources (e.g., time, energy) to meet the demands, thus they experience increased anxiety, leading to less rest and more susceptibility to injury. Consequently, the swimmer fails to complete class assignments and also gets pulled from individual events and relays due to performance decrements in the pool.

Arousal is a combination of physiological and psychological activation that varies on a continuum from very un-aroused (e.g., sleeping) to very aroused (e.g., highly excited, animated; Taylor and Wilson, 2002). Arousal is not inherently labeled as good or bad, as an individual might become highly aroused (e.g., increased respiration and heart rate) when hearing the national anthem at the start of a soccer game due to nervousness *or* due to excitement. Easterbrook's (1959) **cue utilization theory** describes the influence of physiological and psychological arousal on attention, and how the intersection of arousal and attention may influence performance. When arousal is too high, individuals have a narrowed attentional focus whereby they miss relevant cues in the environment. For example, a soccer player who is highly anxious might miss an opponent slide tackling them from the left. When arousal is too low, individuals have a broad attentional focus whereby focus might be on irrelevant cues in the environment. For example, a bored soccer defender is observing activities happening off field when their attention should be on watching for approaching forwards. When arousal is optimal or just right, individuals can scan the environment for relevant cues whereby they ignore irrelevant cues and focus on cues most germane to successful task completion. In the case of the above soccer player, optimal arousal enables them to scan the environment to accurately pass the ball (and ignore the irrelevant cheering from the stands), and to protect themselves from the slide tackle.

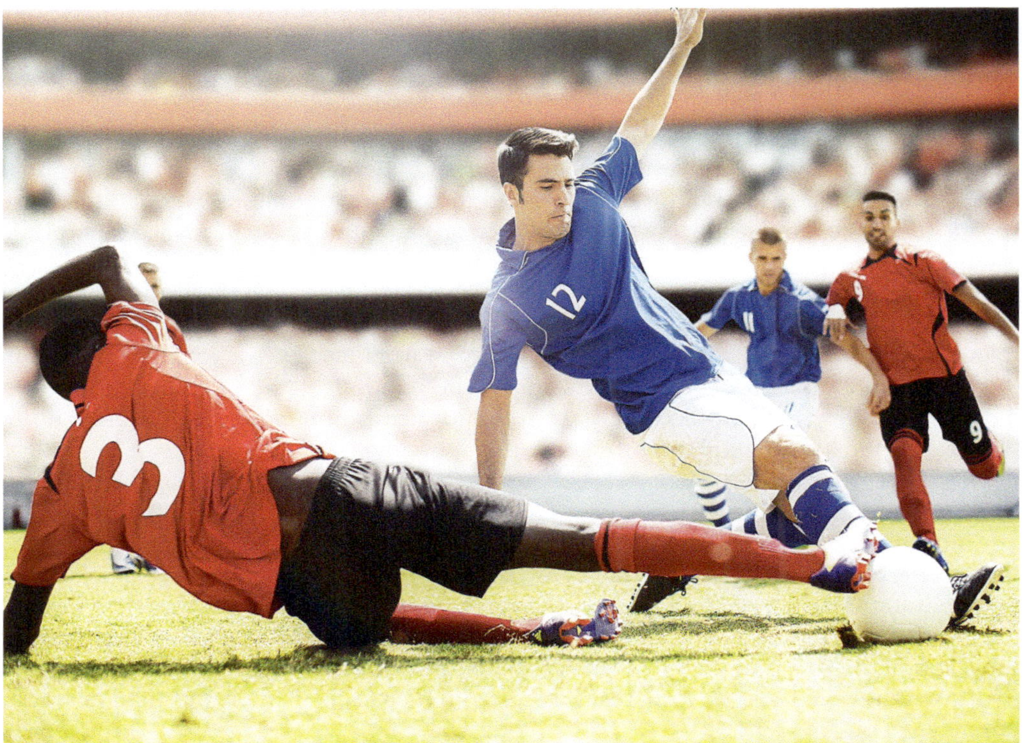

Finally, **anxiety** is described as a negative emotional state and is associated with physiological and/or psychological responses (Martens, Vealey, and Burton, 1990). Anxiety can manifest cognitively (e.g., rumination, worry, apprehension) and/or somatically (e.g., increased heart rate and respiration, gastrointestinal distress, perspiration). An athlete might be nervous about an upcoming tournament, in which they worry about their performance and also have sweaty palms and an upset stomach as university scouts are observing their skills. Furthermore, an individual might have state anxiety, whereby cognitive and somatic symptoms are ever-changing and dependent on the situation. State anxiety is unstable, or not permanent. Trait anxiety, on the other hand, is part of an individual's personality and *is* stable and permanent. An individual with trait anxiety may perceive a non-threatening situation to be threatening and have a disproportionate cognitive and/or somatic reaction to the situation.

Several theories exist to help scholars understand how stress, arousal, and anxiety influence performance; however, three main theories are currently used by today's scholars. Hanin's (1997) individualized zones of optimal functioning (IZOF) model is used to describe how athletes have a "zone" of optimal state anxiety in which their best performance occurs. When athletes are outside this zone, poor performance occurs. These zones operate on a continuum from low state anxiety to high state anxiety. An athlete who has a low IZOF will perform best when their state anxiety level is low (e.g., low heart rate and respiration rate, calm). Accordingly, an athlete who has a moderate IZOF will perform best when their state anxiety level is moderate (e.g., not too calm, not too excited). An athlete who has a high IZOF will be expected to perform best when their state anxiety level is high (e.g., highly excited). It is important for practitioners to help athletes identify their optimal zone of functioning by recalling their best previous performances. Subsequently, practitioners will use various strategies to help an athlete shift into their optimal zone to be prepared for performance.

Hardy's (1996) catastrophe model is used to understand the interaction between physiological arousal and cognitive anxiety. If cognitive anxiety is low (i.e., not worried about performance), increases in arousal are related to performance in an inverted-U pattern. As an athlete's cognitive anxiety increases, arousal can improve performance to a certain point, after which performance systematically decreases. If cognitive anxiety is high (i.e., very worried about performance), the increases in arousal reach a threshold of optimal performance, after which performance deteriorates rapidly—or catastrophically. Physiological arousal and/or cognitive anxiety will then need to decrease for performance to increase. Taken together, practitioners should be mindful of the relationship between cognitive anxiety and physiological arousal and incorporate strategies accordingly to facilitate optimal individual performance.

Kerr's (1997) reversal theory is used to explain how an athlete's interpretation of their arousal influences performance. One athlete might perceive high arousal to be an indicator of feeling nervous, while another athlete might perceive high arousal to be an indicator of excitement. Athletes are thought to make "reversals," or quick shifts, in their interpretation of arousal levels. Therefore, an athlete might perceive their arousal as positive one moment, and then quickly shift to perceive the arousal as negative the next moment. To optimize performance, practitioners consulting with athletes should work with them to be able to perceive high arousal as excitement rather than nerves or anxiety.

Motivation

Another area in exercise and sport psychology is **motivation**, described as the direction and intensity of one's effort (Sage, 1977). Direction of effort refers to starting or stopping a behavior. For example, a golfer might begin private lessons to lower their overall score, or a mixed martial arts athlete might reduce their late-night eating to make weigh-in at an upcoming fight. Intensity of effort refers to how much effort an individual puts forth. For example, while two youth athletes might start ice hockey camp for the first time, one athlete might put forth considerably more effort than the other athlete during practice.

The direction and intensity of an individual's motivation is determined in part by their approach to the situation. Three approaches to motivation are described below.

- A person-centered approach identifies the personal characteristics of individuals (e.g., personal interests, goals, personality traits) as the determinants that influence direction and intensity of a behavior. For example, an athlete who has global self-esteem may not hesitate before starting a new sport such as pickleball.
- A situation-centered approach characterizes the environment (e.g., social support, weather, facilities) as the determinants that influence direction and intensity of a behavior. For example, a youth gymnast might be motivated to apply effort during practice, but not during a competition.
- An interactional approach characterizes both the personal and the situational factors as the determinants that influence direction and intensity of a behavior. This approach to motivation is the most widely accepted by exercise and sport psychology professionals. Using the aforementioned pickleball example, an athlete who does not have global self-esteem might hesitate to start playing pickleball unless they are playing with their best friends, at which point they are highly motivated to begin.

Several theories of motivation exist to help scholars understand how motivation can be applied to individuals and groups to improve motivation; however, three main theories are currently used by today's scholars. According to the achievement goal theory (Nicholls, 1989), an individual is motivated by their perception of what it takes to achieve success. The two goal orientations are ego orientation and task orientation. When an individual is ego oriented, they have a desire to demonstrate superior competence relative to others and/or normative standards. These individuals are motivated by the outcome, and winning or beating others is the goal. For example, an ego-oriented basketball player will perceive the game as a success if they have the highest free throw percentage in a game, even if it wasn't their best game or their team lost. When an individual is task oriented, they have a desire to meet the demands of the task, exerting effort, and developing their own competence with the task. These individuals are motivated by mastering the task, and improving their own past performance is the goal. For example, a task-oriented basketball player will perceive the game as a success if they have their personal best highest free throw percentage during a game, even if it wasn't the best free throw percentage on the team. These two goal orientations are independent of one another, meaning that one or both orientations may exist within an individual.

According to self-determination theory (Deci and Ryan, 1985), an individual is motivated in part by the three basic needs of competence (i.e., the ability to successfully complete a task), autonomy (i.e., control over choices being made), and relatedness (i.e., feeling supported and understood by others). When an individual does not have competence, autonomy, and/or relatedness as they approach a task, the propensity for that individual to discontinue or experience burnout is greater. For example, an athlete rehabilitating a knee injury will feel motivated if they perceive that they can complete their at-home exercises successfully, if they have a choice in the exercises they are completing, and if they feel understood and supported by the practitioner providing oversight of their physical rehabilitation.

According to Dweck and Leggett's (1988) theories of intelligence, an individual's motivation is influenced by their perception of ability as stable or dynamic. When an individual has an entity perspective on ability, they perceive that their abilities (e.g., intelligence, athleticism) are fixed and cannot change over time. These individuals focus on performance-oriented goals in which they know they can win, and they attribute failure to lack of ability, rather than lack of effort. It is not unusual for individuals with an entity view on ability to discontinue their participation in activities in which they have little initial success. Conversely, when an individual has an incremental perspective on ability (i.e., growth mindset), they perceive that their abilities are malleable and can be changed over time with effort. These individuals focus on mastery-oriented goals where they can develop skills, and they attribute failure to situational factors. Ideally, athletes learn to foster a growth mindset whereby they persist in the face of setbacks (rather than give up), embrace challenging situations (rather than avoid challenges), and learn from critical feedback (rather than ignore feedback).

Confidence and Self-Efficacy

Confidence is described as an individual's belief in their ability to be successful. Research by Vealey and Chase (2008) suggests that confidence can take the form of a state (i.e., perceived in the moment and dynamic) or a trait (i.e., part of one's personality and stable). It is beneficial for athletes to feel confident, as confidence enhances concentration, increases effort, regulates positive emotions, affects goals, and has an overall impact on performance. **Self-efficacy** refers to an individual's belief in their ability to accomplish a specific task (Bandura, 1977). Several theories of confidence and self-efficacy exist to help scholars understand how confidence plays a role in athlete success. Two main theories used by scholars today are the self-efficacy theory and the multidimensional model of self-confidence.

Self-efficacy theory (Bandura, 1986) is used to describe the four sources of an individual's confidence in a specific task. The task is situation-specific and one's confidence relevant to the task can change across time. The four sources of self-efficacy are listed below in order of importance.

- Performance accomplishments include previous successful attempts at a task and are the primary source of self-efficacy. For example, an athlete who successfully swims 100 meters of freestyle is likely to feel confident in achieving this task again in the future. To improve the confidence of novice athletes, it is important to start with tasks where the probability of success is high (i.e., swimming 25 or 50 meters of freestyle).
- Vicarious or imaginal experiences include watching others or imagining oneself successfully performing a task. For example, observing a diving teammate complete a back somersault tuck can reduce anxiety and improve confidence in believing they too can complete the back somersault tuck.

- Verbal persuasion includes verbal encouragement in the form of self-talk or positive feedback from others. Elite athletes often utilize self-talk to improve their confidence, and subsequently their performance. For example, an athlete might tell themselves, "You can do it; trust your training."
- Physiological and affective states include physical arousal and emotions. Heart rate, respiration rate, perspiration, and mood can influence how one performs at a given task. For example, an athlete's confidence can decrease if they normally feel calm before hitting a golf ball off the tee, yet now feel their heart rate increase and tension building in their shoulders.

The multidimensional model of sport confidence (Vealey, 2002) is used to describe the multiple sources of sport confidence and the influence these sources have on performance. Demographic factors (e.g., age, race), personality (e.g., goal orientation), and organizational culture (e.g., motivational climate, goals, competitive standard) influence three sources of sport confidence: (a) achievement (i.e., mastery and ability), (b) self-regulation (i.e., physical and mental preparation), and (c) social climate (i.e., social support, leadership, and environmental factors). These three sources, in turn, influence and are influenced by three types of sport confidence (i.e., decision-making skills, physical training, and resilience). How confident an athlete perceives themself to be in their decision-making skills, physical training, and resiliency, subsequently influences their affect, behavior, and cognition, which ultimately affects performance. For example, a volleyball player who has an optimistic personality and a mastery-oriented coach will feel confident in her ability to block the volleyball, be mentally prepared before games, and communicate effectively with her teammates during games. Consequently, she has good

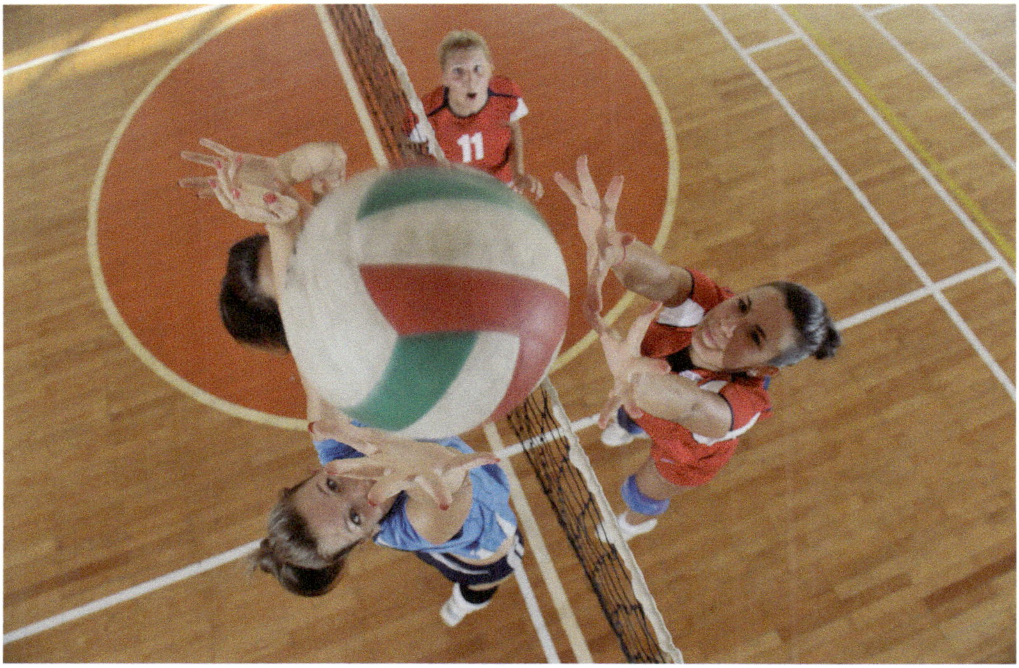

decision-making skills, trusts her physical training, and can refocus after making an error. She then has solution-focused and positive affect, behavior, and cognitions. Taken together, she is confident in her ability to play as a middle blocker.

Team Dynamics

A **team** is described as any group of individuals who interact with one another to achieve a superordinate goal (Carron and Hausenblas, 1998). **Team dynamics** involves the process of developing roles, establishing norms, and utilizing a shared communication method to achieve the collective goal (Carron and Eys, 2012).

Tuckman (1965) proposed that teams go through four stages as they develop and strive to achieve the superordinate goal.

- The "forming" stage occurs when athletes are familiarizing themselves with each other, understanding their similarities and differences.
- The "storming" stage occurs when athletes begin to have interpersonal conflict. Conflict can ensue as individuals determine their role and status within the team.
- The "norming" stage occurs when conflict is replaced by cooperation and a sense of unity forms. The athletes begin to work together to reach their superordinate goal.
- The "performing" stage occurs when athletes understand and embrace their roles, relationships are solidified, and progress is made toward achieving the superordinate goal.

For a team to function optimally, athletes need to have clarity in their roles, accept their roles, and execute their roles. Roles might be formal (e.g., appointed, organized) such as team captain or quarterback, or informal (e.g., unappointed, unorganized) such as team comedian or star player. To function optimally, a team should also have norms, or expectations for the standards of behavior for all athletes. Norms on an athletic team might include showing up for all team events 10 minutes in advance, wearing team athletic apparel in the strength and conditioning room, or consistently checking the team chat every morning. Taken together, for optimal team dynamics, and to subsequently improve team performance, it is essential that strong communication exists between athletes, coaches, support staff, and administrators so that all members of a team are working cooperatively and cohesively toward the same superordinate goal.

Burnout and Recovery

Burnout is a psychological syndrome caused by a prolonged response to stress (Raedeke and Smith, 2001) and often coincides with the physiological symptoms of overtraining. Three characteristics are consistent with sport burnout: emotional exhaustion (i.e., a feeling of being emotionally overextended by sport), depersonalization (i.e., a feeling of detachment or indifference towards sport), and reduced personal accomplishment (i.e., a feeling of negative evaluation of one's achievements in sport). For example, a tennis player who is experiencing symptoms of burnout might feel joyless or frustrated when playing, find excuses to avoid going to practice, and feel less successful during games.

To reduce the risk of developing burnout, researchers and practitioners have begun to encourage engagement in recovery strategies. **Recovery** has been conceptualized as a restorative process occurring after a psychophysiological stressor arises and/or as a proactive process before the stressor arises (Kallus and Kellmann, 2016; Kellmann et al., 2018). Currently, the best practice in facilitating recovery is a multidimensional approach comprised of physical recovery activities (e.g., foam rolling, ice baths), psychological recovery activities (e.g., journaling, reading), and social recovery activities (e.g., positive interactions with friends). To optimize recovery, athletes should match the recovery mechanism to the stressor. For example, a basketball player might take proactive steps to mitigate the risk of sport overtraining and burnout by thoroughly stretching after every practice to reduce soreness, spending 30 minutes each day mentally detaching from basketball by drawing, and calling family each week to interact with non-sport individuals.

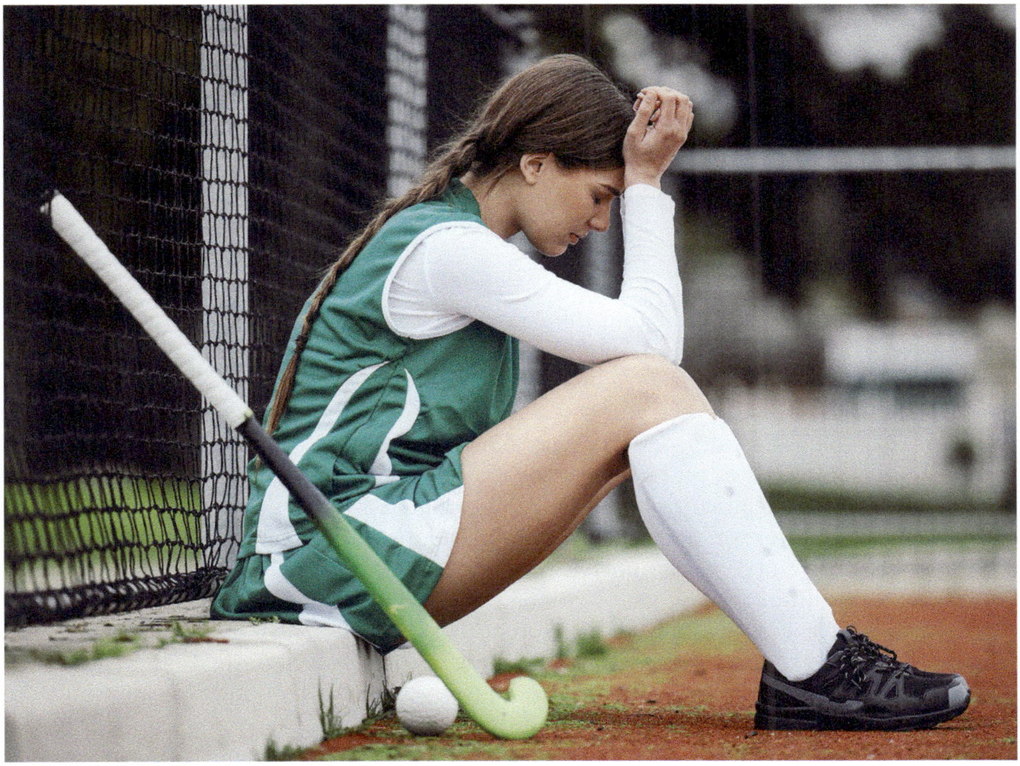

To better conceptualize the relationship between recovery and stress, two main athlete recovery models have been proposed. Kenttä and Hassmén (1998) developed the overtraining and recovery conceptual model, asserting that the recovery process must include engagement in recovery activities which match the source and magnitude of the stress to counterbalance the deleterious effects of stress. For example, stressors of a psychological origin should be matched with recovery interventions that alleviate the psychological stress (e.g., meditation, journaling). As in the aforementioned example, the basketball player is balancing the source of the stress with an appropriate, matched recovery strategy.

Kellmann and Kallus (2001) developed the scissors-model of the interrelation of stress-states and recovery demands, describing that increases in recovery must simultaneously occur as stress increases if the stress-recovery balance is to remain stable. The stress states and recovery demands affect one another such that if an athlete is unwilling or unable to take the time to recover, more stress will accumulate which can lead to symptoms of overtraining (Kellmann, 2002). When an athlete does make time to regularly engage in quality recovery activities, an increase in stress will not necessarily impact their performance and health. Thus, when an athlete perceives an event or day(s) to be particularly stressful, they should prioritize time to engage in recovery activities to counterbalance the stress and avoid the accumulated effects of the stress symptoms. For example, in the days leading up to a competition, athletes should devote extra time to rest and engage in physical recovery strategies, even if they perceive they cannot make the time. When they do prioritize the time to rest, a continued increase in stress during competition will not necessarily impact their performance.

TECHNOLOGY AND RESEARCH TOOLS

Technology used to advance research and application has been a game changer in the 21st century, impacting not only the field of exercise science but the discipline of exercise and sport psychology as well. The most widely utilized methods of collecting data and advancing practical knowledge are discussed below.

Assessments

The use of assessments for eliciting information from athletes is commonplace in exercise and sport psychology research and applied practice (Taylor, 2017). Assessments are used in research to quantitatively assess performance-related variables, whereby statistics are applied to the data to infer outcomes. Assessments are also used in research and applied practice to collect information about an athlete client; conceptualize their case; and develop, deliver, monitor, and assess interventions (Vealey et al., 2019). Due diligence by the researcher and practitioner should be completed to ensure that assessments are psychometrically appropriate for the target population. Furthermore, not only should practitioners be trained to administer, score, and interpret assessments (AASP, 2024), and thus work within their scope of competence to do no harm, it is also worth noting additional impacts assessments can have on athletes. When distributing assessments to a sample of athletes for research or applied practice purposes, providing them with results and/or feedback is a way to extend gratitude to the athletes for their time as well as to possibly improve their performance.

Biofeedback

Biofeedback technology allows individuals to utilize live physiological feedback to facilitate psychophysiological awareness (Sime, 2003), thus ideally leading to optimal performance. Common forms of biofeedback include neurofeedback, thermal biofeedback, electromyography, and the most widely used biofeedback in exercise and sport psychology—heart rate variability biofeedback (Gross et al., 2019). This biofeedback method involves placing sensors on the body such that heart rate variability, a physiological measure of the autonomic nervous system, is captured and displayed on a monitor. Individuals are then tasked with following various breathing protocols to align their heart and respiratory rates with the overall aim of reducing these rates and subsequently promoting relaxation. In exercise and sport psychology, biofeedback is most often used to manage anxiety and pre-performance competitive stress, enhance sleep quality, manage pain during injury rehabilitation, and develop mindfulness (Gross et al., 2019; Morgan and Mora, 2017).

Virtual Reality

Virtual reality is a computer-based system that offers an immersive and interactive simulation experience for exercisers and athletes (Katz et al., 2006). The most common type of virtual reality system is a head-mounted display, whereby an individual wears headgear in which two digital screens relay images to the user. The advanced technology of virtual reality systems allows for individuals to experience live sensory information, thus enabling them to practice appropriate responses that can prepare them for actual scenarios. Virtual reality is one of the most promising technologies in exercise, sport, and performance settings. Within an exercise and sport setting, virtual reality is used for a variety of reasons, including to improve perceptual-cognitive skills, promote relaxation, facilitate injury rehabilitation, and achieve more repetitions with reduced risk of injury (Bird, 2020).

Research Abstract

Research methodologies for exercise and sport psychology include both quantitative and qualitative approaches. The published abstract below serves as an example of a quantitative approach to studying sport psychology using a tactical population.

Exhibit 9.2 Abstract of a quantitative research study in exercise psychology

Wahl, C.A., Meyer, B.B., & Ebersole, K.T. (2024, July). *Differences in stress, recovery, and engagement in recovery activities between ranks of active-duty firefighters* [Conference presentation]. National Strength and Conditioning Conference, Baltimore, MD, United States.

To optimize workplace functioning and reduce chronic stress, burnout, and poor health throughout an organization, sport and occupational health researchers have recently begun to examine the importance of recovery for both the individual (e.g., athlete) as well as the staff and leaders (e.g., athletic trainers, coaches) around the individual. Similar organizational structures exist within the fire service, whereby the recovery needs for staff or those at higher ranks (e.g., Lieutenant [Lt]) are just as important to consider as those at lower ranks (e.g., firefighters [FF]) due to their unique job duties and stressors. This organization-wide approach to recovery, however, has not previously been examined in the fire service. Failure to examine differences in perceptions of stress and recovery or the specific recovery activities engaged in by FFs of various ranks precludes recommendations of rank-specific recovery interventions.

Purpose: To examine the differences in perceived stress and recovery status and recovery activities between FFs of a lower rank and FFs of a higher rank.

Methods: 261 (239 male, 22 female) active-duty FFs (age: 39.2 ± 9.4 yrs) completed the FF-adapted version of the Assessment of Recovery Activities for Athletes (ARAA-FF) to measure type and frequency of recovery activities engaged in over a 7-day period, as well as perceptions of stress and recovery status. 154 FFs reported being of a lower rank (i.e., FF and Heavy Equipment Operator [HEO]), while 107 FFs reported being of a higher rank (i.e., Lt, Captain [Cpt], and Battalion Chief [BC]). Independent t-tests ($p < 0.05$) were used to examine the differences between FF ranks in ARAA-FF subscales and perceptions of stress and recovery status.

Results: Results indicated that lower rank FFs had significantly lower scores on the *Sleep* ($t(259) = -2.06$, $p = 0.041$) and significantly higher scores on the *Training Breaks* ($t(259) = 2.53$, $p = 0.012$) subscales of the ARAA-FF. No significant differences ($p > 0.05$) existed between ranks on perceptions of physical, psychological, or social stress or recovery status. While not statistically significant, FFs of a lower rank engaged in recovery activities to promote *Psychological Detachment*, *Community*, *Firefighter Interactions*, and *Non-Firefighter Interactions* more than FFs of a higher rank, whereas FFs of a higher rank engaged in recovery activities to promote *Readiness, Relaxation, Mastery,* and *Autonomy* more than FFs of a lower rank.

Conclusions: Higher FF rank is associated with higher levels of sleep-promoting activities (e.g., sleeping in a cool, dark environment), yet lower levels of perceived training breaks (e.g., using off-duty time to physically relax and recover, saving energy for oneself).

Practical Applications: While rank might not influence a FF's ability to detach from work, implement adequate nutrition strategies, or engage in social recovery activities, significant differences emerged that warrant practical application. Developing sleep hygiene protocols for FFs or HEOs might be beneficial to promote recovery, especially when considering that these FFs often have communal bunking while on-duty. In contrast, discussing the importance of utilizing off-duty time to physically relax may be beneficial for "bosses", or those FFs of the Lt, Cpt, or BC rank. Implementation of these protocols may improve on- and off-duty recovery for individuals across all ranks.

CAREER AND EMPLOYMENT OPPORTUNITIES

General Description of Career Opportunities

Employment opportunities in exercise and sport psychology are continuously evolving and expanding. Contemporary exercise and sport psychology professionals can pursue a variety of careers beyond those traditionally found in higher education, including working as consultants to clients in the health and wellness, elite sport, tactical, and other performance domains. Individuals consulting with clients may work as an employee of a corporation, or as an employee of their own private consultancy. Whether operating independently or as an employee within a larger firm or academic institution, exercise and sport psychology professionals may possess the credentials and competencies to work in the domains described below.

Consultants Working Within a Health and Wellness Domain

Exercise psychology professionals work within corporate wellness, applying motivational and adherence strategies to improve the health and wellness of employees. Sport and performance psychology professionals work with companies such as Peloton or Polar to improve holistic performance parameters including heart rate variability and other recovery metrics. Exercise and sport psychology professionals might also consult independently with individuals trying to adapt or adhere to a program of regular physical activity as well as those working toward a specific exercise or fitness goal. These professionals might be dual credentialed so that they can legally and ethically work within performance parameters as well as assist in cases where there are clinical mental health concerns.

Consultants Working Within an Elite Sport Domain

Sport psychology professionals work within elite sport helping athletes, teams, coaches, and sport organizations to optimize mental performance and/or mental health. Since the National Collegiate Athletic Association (NCAA) placed an emphasis on monitoring and improving student-athlete mental health and well-being, it has become common for larger universities to employ a full-time sport psychologist to oversee the mental health and wellness of the athletic department. Many of these positions require a dual credentialed professional, such that the staff member possesses the competencies required to provide service in both mental performance and clinical mental health. Sport psychology professionals may find similar work within Olympic and professional sport organizations and, pending formal training and experience, they may progress into various performance management and/or front office roles.

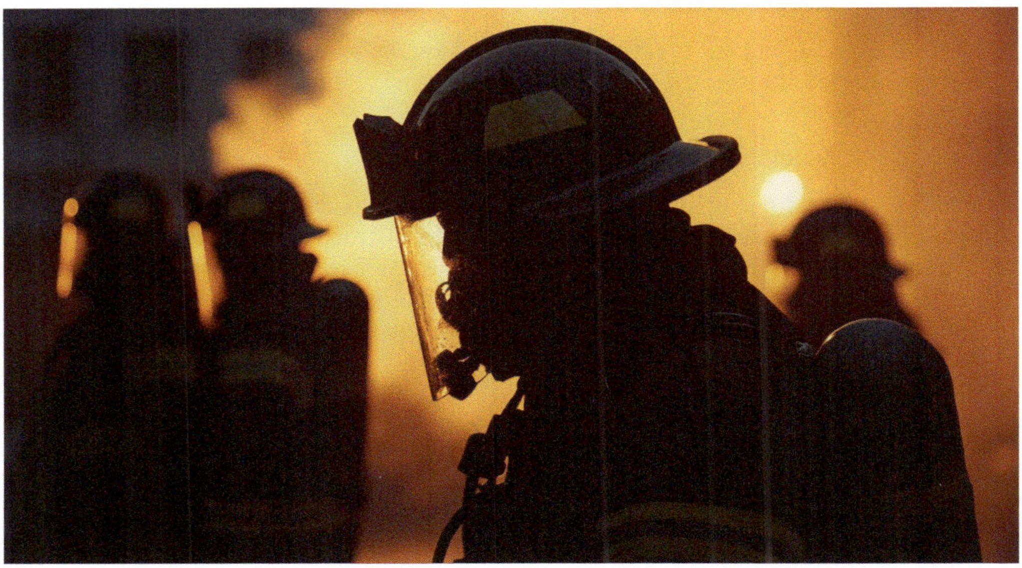

Consultants Working Within a Tactical Domain

The military is currently the second largest employer of sport and performance psychology professionals (AASP, 2021). These professionals help prepare military members for peak performance and resiliency or work with them to reduce post-traumatic stress disorder symptoms. Concurrently, sport and performance psychology professionals work with military personnel on self-regulation, team dynamics, and communication, all of which have the potential to optimize their performance in training and combat. Other tactical populations such as firefighters, police officers, and first responders have also begun to employ sport and performance psychology professionals to optimize individuals' health, wellness, and performance in the line of duty.

Consultants Working Within Other Performance Domains

Doctors perfecting their surgical skills, singers and actors preparing for long tours and performances, and corporate managing directors or partners working to improve their leadership skills are further examples of sport and performance psychology services being utilized, and where consulting opportunities exist.

Higher Education

Historically, careers within higher education have predominated among individuals with training in exercise and sport psychology. Some sport and exercise psychology professionals choose to work in academia, where they teach classes and engage in research. Research opportunities exist within colleges and universities, sport research institutes, medical research laboratories, and other settings. Furthermore, and consistent with the trend toward consulting in applied exercise and sport psychology, academicians working within a university setting might also seek collaborations embedded as a mental performance consultant within an athletic department.

EDUCATION REQUIREMENTS

For future exercise and sport psychology professionals, several educational tracks exist. The track selected is informed primarily by career goal.

Clinical Mental Health Exercise and Sport Specialist

Clinical mental health specialists have extensive training in clinical or counseling psychology, counseling, or social work, supporting the diagnosis and treatment of individuals with clinical mental health concerns. These professionals are licensed by state boards and are ethically and legally able to treat individuals with emotional disorders. Just as the population at large can develop clinical mental health concerns, so too can exercisers and athletes.

Educational Exercise and Sport Specialists

Educational specialists have extensive training in exercise science and have secondary training in the biopsychosocial aspects of human movement. Consistent with their training and competencies, educational specialists are not licensed mental health providers. Instead, educational specialists must refer to licensed providers if a client presents with an emotional disorder. Educational exercise and sport specialists are often described as "mental coaches," whereby they possess the graduate level training to educate individuals and teams on psychological skills to improve their health, wellness, and performance. For example, these professionals might discuss how to facilitate a mastery oriented motivational climate with a youth sport coach or parent, introduce goal setting strategies to maximize exercise adoption and adherence with an older adult, or teach breathing strategies to decrease pre-performance anxiety in a softball player.

Dual Credentials

Given the emphasis on improving clinical mental health and wellness among athletes and exercisers, it is not uncommon for professionals to be dual credentialed, meaning they have advanced degrees and training in both clinical mental health and educational exercise and sport psychology. Degree options, licensure, and certifications for careers are discussed below.

CERTIFICATIONS AND LICENSURE

Over 100 graduate degree programs around the world exist in sport and exercise psychology. Some of these programs prepare students for clinical mental health careers, while others prepare students for educational careers.

Clinical Mental Health Graduate Programs

Students interested in a career that allows them to work with exercisers, athletes, and other performers within a clinical mental health setting may pursue a Doctor of Philosophy (PhD) in Counseling or Clinical Psychology or a Doctor of Psychology (PsyD). These programs are licensed by the American Psychological Association (APA), and the student must complete extensive educational and internship supervision requirements before sitting for a state licensure examination. The term *psychologist* is a legally protected term, whereby only individuals who complete all APA requirements can title themselves as a psychologist. If a student is not interested in pursuing a doctoral degree to become a licensed mental health provider, two master's level degree programs exist: Licensed Professional Counselor (LPC) and Clinical Social Worker (LCSW). Both LPCs and LCSWs can diagnose and treat a variety of mental, emotional, and behavioral concerns, while LCSWs are also trained to help clients with other aspects of life (e.g., housing, employment). Few clinical mental health graduate programs currently offer additional education in exercise and sport psychology. As such, students working in mental health who want to specialize with exercise, sport, and other performance populations must seek additional educational opportunities to ensure they are knowledgeable in other exercise science disciplines such as exercise physiology, motor learning, and biomechanics, among others.

Educational Graduate Programs

Students interested in a career that allows them to work with exercisers, athletes, and other performers on mental performance exclusively may pursue a PhD, Doctor of Education (EdD), or master's degree in a non-psychology-related discipline (e.g., kinesiology, health sciences). Each of the above degree options should be accompanied by a specific emphasis, track, or specialization in sport, performance, and/or exercise psychology so that the student receives additional training in sport and exercise psychology.

Dual Credentials

Students interested in a career within both clinical mental health and mental performance settings may pursue an educational path that results in dual credentialing (i.e., a combination of degree options that leads to competence in both clinical mental health and educational exercise and sport psychology). For example, they might have a master's degree in kinesiology with an emphasis in sport and performance psychology and a PhD in counseling psychology; or, they might have two master's degrees, one in clinical social work and the other in kinesiology with an emphasis on psychosocial sport studies. A variety of educational pathways exist for students who want to work with exercisers, athletes, and other performers on both mental health and mental performance.

Certification

The only certification approved by the AASP is the Certified Mental Performance Consultant (CMPC®). To hold this certification, professionals must possess a graduate degree and (a) complete designated graduate-level coursework in both exercise science and psychology; (b) complete a minimum of 400 hours of applied work with athletes, exercisers, or performers; (c) pass a certification exam; and (d) engage in continuing education. Today, and regardless of the degree(s) one holds, employers often seek professionals who possess the CMPC credential, which signifies their holistic expertise, education, and training in both exercise science and psychology.

PROFESSIONAL ORGANIZATIONS

Exercise and sport psychology researchers and professionals may be members of one or more professional organizations. The following is a list of the most recognized organizations.

Exhibit 9.3 Professional organizations

Association for Applied Sport Psychology (AASP)
https://appliedsportpsych.org/

American Psychological Association Division 47 (Exercise and Sport)
https://www.apa.org/about/division/div47

British Association of Sport and Exercise Sciences (BASES)
https://www.bases.org.uk/

Canadian Sport Psychology Association (CSPA)
https://www.cspa-acps.com/

European Federation of Sport Psychology (FEPSAC)
https://fepsac.com/

International Society of Sport Psychology
https://issponline.org/

North American Society of Sport Psychology (NASPSPA)
https://www.naspspa.com/

JOURNALS

Exercise and sport psychology-related research can be found in various journals and related publications. The following list includes journals that are most prominent in the discipline.

- *Journal of Applied Sport Psychology*
- *Journal of Sport Psychology in Action*
- *Sport, Exercise, and Performance Psychology*

- *International Journal of Sport and Exercise Psychology*
- *Journal of Sport and Exercise Psychology*
- *The Sport Psychologist*
- *Journal of Counseling and Clinical Psychology*
- *Frontiers in Psychology: Movement Science and Sport Psychology*

FUTURE DIRECTIONS

While scholars have made great strides over the past 150 years in understanding and applying exercise and sport psychology to athletes, exercisers, performers and others, the need for continued research is ongoing. Below are three areas in need of future research.

Use of Technology in Sport Psychology

The AASP published a special edition on the use of technology in applied sport psychology featuring biofeedback, virtual reality, and eye tracking devices (Watson and Coker-Cranney, 2019). Just as technology is always advancing, so too is the need for research on the application to and advancement of sport psychology. Coaches and athletes have been using technology to gain a physical, technical, or tactical edge for decades, whereas using technology to gain a psychological edge has only recently begun. As consumers are constantly within reach of their smartphones, development of application-based programs and research on the efficacy of those programs is one specific area of future research.

Integrated Approach to Improving Health and Performance

Within a sport environment, the use of an integrated approach (e.g., interdisciplinary, transdisciplinary; Hess, Gnacinski, and Meyer, 2019) to create solutions is increasingly common. For example, within an athletic department, sports medicine professionals, sport dieticians, strength and conditioning coaches, and sport psychology consultants often work collaboratively with coaches and athletes to improve athlete health, well-being, and performance. Yet, this integrated approach to improving health and performance is notably missing within military and other tactical populations, as well as with exercisers. For example, a metropolitan fire department might employ an athletic trainer, exercise physiologist, and mental health provider, yet these providers may not collaborate to improve firefighter health and readiness for duty and/or do not include the firefighter in the decision-making process, thus leading to potentially unsuccessful solutions to health concerns. Future research could examine facilitators and barriers to developing a collaborative, integrated approach to improving health and performance in non-sport populations.

Efficacy of Psychological Skills Training

Psychological skills training refers to the systematic rehearsal of mental strategies to enhance performance and/or to increase enjoyment in sport and exercise. Psychological skills include imagery, meditation, breathwork, self-talk, relaxation, goal setting, and concentration. While over 400 peer-reviewed articles have been published on psychological skills training (Park and Jeon, 2023), researchers and practitioners alike have questioned the effectiveness of psychological skills training to enhance performance. Results from meta-analyses have suggested that while psychological interventions can enhance performance, the quality of the research methods is questionable (Lange-Smith et al., 2023) and therefore the results are equivocal (Reinebo et al., 2024). Since implementing psychological strategies is often the foundation for applied practice in sport and exercise psychology, high quality, randomized controlled trials are needed to accurately examine the effectiveness of all psychological strategies.

SUMMARY

Exercise and sport psychology is the scientific study of behavior in exercise and sport environments in both individual and group contexts. Exercise psychology is described as the application of psychology to promote, maintain, and enhance exercise and physical activity, whereas sport psychology is described as a multifaceted discipline, informed by principles of exercise science and psychology, and applied within a sport or performance context. Because psychological factors affect an individual's adoption of and adherence to exercise and performance in sport, and because participation in exercise and sport affects an individual's psychological health and well-being, it is important for exercise science students to develop a clear understanding of the discipline that is exercise and sport psychology.

STUDY QUESTIONS

1. Define exercise psychology. Provide two examples of applied exercise psychology.
2. Define sport psychology. Provide two examples of applied sport psychology.
3. Describe three ways that exercise can improve mental health, quality of life, and/or cognitive function.
4. What is the difference between stress, arousal, and anxiety?
5. How can an athlete improve their self-efficacy in their sport?
6. Describe how recovery can offset the effects of burnout.
7. What career opportunities are available in exercise and sport psychology?
8. What educational tracks are available for students interested in a career in exercise and sport psychology?

LEARNING ACTIVITIES

1. Mental Health and Acute Exercise Activity
   a. Rate the following mental and emotional health dispositions on a scale from 0 (*not at all*) to 10 (*extremely*) with regard to how students currently feel:
      i. Anger
      ii. Stress
      iii. Fatigue
      iv. Enthusiasm
      v. Ability to concentrate
      vi. Contentment
   b. Go on a 30-minute walk outside.
   c. Post-walk, rate the above mental and emotional health dispositions once more.
   d. Did your scores change? Why or why not? Fully explain your rationale.
2. How to Identify Exercise and Sport Psychology Practitioners Activity
   a. Go to the Association for Applied Sport Psychology's "How to Identify the Right Provider" handout. See: Association for Applied Sport Psychology (n.d.b.).

b. Describe the difference between "low" functioning and performance and "high" functioning and performance.
c. A clinically trained/licensed mental health provider would be required to treat which performer(s)?
d. What degree and/or licensure would be required for a professional to be "clinically trained"?

SUGGESTED READING AND RELATED WEBSITES

Association for Applied Sport Psychology. (n.d.a.). Association for Applied Sport Psychology website. Available at: https://appliedsportpsych.org/

Cox, R. H., (2012). *Sport psychology: Concepts and applications* (7th ed.). McGraw Hill.

Eklund, R. C., and Tenenbaum, G. (2020). *Handbook of sport psychology* (4th ed.). Wiley.

Horn, T. S., and Smith, A. L. (2019). *Advances in sport and exercise psychology* (4th ed.). Human Kinetics.

Lox, C. L., Martin Ginis, K. A., Gainforth, H. L., and Petruzzello, S. J. (2019). *The psychology of exercise: Integrating theory and practice* (5th ed.). Routledge.

Weinberg, R. S., and Gould, D. (2024). *Foundations of sport and exercise psychology* (8th ed.). Human Kinetics.

REFERENCES

Anshel, M. (2011). *Applied health fitness psychology*. Human Kinetics.

Association for Applied Sport Psychology. (n.d.b.). How to identify the right provider. Available at: https://appliedsportpsych.org/site/assets/files/33107/aasp_mental_health_services_continuum.pdf

Association for Applied Sport Psychology (AASP). (2021). *2020 compensation report for mental performance work*. University of Western States. Available at: https://www.uws.edu/2021/07/26/aasp-publishes-compensation-report-for-mental-performance-work/

Association for Applied Sport Psychology (AASP). (2024). Association for Applied Sport Psychology ethical principles and standards. Zito, M., Carter, C., Herzog, T., Kerulis, M., Muscat, A., Shigeno,T., Skvarla, L. (Eds.). Available at: https://appliedsportpsych.org/about-the-association-for-applied-sport-psychology/ethics/

Bandura, A. (1977). Self-efficacy: Toward a unifying theory of behavioral change. *Psychology Review, 84*, 191–215.

Bandura, A. (1986). The explanatory and predictive scope of self-efficacy theory. *Journal of Social and Clinical Psychology, 4*(3), 359–373. https://doi.org/10.1521/jscp.1986.4.3.359

Berger, B. G. and Tobar, D. A. (2011). Exercise and quality of life. In T. Morris and P. Terry (Eds.), *The New Sport and Exercise Psychology Companion* (pp. 483–505). Fitness Information Tech.

Biddle, S., and Mutrie, N. (2008). *Psychology of physical activity: Determinants, well-being, and interventions*. Routledge.

Bird, J. M. (2020). The use of virtual reality head-mounted displays within applied sport psychology. *Journal of Sport Psychology in Action, 11*(2). https://doi.org/10.1080/21520704.2018.1563573

Brown, J. D. (1991). Staying fit and staying well: Physical fitness as a moderator of life stress. *Journal of Personality and Social Psychology, 60*, 555–561.

Carron, A. V., and Hausenblas, H. A. (1998). *Group dynamics in sport* (2nd ed.). Fitness Information Technology.

Carron, A. V. and Eys, M. A. (2012). *Group dynamics in sport* (4th ed.). Fitness Information Technology.

Chen, M. D. and Rimmer, J. H. (2011) Effects of exercise on quality of life in stroke survivors: A meta-analysis. *Stroke*, *42*, 832–837. http://dx.doi.org/10.1161/STROKEAHA.110.607747

Colledge, F., Sattler, I., Schilling, H., Gerber, M., Pühse, U., and Walter, M. (2020). Mental disorders in individuals at risk for exercise addiction – A systematic review. *Addictive Behaviors Reports*, *12*, 1–8. https://doi.org/10.1016/j.abrep.2020.100314

Deci, E. L., and Ryan, R. M. (1985). *Intrinsic motivation and self-determination in human behavior.* Plenum Publishing.

Dweck, C. S., and Leggett, E. L. (1988). A social-cognitive approach to motivation and personality. *Psychological Review*, *95*(2), 256–273. https://doi.org/10.1037/0033-295X.95.2.256

Easterbrook, J. A. (1959). The effect of emotion on cue utilization and the organization of behavior. *Psychological Review*, *66*(3), 183–201. https://doi.org/10.1037/h0047707

Ensari, I., Greenlee, T. A., Motl, R. W., and Petruzzello, S. J. (2015). Meta-analysis of acute exercise effects on state anxiety: An update on randomized controlled trials over the past 25 years. *Depression and Anxiety*, *32*(8), 624–634. https://doi.org/10.1002/da.22370

Felce, D., and Perry, J. (1995). Quality of life: Its definition and measurement. *Research in Developmental Disabilities*, *16*(1), 51–74. https://doi.org/10.1016/0891-4222(94)00028-8

Ferrer-Uris, B., Ramos, M. A., Busquets, A., and Angulo-Barroso, R. (2022). Can exercise shape your brain? A review of aerobic exercise effects on cognitive function and neuro-physiological underpinning mechanisms. *AIMS Neuroscience*, *9*(2), 150–174. https://doi.org/10.3934/Neuroscience.2022009

Gill, D. L., Williams, L., and Reifsteck, E. J. (2017). *Psychological dynamics of sport and exercise psychology* (4th ed.). Human Kinetics.

Granito, V. J. (2017). History of sport, exercise, and performance psychology in North America. *Psychology*. https://doi.org/10.1093/acrefore/9780190236557.013.133

Gross, M. J., Bringer, J. D., Kilduff, L. P., Cook, C. J., Hall, R., and Shearer, D. A. (2019). A multimodal biofeedback protocol to demonstrate physiological manifestations of psychological stress and introduce heart rate variability biofeedback stress management. *Journal of Sport Psychology in Action*, *9*(4), 216–226. https://doi.org/10.1080/21520704.2018.1496210

Hanin, Y. L. (1997). Emotions and athletic performance: Individual zones of optimal functioning model. *European Yearbook of Sport Psychology*, *1*, 29–72.

Hardy, L. (1996). Testing the predictions of the Cusp Catastrophe Model of anxiety and performance. *The Sport Psychologist*, *10*(2), 140–156.

Heissel, A., Heinen, D., Brokmeier, L. L., Skarabis, N., Kangas, M., Vancampfort, D., Stubbs, B., Firth, J., Ward, P. B., Rosenbaum, S., Hallgren, M., and Schuch, F. (2023). Exercise as medicine for depressive symptoms? A systematic review and meta-analysis with meta-regression. *British Journal of Sports Medicine*, *57*(16), 1049–1057. https://doi.org/10.1136/bjsports-2022-106282

Henriksen, K., Schinke, R., Moesch, K., McCann, S., Parham, W. D., Larsen, C. H., and Terry, P. (2020). Consensus statement on improving the mental health of high-performance athletes. *International Journal of Sport and Exercise Psychology*, *18*(5), 553–560. https://doi.org/10.1080/1612197X.2019.1570473

Herbert, C., Meixner, F., Wiebking, C., and Gilg, V. (2020). Regular physical activity, short-term exercise, mental health, and well-being among university students: The results of an online and a laboratory study. *Frontiers in Psychology*, *11*, 1–23. https://doi.org/10.3389/fpsyg.2020.00509

Hess, C. W., Gnacinski, S. L., and Meyer, B. B. (2019). A review of the sport injury and rehabilitation literature: From abstraction to application. *The Sport Psychologist*, *33*, 232–243. https://doi.org/10.1123/tsp.2018-0043

Hess, C. W., and Meyer, B. B. (2021). The lived experiences of an elite athlete performance management team through injury rehabilitation: An interpretative phenomenological analysis. *Journal of Sport Rehabilitation*, *31*(2), 199–210. https://doi.org/10.1123/jsr.2021-0072

Jeunet, C., Hauw, D., and Millán, J. R. (2020). Sport psychology: Technologies ahead. *Frontiers in Sports and Active Living*, *2*, 1–3. https://doi.org/10.3389/fspor.2020.00010

Juwono, I. D., Tolnai, N., and Szabo, A. (2022). Exercise addiction in athletes: A systematic review of the literature. *International Journal of Mental Health and Addiction*, *20*, 3113–3127.

Kallus, K. W., and Kellmann, M. (2016). *The recovery-stress questionnaires: User manual.* Pearson.

Katz, L., Parker, J., Tyreman, H., Kopp, G., Levy, R., and Chang, E. (2006). Virtual reality in sport and wellness: Promise and reality. *International Journal of Computer Science in Sport*, *4*(1), 1–16.

Kellmann, M., Bertollo, M., Bosquet, L., Brink, M., Coutts, A. J., Duffield, R., Erlacher, D., Halson, S. L., Hecksteden, A., Heidari, J., Kallus, K. W., Meeusen, R., Mujika, I., Robazza, C., Skorski, S., Venter, R., and Beckmann, J. (2018). Recovery and performance in sport: Consensus statement. *International Journal of Sports Physiology and Performance*, *13*(2), 240–245. https://doi.org/10.1123/ijspp. 2017–0759

Kellmann, M., and Kallus, K. W. (2001). *The recovery-stress questionnaire for athletes: User manual.* Human Kinetics.

Konttä, G., and Hassmén, P. (1998). Overtraining and recovery. A conceptual model. *Sports Medicine*, *26* (1), 1–16. https://doi.org/10.2165/00007256-199826010-00001

Kerr, J. H. (1997). *Motivation and emotion in sport: Reversal theory.* Psychology Press. https://doi.org/10.4324/9781315784908

Kim, I., and Ahn, J. (2021). The effect of changes in physical self-concept through participation in exercise on changes in self-esteem and mental well-being. *International Journal of Environmental Research and Public Health*, *18*(10). https://doi.org/10.3390/ijerph18105224

Knobf, M. T., Musanti, R., and Dorward, J. (2007). Exercise and quality of life outcomes in patients with cancer. *Seminars in Oncology Nursing*, *23*(4), 285–296. https://doi.org/10.1016/j.soncn.2007.08.007

Landolfi, E. (2013). Exercise addiction. *Sports Medicine*, *43*(2), 111–119.

Lange-Smith, S., Cabot, J., Coffee, P., Gunnell, K., and Tod, D. (2023). The efficacy of psychological skills training for enhancing performance in sport: A review of reviews. *International Journal of Sport and Exercise Psychology*. https://doi.org/10.1080/1612197X.2023.2168725

Lox, C. L., Martin Ginis, K. A., and Petruzzello, S. J. (2017). *The psychology of exercise: Integrating theory and practice* (4th ed.). Routledge.

Martens, R., Vealey, R. S., and Burton, D. (1990). *Competitive anxiety in sport.* Human Kinetics.

Martin, C. K., Church, T. S., Thompson, A. M., Earnest, C. P. and Blair, S. N. (2009). Exercise dose and quality of life: A randomized controlled trial. *Archives of Internal Medicine*, *163*(3), 269–278. https://doi.org/10.1001/archinternmed.2008.545

Markland, D., and Ingledew, D. K. (2007). The relationship between body mass and body image and relative autonomy for exercise among adolescent males and females. *Psychology of Sport and Exercise*, *8*, 836–853.

Morgan, S. J., and Mora, S. A. M. (2017). Effect of heart rate variability biofeedback on sport performance, a systematic review. *Applied Psychophysiological Biofeedback*, *42*, 235–245. https://doi.org/10.1007/s10484-017-9364-2

Morley, J. E. (2018). An overview of cognitive impairment. *Clinics in Geriatric Medicine*, *34*(4), 505–513. https://doi.org/10.1016/j.cger.2018.06.003

Nicholls, J. G. (1989). *The competitive ethos and democratic education.* Harvard University Press.

Park, I., and Jeon, J. (2023). Psychological skills training for athletes in sports: Web of science bibliometric analysis. *Healthcare*, *11*, 1–15.

Ransford, C. P. (1982). A role for amines in the antidepressant effect of exercise: A review. *Medicine and Science in Sports and Exercise*, *14*, 1–10.

Raedeke, T. D., and Smith, A. L. (2001). Development and preliminary validation of an athlete burnout measure. *Journal of Sport and Exercise Psychology*, *23*(4), 281–306. https://doi.org/10.1123/jsep.23.4.281

Reinebo, G., Alfonsson, S., Jansson-Fröjmark, M., Rozental, A., and Lundgren, T. (2024). Effects of psychological interventions to enhance athletic performance: A systematic review and meta-analysis. *Sports Medicine*, *54*, 347–373.

Sachs, M. L. (1984). The runner's high. In M. L. Sachs and G. W. Buffone (Eds.), *Running as therapy: An integrated approach* (pp. 273–287). University of Nebraska Press.

Sage, G. (1977). *Introduction to motor behaviour: A neurophysiological approach* (2nd ed.). Addison-Wesley.

Schmidt, R. J. (2018). Exercise and sport psychology. In D. J. Housh, T. J. Housh, and G. O. Johnson (Eds.), *Introduction to exercise science* (5th ed., pp. 263–285). Routledge.

Sime, W. (2003). Sport psychology applications of biofeedback and neurofeedback. In M. S. Schwartz and F. Andrasik (Eds.), *Biofeedback: A practitioner's guide* (3rd ed., pp. 560–588). The Guilford Press.

Smith, R. E. (1986). Toward a cognitive-affective model of athletic burnout. *Journal of Sport Psychology*, *8*(1), 36–50.

Smith, P. J., and Merwin, R. M. (2021). The role of exercise in management of mental health disorders: An integrative study. *Annual Review of Medicine*, *72*, 45–62. https://doi.org/10.1146/annurev-med-060619-022943

Steinberg, H., and Sykes, E. A. (1985). Introduction to symposium on endorphins and behavioral processes: Review of literature on endorphins and exercise. *Pharmacology, Biochemistry Behavior*, *23*, 857–862.

Taylor, J. (2017). Importance of assessment in sport psychology consulting. In J. Taylor (Ed.). *Assessment in Applied Sport Psychology* (pp. 3–14). Human Kinetics.

Taylor, J., and Wilson, G. S. (2002). Intensity regulation and sport performance. In J. L. Van Raalte and B. W. Brewer (Eds.), *Exploring sport and exercise psychology* (2nd ed., pp. 99–130). American Psychological Association. https://doi.org/10.1037/10465-006

Tuckman, B. W. (1965). Developmental sequence in small groups. *Psychological Bulletin*, *63*(6), 384–399. https://doi.org/10.1037/h0022100

Vealey, R. S. (2002). Personality and sport behavior. In T. S. Horn (Ed.), *Advances in sport psychology* (2nd ed., pp. 43–74). Human Kinetics.

Vealey, R. S., and Chase, M. A. (2008). Self-confidence in sport. In T. S. Horn (Ed.), *Advances in sport psychology* (3rd ed., pp 66–97). Human Kinetics.

Vealey, R. S., Cooley, R., Nilsson, E., Block, C., and Galli, N. (2019). Assessment and the use of questionnaires in sport psychology consulting: An analysis of practices and attitudes from 2003 to 2017. *Journal of Clinical Sport Psychology*, *13*(4), 505–523.

Watson, J. C., and Coker-Cranney, A. M. (2019). Introduction to the special issue: Using technology in applied sport psychology. *Journal of Sport Psychology in Action*, *9*(4), 213–215. https://doi.org/10.1080/21520704.2018.1552446.

Willis, J. D. and Campbell, L. F. (1992). *Exercise psychology*. Human Kinetics.

10 Sports Injury Prevention and Rehabilitation

Kyle T. Ebersole and David J. Cornell

LEARNING OBJECTIVES

After studying this chapter, the student will be able to:

- identify common healthcare professionals involved in an injury rehabilitation team and describe the preparation pathways for becoming a licensed provider
- explain strategies for mitigating injury risk through safe exercise practices, such as pre-participation screening, warm-up, cool-down, and recovery
- discuss the role of protective equipment, clothing, and footwear in preventing exercise-related injuries
- describe the importance of consulting with trained exercise professionals to ensure safe and effective exercise plans
- outline the ways in which technology and science contribute to rehabilitation techniques and modalities for improving function, mobility, and quality of life following injury or surgery

INTRODUCTION

The risk of injury is associated with participation in any kind of physical activity such as exercise and sport, as well as the occupational demands associated with certain types of jobs. The Consumer Product Safety Commission (CPSC) reported that in 2022, 3.6 million people were treated by emergency rooms for injuries due to sport or participation in recreational activities (National Safety Council, 2024). In addition, the National Health Statistics Report estimated in 2021 that nearly 9% of all adults living in the United States suffered an overuse musculoskeletal injury with nearly 51% seeking a consultation with a healthcare professional (Garnett, Elgaddal, and Spencer, 2023). In many cases, the recovery from a musculoskeletal injury involves some form of rehabilitation including stretching, strengthening, and the restoration of cardiovascular capacity. As such, injury management in the form of mitigation strategies and post-injury rehabilitation have become an essential component to the exerciser, athlete, or occupational worker in support of achieving and maintaining optimum health and performance. Historically, physical rehabilitation of injury has been the primary role of athletic trainers and physical therapists; therefore, these two professions will be the focus of this chapter. However, it is important to note that other members of a rehabilitation or performance team may include occupational therapists, sport psychologists, dietitians, personal trainers, strength and conditioning specialists, and sports scientists, as well as other qualified healthcare providers such as medical doctors and chiropractors.

DOI: 10.4324/9781032697185-10

HISTORICAL PERSPECTIVES

Athletic Training

The current version of the athletic trainer first evolved in association with the growth of intercollegiate athletes in the late 19th and early 20th centuries in the United States. As intercollegiate athletic programs grew in popularity during the first half of the 20th century, there was parallel growth in the number of athletic trainers associated with these programs. Because no formal professional education programs for athletic trainers existed, much of their knowledge was learned on the job and borrowed from the medical community. The need for a professional association for athletic trainers became apparent during the 1940s, when several regional athletic training associates began to meet on a regular basis (Ebel, 1999). Thus, the stage was set for the establishment of a professional association of athletic trainers at the national level and in June 1950 the first national meeting of athletic trainers was held in Kansas City, Missouri, at which the National Athletic Trainers' Association (NATA) was formed (Ebel, 1999). This first meeting was attended by 101 athletic trainers from across the United States (O'Shea, 1980). Five years later, the NATA approved the publication of its professional journal, *The Journal of the National Athletic Trainers' Association*, which was published quarterly. The publication is now called *Journal of Athletic Training*.

On June 21, 1967, the American Medical Association (AMA) first recognized the role of the athletic trainer as an important part of an athlete's healthcare team, but it wasn't until June 1990 that the AMA's Council on Medical Education (CME) formally recognized athletic training as an allied health profession (Delforge and Behnke, 1999; Ebel, 1999). The AMA recognition brought with it a significant amount of prestige for the athletic training profession. Today, the NATA has grown to over 45,000 members across the world.

Physical Therapy

Physical therapists were originally called reconstruction aides who assisted physicians in meeting the needs of soldiers preparing for and returning from World War I. In 1918, Mary McMillan, a reconstruction aide working in the Walter Reed program, began to formalize the training for physiotherapists (American Physical Therapy Association [APTA], 2020; Moffat, 2003). By 1919, hospitals began employing nearly 700 reconstruction aides, who focused on the rehabilitation of the nearly 50,000 wounded soldiers returning from World War I. Shortly after this rise in healthcare need for military veterans, the American Women's Physical Therapeutic Association (AWPTA) was formed in January 1921 at a gathering of approximately 30 women at Keens Chophouse in New York City (APTA, 2020). At this inaugural meeting, Mary McMillan was elected as the first AWPTA president and she would lead the AWPTA to admitting men into the profession in 1922 and changing the association name to the American Physiotherapy Association (APA) (Moffat, 2003). Concurrent with the increased military demand for physiotherapists, the United States also experienced the poliomyelitis epidemic from the 1920s to the 1940s. Perhaps the most well documented case of polio was that of President Franklin Delano Roosevelt, who benefited greatly from the physical rehabilitation provided by physiotherapists. Collectively, the military and polio-related physical rehabilitation needs helped establish a national presence for the APA, leading to the writing of the first *Code of Ethics* in 1935. In 1946, the APA officially changed its name to the American Physical Therapy Association (APTA), which currently has over 100,000 members (APTA, 2020).

FUNDAMENTALS CONCEPTS

Athletic Training

According to the Board of Certification for Athletic Trainers (n.d.), athletic trainers (ATs) are described as "healthcare professionals who render service or treatment, under the direction of or in collaboration with a physician, in accordance with their education and training and the states' statutes, rules and regulations." The scope of practice of athletic training is defined within the *Athletic Training Practice Analysis*, which identifies essential knowledge and skills for the athletic training profession, informs the development of the national certification exam, and guides expectations for continuing competence programming. According to the most recent eighth edition of the *Athletic Training Practice Analysis (BOC PA)*, ATs function within five practice domains: (1) risk reduction, wellness and health literacy; (2) assessment, evaluation and diagnosis; (3) critical incident management; (4) therapeutic intervention; and (5) healthcare administration and professional responsibility (Board of Certification, 2021). The activities of the AT will vary across each domain but may include:

- **Risk reduction, wellness, and health literacy**: the AT will utilize process (e.g., clinical measurements, pre-participation screening, and surveys) to identify non-modifiable intrinsic (e.g., prior medical history) and modifiable extrinsic (e.g., nutrition, training load, and biomechanics) risk factors for injury and then create solutions to reduce the risk for injury. The multi-factorial aspect of risk reduction creates an opportunity within this domain for the AT to educate the athlete or patient for the value of the holistic components of health and wellness as well as the use of protective equipment.
- **Assessment, evaluation and diagnosis**: the AT will often perform the activities of this domain at an external site (e.g., playing field, basketball court, and weight room) as well as within a clinical room setting. The AT will use information gathered from a subjective (e.g., asking questions) and objective (e.g., tests and measurements) evaluation to complete a differential diagnosis and develop a plan of care.
- **Critical incident management**: at the center of this domain is the development and implementation of an emergency action plan (EAP) for emergent situations across all potential venues within an organization or institution. Effective execution of the EAP requires the AT to act quickly, often in a stressful environment, to identify the best course of care including primary and secondary survey for immediate safety concerns and injury triage.
- **Therapeutic intervention:** this domain often represents a traditional definition of rehabilitation where best practices are used to select therapeutic modalities (e.g., ultrasound, electrical stimulation, manual therapy), exercise, and education to meet the injury care needs of the patient.
- **Healthcare administration and professional responsibility**: the AT will often work as part of an integrated medical team of other professionals (e.g., orthopedic surgeon, strength and conditioning specialist, nutritionist, sport psychologist) to deliver high quality, patient-centered care that meets that expectations of the local laws, regulations, and professional ethical standards that define patient care.

Physical Therapy

According to the Federation of State Boards of Physical Therapy (n.d.), physical therapists (PTs) are movement experts who aim to improve quality of life by promoting the patient's ability to move, reduce pain, restore function, and prevent disability through hands-on care and patient education. The APTA defines the PT's scope of practice as falling within three areas: professional, jurisdictional, and personal. The professional area is informed from the knowledge and scientific literature that shapes the education and evidence which drives the practice of physical therapy. Jurisdiction refers to the legal boundaries set by a state's governing body through its practice act, which defines the scope and regulation of physical therapy practice. The personal scope of practice for a PT refers to the education and competency standards required for the activities they perform. The practices that fall under the scope of a physical therapist and developed as part of an accredited education program are guided by the *APTA Guide to Physical Therapist Practice*, currently in its fourth version (APTA, n.d.b). The PT will practice across a continuum of care that includes acute and chronic injuries, illnesses, and pathologies. In general, PT practice will restore, maintain, and promote optimal physical function by using an examination process, including subjective and objective findings from tests and measures, to determine a diagnosis and develop a subsequent treatment plan incorporating a variety of therapeutic agents and exercise techniques. Within this scope of practice and beyond traditional treatment for the patient, the PT may be involved with instruction and fitting for assistive devices (e.g., crutches, walkers, wheelchairs), educating on lifestyle factors (e.g., stress, nutrition, body weight), and supporting the implementation of exercise programs. PTs and ATs have several practice overlaps; however, a common distinction between the two professions is that ATs, depending on job environment, may focus more on prevention and acute injury management, whereas PTs may work with a broader patient population with longer term rehabilitation needs.

APPLICATIONS TO EXERCISE SCIENCE

A basic understanding of sports injury and rehabilitation is essential for exercise science students, since it gives them the knowledge and skills that help prevent injuries, support rehabilitation, and design safe training programs. Having this foundation is also necessary to support both physical and mental aspects of recovery and to implement modified exercises that aid in a gradual return to physical activity. It also enhances their ability to collaborate with ATs, PTs, and medical staff, fostering effective interdisciplinary care. While the following information is described with reference to ATs and PTs, much of the information also applies to exercise science students interested in careers, such as personal training and strength and conditioning, in which expertise in injury prevention and management is critical for promoting safe and sustainable fitness and performance outcomes.

The International Classification of Functioning, Disability, and Health

Athletic training and physical therapy are closely aligned with the disciplines of kinesiology and exercise science, since they are grounded in foundational principles such as bioenergetics, biomechanics, exercise physiology, motor behavior, and sport psychology. At the center of practice for athletic training and physical therapy is the International Classification of Functioning, Disability and Health (ICF), developed by the World Health Organization (WHO) in 2001 (WHO, 2001). The ICF is a framework to create a common language for disability that better aligns with the WHO definition of health: "A state of complete physical, mental, and social well-being and not merely the absence of disease or illness" (WHO, 2001). The ICF attempts to reshape how health is defined to be more enabling vs. disabling in language and align with a biopsychosocial approach to health.

The ICF model (Exhibit 10.1) is based on a broad definition of "health condition" as a term for disease, disorder, injury, or trauma, but could also include aging and stress or the etiological underpinnings to an illness. The framework for exploring the health condition is based on an integrative relationship between body structure and function, activity, and participation, as well as contextual considerations, such as environmental and personal factors. These components rely on a sound knowledge of anatomy, physiology, physiological and psychological responses to exercise and activity, as well as physiological, psychological, biomechanical, and motor behavior factors, which may explain impairments to movement and function. As such, the ICF is fundamentally informed from the exercise science disciplines, creating a common basis for the way in which many healthcare professionals approach rehabilitation with a patient (Snyder, 2008).

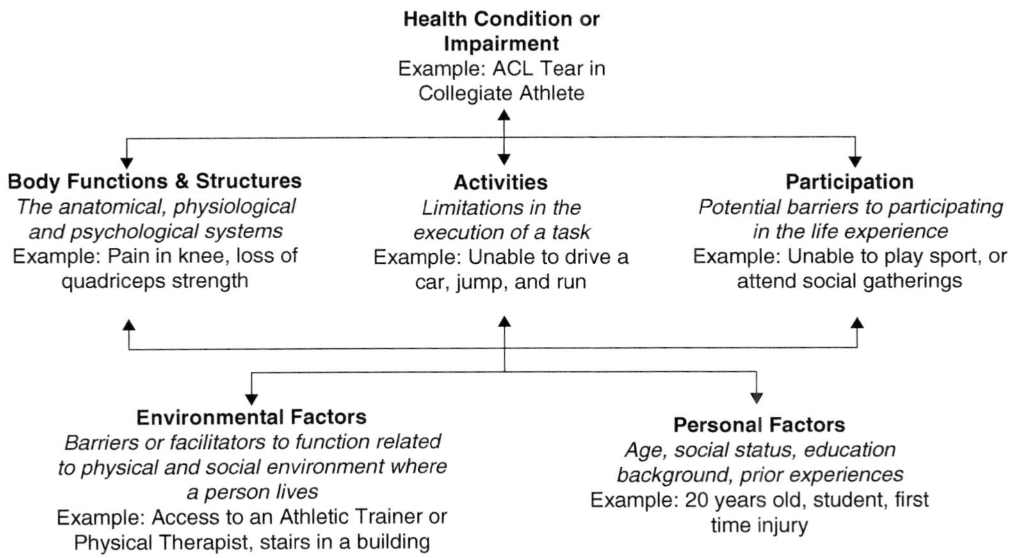

Exhibit 10.1 Example application of the ICF model to an injury

Injury and Performance Continuum

Musculoskeletal injuries are often categorized as acute (i.e., sudden onset) or chronic (i.e., gradual onset related to overuse) and by severity (i.e., first degree, second degree, or third degree) (Wang et al., 2024). The rehabilitation of an injury is grounded in the pathobiology of soft-tissue (i.e., muscle, ligament, tendon, joint capsules) repair that involves a cascade of events, including an inflammatory phase, a proliferative or repair phase, and a remodeling phase (Wang et al., 2024). The amount of time spent in each phase, and therefore, the total amount of time for recovery, is tissue and injury severity dependent. ATs and PTs are trained healthcare professionals with expertise in injury care due, in part, to their educational preparation in basic sciences and the disciplines of exercise science and kinesiology.

The end point of injury rehabilitation has historically been identified as the return to sport participation by an athlete or preinjury activities by a patient (Draovitch et al., 2022). In recent years, the growth of sport and performance science as a discipline, as well as post-professional certification opportunities, has evolved the injury rehabilitation continuum to emphasize both recovery and high performance. This paradigm shift highlights the need for continued care and performance training after an athlete or patient is cleared to return to play, to ensure that they meet the high demands of their sport, occupation, or activity. As a result, ATs and PTs often collaborate with other healthcare and exercise professionals to optimize a patient's return to full participation.

A unique consideration for injury management in sport and occupation involves key elements related to screening and monitoring, as well as foundational exercise principles related to preparation for and recovery from a sport, job, or activity. Developing a warm-up and cool down protocol specific to the activity and establishing appropriate periodized fitness and training plans are extremely important to injury prevention and recovery. ATs and PTs may be responsible for contributing to pre-participation health screening, recommending and managing protective equipment, and considering the impact that clothing and footwear may have on an individual's ability to optimize recovery and performance.

HEALTH/CLINICAL ASPECTS

Both ATs and PTs are part of the traditional clinical rehabilitation model, and entry level professionals can find employment in health or clinical settings upon graduation. However, advanced education and training have recently become a popular pathway for gaining specialized expertise to enhance patient care.

Athletic Training

The Commission on Accreditation of Athletic Training Education (CAATE) program is responsible for the administration of the residency and fellowship programs for ATs. The residency program aims to serve as a professional development pathway between graduate education and autonomous clinical practice, with an emphasis on one of eight specialty areas: prevention and wellness, urgent and emergent care, primary care, orthopedics, rehabilitation, behavioral health, pediatrics, and performance enhancement (CAATE, n.d.). Athletic training residency education occurs in clinical settings and emphasizes the development of patient care skills that complement the medical knowledge and expertise for a chosen area of specialty practice. The fellowship program is designed to provide advanced education and intensive programming beyond a core residency program for certified ATs with an interest in developing expertise within a subspecialty area. Athletic trainers applying for the fellowship program have the opportunity to define the subspeciality area of interest, provided it meets the following criteria (CAATE, n.d.):

- the clinical care and safety of patients will be improved through the recognition of the subspecialty
- the proposed subspecialty area demonstrates the existence of a body of scientific medical knowledge underlying the subspecialty that is (a) focused on a body system or population within the larger specialty area, (b) clinically distinct from other areas in

which accreditation is already offered, and (c) sufficient for educating individuals in a clinical field and not simply educating more techniques
- the proposed subspecialty area has an established presence in healthcare at a national level and it falls within the domains of athletic training
- the educational program is primarily clinical in accordance with the accreditation standards for fellowship programs

One clinical area that continues to see growth is the physician practice setting. Athletic trainers in physician practice improve productivity, patient outcomes, and satisfaction by providing value to the practice through skills in triage, taking patient histories, performing evaluations, and providing instruction on exercise prescription and rehabilitation, as well as general patient education.

Physical Therapy

In 1978, the APTA's House of Delegates established the framework for specialist certification by publishing the *Essentials for Certification of Advanced Clinical Competence in Physical Therapy*. This program allows PTs to develop expertise in specific areas of practice and formally recognizes those with advanced clinical knowledge, experience, and skills. It also helps consumers and the healthcare community to identify these specialists. Today, the certifications are overseen by the American Board for Physical Therapy Specializations (ABPTS) (ABPTS, n.d.) and only PTs licensed to practice in the United States are eligible to sit for a specialty exam. As of June 2024, over 40,000 PTs have obtained a specialist certification in one of the ten specialty areas including cardiopulmonary, clinical electrophysiology, geriatrics, neurology, oncology, orthopedics, pediatrics, sports, women's health, and wound management (ABPTS, n.d.). The number of PTs certified in these specialty areas is dependent on the specialty and varies greatly. For example, there are currently only 549 certified cardiopulmonary specialists, whereas there are over 22,000 PTs who are board certified orthopedic clinical specialists (OCS) (ABPTS, n.d.).

SPORTS/PERFORMANCE ASPECTS

Both ATs and PTs work in sport and performance settings. However, because these environments are historically in the discipline of athletic training many ATs work in a sports-related setting. Even so, the rise of sport and performance science in professional and collegiate sports has created new opportunities for both ATs and PTs.

Athletic Training

Many ATs are employed in a collegiate setting, serving more than 460,000 student athletes across the United States, at all levels of competition and including all NCAA divisions (i.e., DI, DII, DIII), NAIA, two-year institutions, as well as intramural and club sport programs (NATA, n.d.b.). Secondary schools are the second largest employment setting for certified ATs (NATA, n.d.b.). Many ATs in this setting are members of the NATA Secondary School Athletic Trainers' Committee, which supports the advancement of secondary school athletic training and develops resources to enhance the effectiveness and marketability of ATs in these roles. While professional sports employ the least number of ATs, they play a significant role in the profession (NATA, n.d.b.). Each major US sport (e.g., baseball, basketball, football, hockey, and soccer) employs teams of professionals dedicated to improving athlete care and advancing the athletic training profession (NATA, n.d.b.).

Although not traditional sports, many occupational roles, such as those in public safety (fire, police, public works) and the military, involve physically demanding tasks, creating new employment opportunities for ATs. These occupations often experience similar injuries as seen in traditional sport. The unique job and task demand of the occupations require the AT to evaluate and rehabilitate an injury with a focus on job-specific demands and tasks. For example, a firefighter with a shoulder injury will need to be able to successfully use the tools of the job like an axe and carry heavy loads like a charged hose. In these settings, the AT often applies foundational exercise science knowledge to develop unique rehabilitation plans. ATs in occupational settings often have access to facilities similar to those in a collegiate sport setting. To address the growing demand and health concerns in these fields, the Public Safety Athletic Trainers' Society (PSATS) (PSATS, n.d.) was established within the NATA.

Physical Therapy

Physical therapists interested in sports often pursue the Sport Clinical Specialist (SCS) board certification, which acknowledges their advanced clinical skills and comprehensive understanding of the physiological, psychological, and pathological challenges athletes face, as well as the strategies to prevent or address these performance barriers. The SCS training provides the PT with sport-focused training far greater than what occurs in most generalist-focused DPT degree programs. PTs pursuing the SCS will gain experience in advanced diagnosis and care for athlete injuries, including acute care on-site of a sport competition. PTs holding the SCS credential are viewed as experts in sport injury and therapy. As of June 2023, there were approximately 3,210 board certified SCS PTs in the United States (NATA, n.d.b.). The American Academy of Sports Physical Therapy (AASPT) is a section of the APTA and is aimed at advancing the research and clinical practice of sports physical therapy. The interests of AASPT often overlap with the Academy of Orthopaedic Physical Therapy (AOPT). Accordingly, the AASPT and AOPT work together to publish a journal that reflects the interests of these two specialists: *The Journal of Orthopaedic and Sports Physical Therapy*. In addition to the overlap between the AASPT and AOPT, the AASPT and the NATA also collaborate with the American Orthopaedic Society for Sports Medicine (AOSSM) and the American Medical Society for Sports Medicine (AMSSM) to publish the journal *Sports Health*, ultimately showcasing the interprofessional collaboration between PTs, ATs, and sports medicine physicians.

TECHNOLOGY AND RESEARCH TOOLS

An exciting aspect of the job of an AT and PT is the use of technology as part of direct patient care, monitoring of rehabilitation, and conducting research. It is not unusual for an athlete or patient to ask questions regarding the length of time until they are able to return to their sport, job, or activity. A clinician's ability to provide a reasonable response to questions like those is, in part, due to the clinician's ability to employ the technology and tools that are found in the clinic and grounded in scientific literature. The current technology-based tools for ATs and PTs generally fall into three categories: physical agents, assessment and measurement tools, and wearable trackers.

Physical Agents

Physical agents, sometimes called treatment modalities, are often used to manage the signs and symptoms of an injury, such as pain and inflammation, as well as to help promote tissue healing. Therefore, they are often key components of a patient's rehabilitation plan. Based on their underlying scientific properties, physical agents are frequently categorized into the groups listed below (Prentice, 2020).

- **Electrical agents** (e.g., transcutaneous and interferential electrical stimulation [Exhibit 10.2a], neuromuscular electrical stimulation [Exhibit 10.2b], iontophoresis [Exhibit 10.2c], dry needling [Exhibit 10.2d], and biofeedback [Exhibit 10.2e]) leverage basic physics and principles of electricity to augment tissue healing including management of pain and inflammation as well as support for restoration of muscle activation and strength.
- **Sound energy agents** (e.g., ultrasound [Exhibit 10.2f] and shock wave therapy [Exhibit 10.2g]) utilize mechanical energy across a variety of frequencies and wavelengths to provide a deep-penetrating tissue healing effect. These agents are frequently used early in injury rehabilitation but have applications along the entire tissue healing continuum.
- **Light therapy** (ultraviolet, low-level laser therapy [Exhibit 10.2h]) incorporates electromagnetic energy from the light spectrum to generate deep tissue photochemical effects to support tissue repair and pain management.
- **Thermal agents** (e.g., cryotherapy [Exhibit 10.2i] and thermotherapy [Exhibit 10.2j]) use the relationship between tissue type and temperature to decrease (cold) or increase (heat) the metabolic rate of the tissue to manage inflammation and pain.
- **Hydrotherapy** (e.g., aquatic therapy [Exhibit 10.2k], such as cold and warm whirlpool, [Exhibit 10.2l]) incorporates the thermal effects (warm or cold) of energy transfer, along with the physical properties of water (buoyancy, resistance, and hydrostatic pressure), to help manage pain, increase blood flow, reduce edema, and improve range of motion.
- **Electromagnetic energy agents** (e.g., shortwave and microwave diathermy) use high-frequency electrical currents, coupled together with variations in pulse outputs, to generate thermal and nonthermal effects on deep tissues. These agents support the reduction of inflammation, pain control, and improvements in tissue length.
- **Mechanical energy agents** (e.g., traction, soft tissue mobilization and massage) (Exhibit 10.2m), instrument assisted soft tissue mobilization (Exhibit 10.2n), cupping (Exhibit 10.2o), vibration, percussion (Exhibit 10.2p) and pneumatic compression devices (Exhibit 10.2q) apply various forms of force and pressure to a tissue or joint to manage pain, increase blood flow, increase tissue length, and improve range of motion. Mechanical agents can also be used to selectively restrict blood flow to manipulate metabolic demand and facilitate tissue healing and growth (e.g., blood flow restriction [Exhibit 10.2r]).

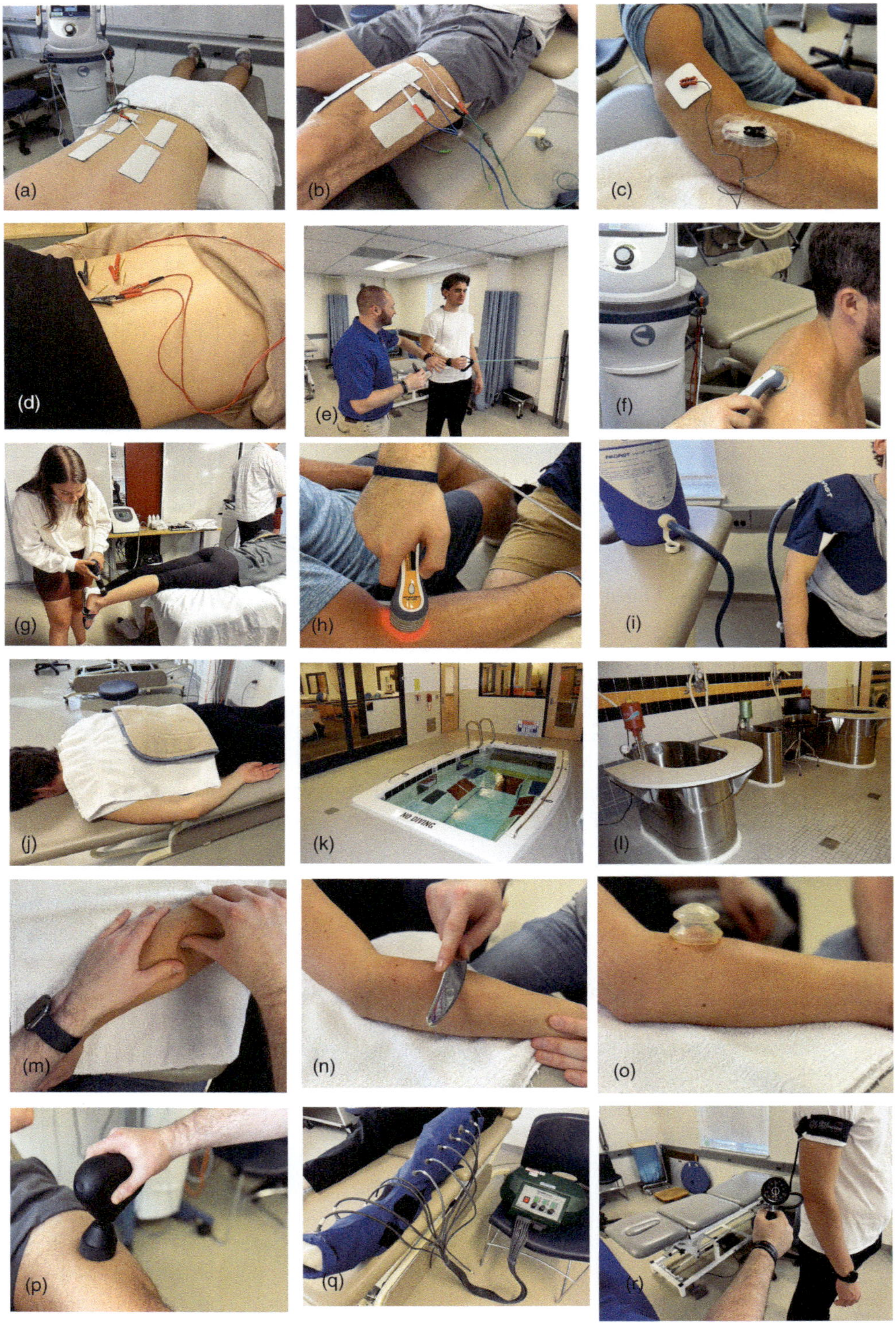

Exhibit 10.2 Examples of physical agents

Assessment and Measurement Tools

Following an injury, each tissue healing phase is associated with key clinical outcomes. For example, during the initial phases of rehabilitation, range of motion and muscle strength are often measured with handheld tools and the data becomes a key component in determining the progression of the healing process. As the injury advances along the healing continuum, different tools are employed to obtain more functional and dynamic measures. In addition, since ATs and PTs are frequently involved with preparticipation screening or pre-season testing of athletes, these same tools can be used to determine an athlete's baseline for a particular measure. These data could then be used to determine areas of strength and weakness for an individual and aid in the development of an exercise or training plan. The common assessment and measurement tools include the following:

- goniometers (Exhibit 6.22a) and inclinometers for evaluation of range of motion and muscle length
- handgrip (Exhibit 6.18c) and handheld manual muscle (Exhibit 6.18b) dynamometers for quantification of muscle strength
- postural balance trainers and machines to quantify balance deficits as well as support the restoration of balance
- isokinetic machines (Exhibit 6.18a), which determine maximal strength and power and can serve as a velocity-specific rehabilitation exercise for building muscle function in specific muscle groups

An area of recent technological advancement that has created unique applications for rehabilitation, as well as in pre-participation evaluations for athletes, is motion capture systems. Motion capture systems include both marker and markerless systems, as well as low-cost and low-tech options that use handheld video devices, including a mobile device. Motion capture (Parks, Wang, and Siu, 2019) provides a unique biomechanical assessment of an individual's movement pattern during a task (e.g., walking, running, jumping, and throwing a ball). The data can then help identify individuals at risk for an injury based on the biomechanical patterns around a joint.

Wearable Trackers

Perhaps the most rapid area of technology advancement that has impacted the AT and PT is wearable trackers. The growth in the health-related wearable industry has been attributed to advancements in data analytics, sensor fabrication technologies, and the emergence of sports science as a discipline (Seshadri et al., 2019). Wearables measure many different types of variables, including heart rhythm, heart rate, heart rate variability, muscle oxygen saturation, respiration rate, activity and movement, sleep quantity and quality, and self-reported perception of effort or fatigue (Seshadri et al., 2019). These devices are widely available to consumers and offer valuable information to help optimize the overall health and wellness of patients. Currently, clinicians are exploring ways to integrate the data into the rehabilitation plan for a patient to determine a relative level of recovery and their response to treatment.

In many cases, the wearable technology growth has occurred in conjunction with the emergence of sports science as a discipline. The NATA (Sizler, 2022) defines sports science as "the analysis and application of scientific principles, theories and data used in a collaborative approach to enhance decision-making associated with injury risk mitigation, objective return-to-play criteria and other health and performance outcomes." This definition clearly identifies the potential role that an AT and PT can play in collecting, interpreting, and/or using such data with an athlete or patient. Much of the literature around wearable technology can be collectively linked to the concept of load monitoring in an athlete or occupational worker. Load monitoring involves utilizing wearable technology and other tools to create a data-informed perspective on the internal response (e.g., changes in heart rate variability (HRV), peak strength, perceived exertion) to the external load (i.e., the actual work such as total distance, time, or weight) an individual performed (Seshadri et al., 2019; Draovitch et al., 2022). ATs and PTs may use the load monitoring approach to differentiate expected from unexpected responses to training, as well as to potentially mitigate overuse injuries.

Exhibit 10.3 Example of a research study in sports injury and rehabilitation

Ebersole, K. T., Cornell, D. J, Flees, R. J., Shemelya, C. M., and Noel, S. E. (2020). Contributions of the autonomic nervous system to recovery in firefighters. *Journal of Athletic Training*, 55, 1001–1008.

Context: Sudden cardiac deaths (SCDs) accounted for nearly half of the line-of-duty deaths among US firefighters over the past ten years. In 2018, 33% of all SCDs occurred after the end of a fire service call. The literature suggests that an imbalance in autonomic nervous system (ANS) regulation of heart rate post-call may interfere with recovery in firefighters.

Objective: To utilize heart rate recovery (HRR) and heart rate variability (HRV), two non-invasive markers of ANS function, to examine the ANS recovery profiles of firefighters.

Design: Cross-sectional study.

Setting: Firehouse and research laboratory.

Patients or Other Participants: Thirty-seven male career active-duty firefighters (mean ± SD, 39.1 ± 8.9 yrs; 178.8 ± 5.4 cm; 87.9 ± 11.2 kg).

Main Outcome Measure(s): Percent maximal heart rate (%MHR), HRV (lnRMSSD), and blood lactate (La^-) were collected after both submaximal and maximal exercise protocols. HRR profiles were examined by calculating the asymptote (), amplitude (), and decay (parameters of the mono-exponential HRR curve for each participant.

Results: Significant differences in the HRR parameters (, after 10 minutes of seated recovery were identified following submaximal vs. maximal exercise (*P* <.001). In addition, although ANS was more suppressed post-maximal exercise, HRV metrics indicated incomplete recovery, and that regardless of test, recovery %MHR and lnRMSSD values did not return to pre-test %MHR and lnRMSSD values. Furthermore, blood La^- remained significantly elevated above pre-test values after ten minutes of recovery within both submaximal and maximal protocols (*P* <.001).

Conclusions: The results of this study suggest that the contributions of the PSNS and SNS to recovery in active-duty firefighters are exercise intensity specific and this is likely an important factor when establishing best practice recovery guidelines.

CAREER AND EMPLOYMENT OPPORTUNITIES

Athletic Training

The profession of athletic training continues to see growth in employment settings and opportunities, with the Bureau of Labor and Statistics reporting that the profession will experience a 23% increase in demand by the year 2030 (Bureau of Labor Statistics, n.d.a.). According to the NATA, the current primary employment settings and percentage of ATs in that setting include colleges and universities (26%) (Exhibit 10.4), secondary schools (24%), clinics and hospitals (16%), professional sports (3%), and emerging settings (6%) such as performing arts, public safety, military, and occupational health (NATA, n.d.b.). Regardless of the employment setting, the practice of athletic training by an AT is informed and guided by the practice domains identified by the practice analysis and by state practice acts and regulations. The relative amount of time spent in each practice domain will vary according to the employment setting. The US Bureau of Labor Statistics projects a strong employment outlook for athletic trainers and expects job opportunities to grow by 14% between 2022 and 2032 (Bureau of Labor Statistics, n.d.a.).

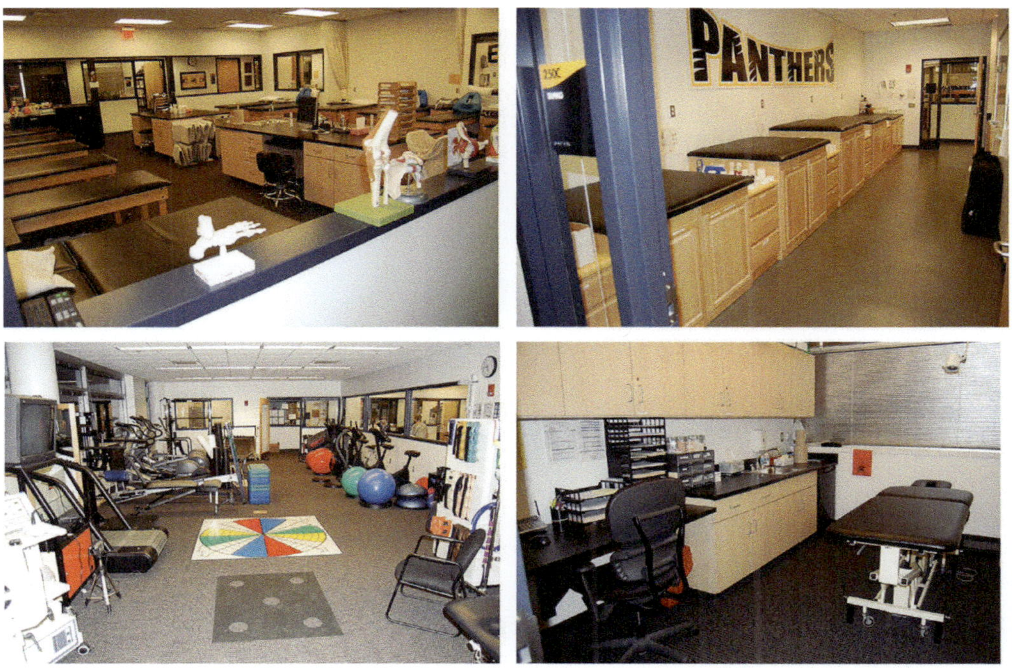

Exhibit 10.4 Examples of university athletic training rooms

Physical Therapy

Physical therapists are experts in movement who work to improve the quality of life in multiple patient populations impacted by disease and injury. They are involved in all phases of injury and disease care—from evaluation and diagnosis to treatment and monitoring of individuals across all ages—and work in a number of settings, including outpatient clinic and rehabilitation facilities (Exhibit 10.5), inpatient hospital and rehabilitation facilities (Exhibit 10.6), skilled nursing facilities, occupational workplaces, and in the homes of patients. The job of a PT is physically demanding, as patient care often requires extensive manual activity and standing, while working with patients. The US Bureau of Labor Statistics projects a strong employment outlook for PTs between 2022 and 2032, with an expected increase in jobs of 15% (Bureau of Labor Statistics, n.d.b.).

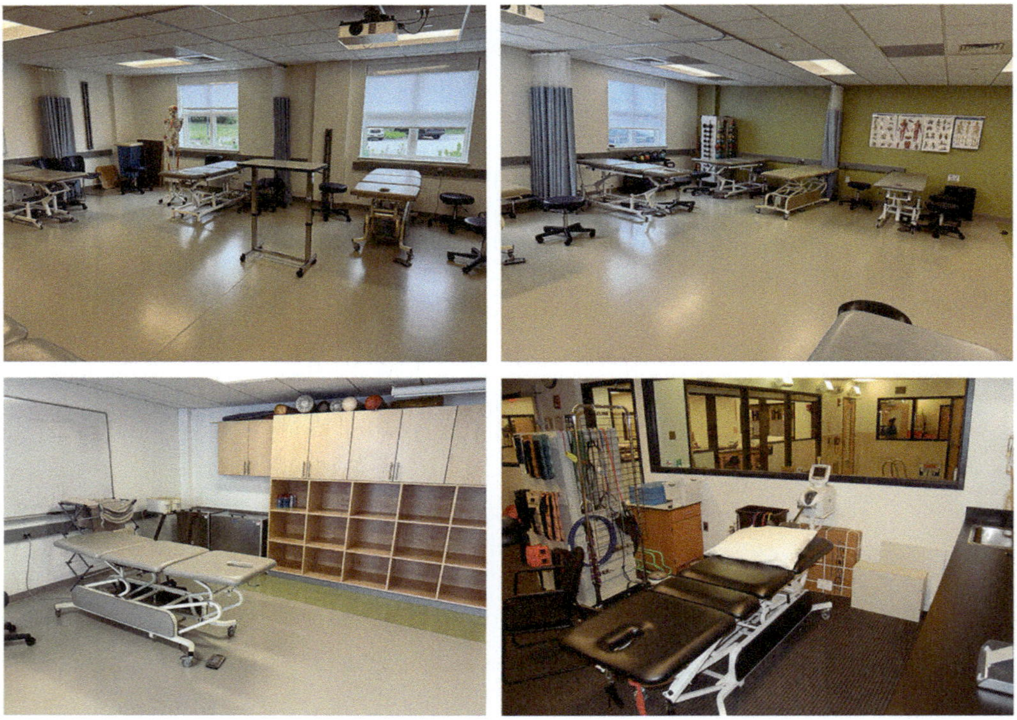

Exhibit 10.5 Examples of outpatient clinic and rehabilitation facilities

EDUCATION REQUIREMENTS

Athletic Training

Professional athletic training degree programs must be accredited by the Commission on Accreditation of Athletic Training Education (CAATE). As of 2022, the only entry point into a professional program was through an entry-level master's degree (CAATE, n.d.). These professional education programs are rooted in a medical-based education model, using a competency-based approach in both the classroom and clinical settings. The educational programs aim to develop comprehensive patient care knowledge and skills based on the five domains of clinical practice: risk reduction; wellness and health literacy; assessment, evaluation, and diagnosis; critical incident management; therapeutic intervention; and healthcare administration and professional responsibility. There are currently 256 accredited professional Master's in Athletic Training programs in the United States (CAATE, n.d.).

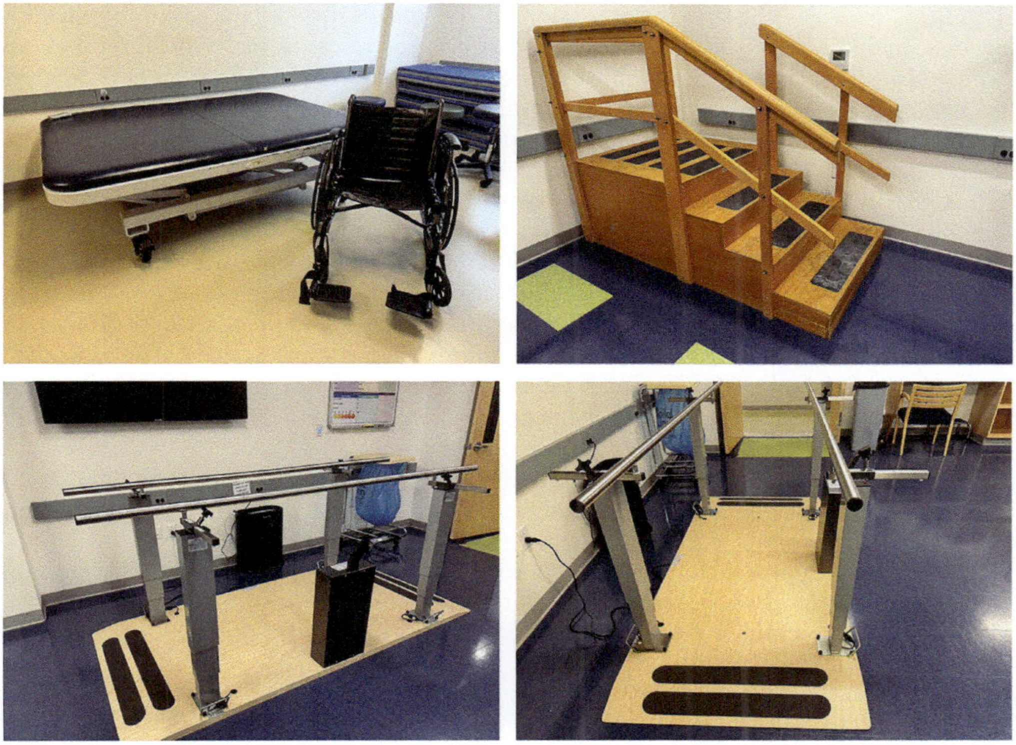

Exhibit 10.6 Examples of inpatient clinic and rehabilitation facilities

Physical Therapy

In the United States, a PT needs a Doctor of Physical Therapy (DPT) degree from a Commission on Accreditation in Physical Therapy Education (CAPTE)-accredited physical therapist education program and must pass the National Physical Therapy Exam (NPTE). There are 279 accredited educational programs in the US, with the average program consisting of 122 credits across 2.5 to 3 years (122 weeks, on average). Coursework follows the standards set forth by CAPTE, which includes many of the foundational disciplines of exercise science (e.g., anatomy and physiology, exercise physiology, biomechanics, motor behavior), clinical and system-based courses (e.g., cardiovascular and pulmonary, endocrine and metabolic, musculoskeletal, neuroscience, psychology, pathology, and pharmacology), and professional values and development courses (e.g., communication, ethics/values, organization and administration, and clinical reasoning). According to the APTA, approximately 77% of the DPT curriculum is classroom (didactic) and lab study and the remaining 23% is dedicated to clinical education, with a minimum of 30 weeks of full-time clinical experience during the length of the program (APTA, n.d.c.).

CERTIFICATIONS AND LICENSURE

Athletic Training

To become an athletic trainer, a student must graduate from an accredited program and then pass the national Board of Certification for Athletic Trainers (BOC-AT) examination.

The BOC provides a detailed description of the certification examination application process, including application criteria and specific requirements, in the *BOC Exam Candidate Handbook*, which is available by visiting the BOC website. The current BOC certification exam consists of 175 scored and unscored (experimental) questions delivered in a combination of multiple-choice items; stand-alone "alternative" items, such as drag and drop, text-based simulation, multi-select, and hot spot; and focused testlets that consist of a scenario followed by key/critical questions related to that scenario. Candidates taking the exam will not know which questions are scored and unscored (experimental). A total of 4 hours is allotted to complete the exam. All 175 test items are presented in one part, and candidates have the ability to move forward or backward throughout the entire exam. Successful completion of the BOC certification exam is the start of a career-long commitment to continuing education. To maintain a current and active Certified Athletic Trainer credential, all ATs must fulfill the recertification requirements. In 2012, the BOC implemented a process that ended the staggered recertification process and moved to a 2-year reporting cycle with common expiration dates for all ATs.

Athletic trainers are licensed in 48 states and the District of Columbia (NATA, n.d.c.). Although Hawaii does not have licensure, ATs are regulated by the state. California remains the only state without licensure or regulation. Each state has its own rules, regulations, and statutes that govern the licensure or regulation of the athletic training profession. To become a licensed or regulated AT, one must pass the BOC-AT exam at minimum and potentially meet state-specific requirements above and beyond that certification examination.

Physical Therapy

All states in the United States require PTs to be licensed. To obtain a license, students must graduate from an accredited DPT Program and pass the NPTE, which is administered by the Federation of State Boards of Physical Therapy (FSBT). The NPTE is designed to assess basic entry-level competence, which is required for the requisite knowledge and skills to be a physical therapist. The FSBT invests considerable time into developing test questions, which are submitted by licensed PTs representing a broad range of practice settings from across the country. The NPTE is administered on set dates four times per year in January, April, July, and October.

The examination consists of 225 stand-alone, multiple-choice questions (five sections of 45 questions) and lasts approximately 5 hours. Some questions may include a graphic or video or may be based on a clinical scenario. The content of the exam is broken into body systems and non-systems. Body system questions fall under the following categories: physical therapy examination; foundations for evaluation, differential diagnosis, and prognosis; and interventions. The defined body systems are: cardiovascular and pulmonary (22–27 questions); musculoskeletal (44–54 questions); neuromuscular and nervous system (39–48 questions); integumentary (8–11 questions); metabolic and endocrine systems (4–6 questions); gastrointestinal system (3–6 questions); lymphatic system (4–7 questions); and system interactions (8–10 questions). Content within the non-body systems includes equipment, devices, and technologies (5–6 questions); therapeutic modalities (4–6 questions); safety and protection (5–7 questions); professional responsibilities (4–5 questions); and research and evidence-based practice (3–5 questions). All licensed PTs are required by the individual state boards of physical therapy to adhere to the statutes and regulations within their state of practice and may include engaging in continuing education.

PROFESSIONAL ORGANIZATIONS

Athletic Training

The NATA is the primary professional organization for ATs. Both the profession and the members benefit from the NATA which works to ensure the advocacy, professional growth, connection, and support needed to keep athletic training essential to healthcare. The NATA headquarters are located in Carrollton, TX, just outside of Dallas. The Annual Clinical Symposia and Athletic Training Expo is held each June and serves as a key opportunity for continuing education and the dissemination of research related to athletic training. Athletic trainers often join other organizations related to their discipline, such as the American College of Sports Medicine (ACSM) and the National Strength and Conditioning Association (NSCA).

Physical Therapy

The APTA is an individual membership professional organization representing over 100,000 members, including physical therapists, physical therapist assistants, and students of physical therapy. The APTA, whose headquarters are located in Alexandria, VA, is led by a board of directors elected from the House of Delegates and includes 51 state chapters and 18 special interest sections and academies. The Annual APTA Combined Sections Meeting is typically held each February and serves as the world's largest conference for continuing education and the dissemination of research related to physical therapy. Many of the APTA sections and academies have their own professional conferences tailored to more specific areas of physical therapy practice, along with state-level conferences organized by state chapters of the APTA. Much like ATs, PTs often join other exercise science-related professional organizations, including the ACSM and the NSCA, as well as professional organizations related to specialty areas.

JOURNALS

Athletic Training

The NATA publishes the *Journal of Athletic Training* monthly, as well as a quarterly journal, *Athletic Training Education Journal*, dedicated to the educational aspects of AT. Members also receive *The NATA News*, a monthly magazine that keeps members current with activities within the profession. In addition, a quarterly newsletter, the *Sports Medicine Legal Digest*, aimed at informing athletic trainers of current legal issues that could affect their daily practice, is available to members. Other research journals that inform the practice of AT include *Journal of Sport Rehabilitation*, *BMC Sports Science, Medicine and Rehabilitation*, *Journal of Orthopaedic and Sports Physical Therapy*, *Medicine and Science in Sports and Exercise*, and *Journal of Strength & Conditioning Research.*

Physical Therapy

APTA members have access to the *PTJ: Physical Therapy & Rehabilitation Journal*, the primary journal of the profession. In addition, each APTA section or academy often has a journal focus on that area of practice. For example, the *Journal of Neurologic Physical Therapy* is available to all Academy of Neurologic Physical Therapy members and the *Journal of Orthopaedic & Sports Physical Therapy* is available to all Academy of

Orthopaedic Physical Therapy members. PTs will also read journals similar to ATs such as *Medicine and Science in Sports and Exercise* and *Journal of Strength & Conditioning Research*.

FUTURE DIRECTIONS

As previously mentioned, employment trends for both ATs and PTs are projected to remain strong through 2032. Both professions are vital to healthcare and often collaborate as part of the same team in many holistic care settings to enhance the overall health and wellness of an individual. In addition, both professions share a commitment to diversity, equity, and inclusion with initiative and efforts aimed at student recruitment and retention. The future growth of the AT and PT professions will likely be driven by technological advancements, changes in general healthcare systems and practice environments, and innovation in research.

Athletic Training

Diakogeorgiou et al. (2021) and Eberman et al. (2019) have suggested that the future of AT will likely include considerations around the growth of emerging practice settings, such as the military and within physicians' offices; the consideration to move toward independent medical models at the collegiate setting where ATs are employed by an external agency versus internally by an institution; expansion of residencies and fellowship programs; and greater contributions to public health and population-specific initiatives. Research will likely focus on the following priorities:

- healthcare competency
- vitality of the profession
- health professions education
- healthcare economics
- health information technology

Physical Therapy

The research agenda for the APTA was developed by a special committee (Scientific and Practice Affairs Committee) and published in 2023. It identifies six key areas of focus for the profession: population health research, mechanistic research, clinical research, education and professional development research, health services research, and workforce research (Stevens-Lapsley et al., 2023). This agenda will likely include questions about the following emerging topics:

- regenerative medicine
- artificial intelligence
- enhanced data analytics
- organizational structure and policy

SUMMARY

Injury management, including both prevention and risk mitigation, as well as treatment and rehabilitation, remains a central aspect of healthcare for many individuals. While rehabilitation from injury involves a diverse team of professionals, ATs and PTs play pivotal roles in the care and recovery process. The future for both the AT and PT is promising, with exciting opportunities in employment and research, as well as continued innovation in techniques, skills, and technology.

STUDY QUESTIONS

1. What are the five practice domains for an athletic trainer as defined by the *Athletic Training Practice Analysis?*
2. According to the APTA and FSBPT, what are the three areas that the practice of a physical therapist falls within?
3. What organization is responsible for accrediting athletic training education programs?
4. What organization is responsible for accrediting physical therapy education programs?
5. How does the International Classification of Function (ICF) inform the practice of athletic training and physical therapy?
6. What is an example of a physical agent, assessment, and measurement tool found in a clinic as part of the rehabilitation of an injury?
7. How can wearable technology inform load monitoring in an athlete?
8. What are the eight specialty areas that define the residency program in athletic training?
9. What are the ten specialist certification areas regulated by the ABPTS for physical therapy?
10. Name the primary journals for athletic training and physical therapy.

LEARNING ACTIVITIES

1. Create a diagram that outlines the pathway to becoming a licensed athletic trainer and physical therapist.
2. Use the information on the NATA website to write a one-page summary of the organization's history.
3. Research (using the internet, AI, and/or written sources) a specific technology or research tool used in athletic training and physical therapy. Create a brief PowerPoint presentation to inform others. You should have a minimum of eight slides, including title and bibliography.
4. Search online for "Athletic Trainer" and "Physical Therapist" jobs. List the common job requirements for application as well as the any recommended criteria.
5. Visit the websites for the NATA (n.d.) and the APTA (n.d.) and explore the schedules for prior conferences. What topics were of interest to you? What surprised you about the topic list?

SUGGESTED READING AND RELATED WEBSITES

American College of Sports Medicine (ACSM). (n.d.). American College of Sports Medicine website, at https://www.acsm.org/ (visited 6 July, 2024).

American Physical Therapy Association (APTA). (n.d.a). American Physical Therapy Association website, at https://www.apta.org/ (visited 6 July, 2024).

American Physical Therapy Association. (2020). *A Century of Movement: Milestones of the American Physical Therapy Association's First 100 Years*. American Physical Therapy Association. Forbes.

Board of Certification (BOC) for the Athletic Trainer. (n.d.). Board of Certification (BOC) for the Athletic Trainer website, at https://bocatc.org/ (visited 6 July, 2024).

Commission on Accreditation of Athletic Training Education (CAATE). (n.d.). Commission on Accreditation of Athletic Training Education website, at https://caate.net/ (visited 6 July, 2024).

Commission on Accreditation in Physical Therapy Education (CAPTE). Commission on Accreditation in Physical Therapy Education website, at https://www.capteonline.org/ (visited 6 July, 2024).

Diakogeorgiou, E., Ray, R. R., Jr., Brown, S., Hertel, J., and Casa, D. J. (2021). The Evolution of the Athletic Training Profession. *Kinesiology Review*, 10(3), 308–318. https://doi.org/10.1123/kr.2021-0027

Eberman, L. E., Walker, S. E., Floyd, R. T., Covassin, T., Nolton, E., Valier, A. R. S., Phan, K., Weiss, L., and Earl-Boehm, J. (2019). The Prioritized Research Agenda for the Athletic Training Profession: A Report from the Strategic Alliance Research Agenda Task Force. *Journal of Athletic Training*, 54(3), 237–244. https://doi.org/10.4085/1062-6050-374-18

Federation of State Boards of Physical Therapy. (n.d.). Federation of State Boards of Physical Therapy website, at https://www.fsbpt.org/ (visited 6 July, 2024).

National Athletic Trainers' Association (NATA). (n.d.). National Athletic Trainers' Association website, at https://www.nata.org/ (visited 6 July, 2024).

National Strength and Conditioning Association (NSCA). National Strength and Conditioning Association website, at https://www.nsca.com/ (visited 6 July, 2024).

Stevens-Lapsley, J., Hicks, G. E., Zimney, K., Slaven, E. J., Manal, T. J., and Jeffries, L. M. (2023). Research Agenda for Physical Therapy from the American Physical Therapy Association. *Physical Therapy*, *103*(10), 126. https://doi.org/10.1093/ptj/pzad126

REFERENCES

American Board for Physical Therapy Specializations: ABPTS. (n.d.). American Board for Physical Therapy Specializations website, at https://specialization.apta.org/ (visited 6 July, 2024).

American Physical Therapy Association (APTA). (2020). *A Century of Movement: Milestones of the American Physical Therapy Association's First 100 Years*. American Physical Therapy Association.

American Physical Therapy Association (APTA). (n.d.b.). *APTA Guide to Physical Therapist Practice 4.0*, at https://guide.apta.org/?_gl=1*qbg3mg*_gcl_au*MTQ1ODg4MjgxMi4xNzU5MTUxMDc3*_ga*MjEyOTczOTgwLjE3NTkxNTEwNzg.*_ga_ZZJK74HXNR*czE3NTkxNTEwNzgkbzEkZzEkdDE3NTkxNTEwODgkajUwJGwwJGgw (visited 6 July, 2024).

American Physical Therapy Association (APTA). (n.d.c.). Becoming a PT, at https://www.apta.org/your-career/careers-in-physical-therapy/becoming-a-pt (visited 6 July, 2024).

Board of Certification for Athletic Trainers. (n.d.) Board of Certification for Athletic Trainers website, at https://bocatc.org/ (visited 6 July, 2024).

Board of Certification (2021). *2021 Practice Analysis Study for Athletic Trainers*. Omaha, NE: James P. Henderson.

Bureau of Labor Statistics. (n.d.a). US Department of Labor, Occupational Outlook Handbook, Athletic Trainers, at https://www.bls.gov/ooh/healthcare/athletic-trainers.htm (visited July 6, 2024).

Bureau of Labor Statistics. (n.d.b.). U.S. Department of Labor, Occupational Outlook Handbook, Physical Therapists, at https://www.bls.gov/ooh/healthcare/physical-therapists.htm (visited July 6, 2024).

Commission on Accreditation of Athletic Training Education (CAATE). (n.d.). Commission on Accreditation of Athletic Training Education website, at https://caate.net/ (visited 6 July, 2024).

Delforge, G. D., and Behnke, R. S. (1999). The History and Evolution of Athletic Training Education in the United States. *Journal of Athletic Training*, 34(1), 53–61.

Diakogeorgiou, E., Ray, R. R., Jr., Brown, S., Hertel, J., and Casa, D. J. (2021). The Evolution of the Athletic Training Profession. *Kinesiology Review*, 10(3), 308–318. https://doi.org/10.1123/kr.2021-0027

Draovitch, P., Patel, S., Marrone, W., Grundstein, M. J., Grant, R., Virgile, A., Myslinski, T., Bedi, A., Bradley, J. P., Williams, R. J., 3rd, Kelly, B., and Jones, K. (2022). The Return-to-Sport Clearance Continuum Is a Novel Approach Toward Return to Sport and Performance for the Professional Athlete. *Arthroscopy, Sports Medicine, and Rehabilitation*, 4(1), e93–e101. https://doi.org/10.1016/j.asmr.2021.10.026

Ebel, R.G. (1999). *Far Beyond the Shoe Box: Fifty Years of the National Athletic Trainers' Association*. Jersey City, NJ: Forbes.

Eberman, L. E., Walker, S. E., Floyd, R. T., Covassin, T., Nolton, E., Valier, A. R. S., Phan, K., Weiss, L., and Earl-Boehm, J. (2019). The Prioritized Research Agenda for the Athletic Training Profession: A Report from the Strategic Alliance Research Agenda Task Force. *Journal of Athletic Training*, 54(3), 237–244. https://doi.org/10.4085/1062-6050-374-18

Federation of State Boards of Physical Therapy. (n.d.). Federation of State Boards of Physical Therapy website, at https://www.fsbpt.org/ (visited 6 July, 2024).

Garnett, M. F., Elgaddal, N., and Spencer, M. R. (2023). Repetitive Strain Injuries in Adults in the Past 3 Months: United States, 2021. National Health Statistics Report, no 189. Hyattsville, MD: National Center for Health Statistics.

Luczak, T., Burch, R., Lewis, E., Chander, H., and Ball, J. (2020). State-of-the-art Review of Athletic Wearable Technology: What 113 Strength and Conditioning Coaches and Athletic Trainers from the USA Said About Technology in Sports. *International Journal of Sports Science & Coaching*, 15(1), 26–40. https://doi.org/10.1177/1747954119885244

Moffat, M. (2003). The History of Physical Therapy Practice in the United States. *Journal of Physical Therapy Education*, 17(3), 15–25.

NATA. (n.d.b.). National Athletic Trainers' Association: Professional Interests, at https://www.nata.org/professional-interests (visited 6 July, 2024).

NATA. (n.d.c.). State Legislative Affairs Advocating for ATs, at https://www.nata.org/advocacy/state (visited 6 July, 2024).

National Safety Council (2024, July 8). Injury Facts, at https://injuryfacts.nsc.org/ (visited 6 July, 2024).

O'Shea, M. E. (1980). *A History of the National Athletic Trainers Association* (2nd ed.). Greenville, NC: NATA.

Ozgok Kangal, M. K. and Regan, J. P. (2025). Physiology, Wound Healing. StatPearls [Internet]. Treasure Island (FL): StatPearls Publishing. Available from: https://www.ncbi.nlm.nih.gov/books/NBK535406/ (visited 29 August, 2025).

Parks, M. T., Wang, Z., and Siu, K. C. (2019). Current Low-Cost Video-Based Motion Analysis Options for Clinical Rehabilitation: A Systematic Review. *Physical Therapy*, 99(10), 1405–1425. https://doi.org/10.1093/ptj/pzz097

Prentice, W. E. (2020). *Rehabilitation Techniques for Sports Medicine and Athletic Training* (7th ed.). Thorofare, NJ: SLACK, Incorporated.

PSATS. (n.d.). Public Safety Athletic Trainers' Society website, at https://www.psatsociety.com/ (visited 6 July, 2024).

Seshadri, D. R., Thom, M. L., Harlow, E. R., Gabbett, T. J., Geletka, B. J., Hsu, J. J., Drummond, C. K., Phelan, D. M., and Voos, J. E. (2021). Wearable Technology and Analytics as a Complementary Toolkit to Optimize Workload and to Reduce Injury Burden. *Frontiers in Sports and Active Living*, *2*, January 2021. https://doi.org/10.3389/fspor.2020.630576

Sizler, B. (2022, June 13). NATA Now: Co-Chair Discusses Sports Science, at https://www.nata.org/nata-now/articles/2022/06/co-chair-discusses-sports-science (visited 6 July 2024).

Snyder, A. R., Parsons, J. T., Valovich McLeod, T. C., Curtis Bay, R., Michener, L. A., and Sauers, E. L. (2008). Using Disablement Models and Clinical Outcomes Assessment to Enable Evidence-based

Athletic Training Practice, Part I: Disablement Models. *Journal of Athletic Training*, 43(4), 428–436. https://doi.org/10.4085/1062-6050-43.4.428

Stevens-Lapsley, J., Hicks, G. E., Zimney, K., Slaven, E. J., Manal, T. J., and Jeffries, L. M. (2023). Research Agenda for Physical Therapy from the American Physical Therapy Association. *Physical Therapy*, 103(10), 126. https://doi.org/10.1093/ptj/pzad126

Wang, C., Stovitz, S. D., Kaufman, J. S., Steele, R. J., and Shrier, I. (2024). Principles of Musculoskeletal Sport Injuries for Epidemiologists: A Review. *Injury Epidemiology*, 11(1), 21. https://doi.org/10.1186/s40621-024-00507-3

WHO. (2001). *International Classification of Functioning, Disability, and Health: ICF*. Geneva: World Health Organization.

Glossary

Abstract A summary of the main elements of a scientific article. Abstracts usually also include a purpose statement, description of the methods, results, and conclusions.

Academy of Nutrition and Dietetics (the Academy) Formerly known as the American Dietetic Association; the world's largest organization of food and nutrition professionals and an excellent resource for individuals interested in becoming an RDN or a DTR.

Acceleration The rate of change of velocity, describing how quickly an object speeds up, slows down, or changes direction.

Accelerometer An electronic device that measures acceleration forces.

Acceptable macronutrient distribution range (AMDR) Guideline specifying the recommended ranges of calories from carbohydrate, fat, and protein in a healthy diet.

Accreditation A formal, independent verification that a program or institution meets established quality standards and is competent to carry out specific conformity assessment tasks.

Action potential An electrical signal that travels along the nerve cells (neurons). It's how messages are transmitted in the nervous system, helping nerves communicate with muscles and other parts of the body.

Acute Of short course; not chronic.

Adaptation Long-term change in the body due to exercise training.

Adenosine triphosphate (ATP) A molecule in which energy (e.g., for muscle contraction) is stored in high-energy phosphate bonds.

Adequate intake (AI) Recommended daily nutrient intake level when there is not enough scientific evidence to establish a Recommended Dietary Allowance (RDA).

Aerobic Requires the use of oxygen for ATP production.

Affordance The reciprocal fit between a person's characteristics and the environment's properties that allow a specific action to occur.

Allied health A field of study and practice that includes hospital and other clinical settings that promote a positive state of well-being. These settings provide a number of employment opportunities for the exercise scientist.

Anaerobic Does not require the use of oxygen for ATP production.

Analysis of variance (ANOVA) Used when comparing the means of three or more groups.

Anatomical position The standard position used to describe the human body where the person is standing, facing forward, arms at the sides, and palms facing forward.

Anatomy The study of the parts of an organism and their relationship to each other.

Anemia Condition where the blood has a lower-than-normal oxygen-carrying capacity due to a deficiency in red blood cells or hemoglobin, which are essential for transporting oxygen.

Angular kinematics Rotational motion around an axis, characterized by angular displacement (change in angular position), angular velocity (rate of change of angular displacement), and angular acceleration (rate of change of angular velocity).

Antioxidant Naturally occurring or synthetic substance that helps protect cells from the damaging effects of oxygen free radicals; highly reactive compounds created during normal cell metabolism.

Anxiety A negative emotional state associated with physiological and/or psychological responses.

Arousal A combination of physiological and psychological activation that varies on a continuum from very un-aroused to very aroused.

Arteries Blood vessels that carry oxygen-rich blood from the heart to the tissues.

Atherosclerosis A disease in which fatty deposits in artery walls lead to a reduction in blood flow through the artery; can lead to heart attack and stroke.

Athletic trainer A healthcare professional who specializes in the prevention, diagnosis, treatment, and rehabilitation of injuries and illnesses related to physical activity.

Augmented feedback Information about a performance provided by an external source that supplements the sensory feedback available to the performer.

Autonomic nervous system Branch of the nervous system that controls the involuntary functions of the body.

Basal ganglia A group of structures deep within the brain that help control movement, coordination, and posture by regulating signals from the motor cortex.

Basal metabolic rate (BMR) The minimal amount of energy required for maintenance of life. The BMR is typically measured under strict laboratory conditions: 12 hours after eating, after a restful sleep, no exercise or activity preceding the test, elimination of emotional excitement, and in a comfortable temperature.

Beta oxidation Catabolic process that breaks down fatty acids into acetyl-CoA, a molecule that enters the citric acid cycle to produce energy.

Bioenergetics The study of how energy is produced, transferred, and used by living organisms, particularly how the body converts food into usable energy to support cellular functions and physical activity.

Biomechanics The study of the forces that act on the body and the effects they produce.

Burnout Psychological syndrome caused by a prolonged response to stress.

Calorimetry The determination of heat loss or gain; a calorimeter is used to measure the amount of heat exchanged in a chemical reaction or by the body under certain conditions.

Cancer A family of diseases, characterized by uncontrolled growth of abnormal cells.

Capillaries The smallest blood vessels that connect arteries to veins and allow the exchange of gases, nutrients, and waste products between the blood and body tissues.

Carbohydrate loading A dietary method used by endurance athletes to increase the carbohydrate (glycogen) stores in the muscles and liver.

Cardiac ischemia Reduced blood flow and therefore oxygen to the heart, often due to atherosclerosis.

Cardiovascular disease Any disease that affects the cardiovascular system; for example, coronary heart disease and peripheral artery disease.

Cartilage A flexible, rubbery tissue found in places like joints, the nose, and ears. It helps cushion joints and provides structure to parts of the body.

Cerebellum A structure located at the base of the brain that is involved in the regulation of coordination and the control of fine movements.

Cerebral localization The mapping of the cerebral cortex into areas and the correlation of the various areas with cerebral function.

Cholesterol A steroid molecule found in the blood that can contribute to lipid deposition and atherosclerosis of artery walls.

Chronic Of long duration; not acute.

Chronic inflammation A systemic, low-level, long-term, inflammatory process that can lead to the development of many chronic diseases.

Cinematography A technique that provides a sequence of images that can be displayed as a motion picture or viewed one by one.

Clinical exercise The use of exercise and physical activity to improve or maintain physical function, manage disease, and enhance overall health and well-being, often prescribed and supervised by qualified healthcare professionals.

Closed-loop control A type of motor control through which sensory feedback from the limbs is used to correct errors in the initial movement plan or program.

Cognitive functioning Process by which individuals take in, use, and respond to information.

Computerized dynamic posturography A process used to measure the control of posture and balance in upright stance.

Concentric contractions Muscle action that involves the production of force while the muscle is shortening, such as when curling a barbell to the chest.

Concurrent training Performing resistance and endurance training in the same session or in close proximity, i.e. within the same day or week.

Confidence An individual's belief in their ability to be successful.

Construct validity The degree to which a test measures an intangible quality or attribute (e.g., sportsmanship or creativity).

Content validity The extent to which the items on a test adequately sample the subject matter and abilities that the test was designed to measure.

Context-conditioned variability Movement variation that results from subtle changes in the performer and the environment.

Contextual interference The degree of performance disruption that results from different amounts of task switching during practice.

Coronary heart disease Narrowing of the coronary arteries, usually caused by atherosclerosis (the build-up of fatty plaques on the artery walls) that prevents adequate blood and oxygen supply to the heart.

Corporate fitness A career opportunity that involves developing and/or supervising fitness programs in various workplaces and community centers.

Correlation Measures the strength and direction of the relationship between two variables.

Criterion validity The extent to which a test correlates with another valid measure of the same concept.

Crosstalk The process by which signaling molecules (such as myokines released from skeletal muscle) can communicate with other organ systems in the body.

Degrees of freedom The number of independent components a control system must regulate.

Densitometry The determination of the density (mass/volume) of the body. Body mass may be measured using an accurate physician's scale, while body volume is commonly measured using the hydrostatic (underwater) weighing technique.

Descriptive statistics Statistical methods used to summarize data (e.g., mean, median, mode).

Developmental biomechanics Focuses on evaluating essential movement patterns across the human life span.

Diabetes A disease in which insufficient insulin is produced (type 1 diabetes) or the body is insensitive to insulin (type 2 diabetes).

Diastole The phase of the heart cycle when the heart relaxes and fills with blood.

Diencephalon Region of the brain located between the brainstem and the cerebral hemispheres that plays a key role in sensory processing, hormonal regulation, and autonomic function. It includes structures such as the thalamus and hypothalamus.

Dietetics The science of applying food and nutrition to health and disease.

Dietitians Experts in nutrition and dietetics who have completed specific education requirements to earn the Registered Dietitian and Nutritionist (RDN) credential and are recognized as medical professionals within the field.

Dual-energy x-ray absorptiometry An imaging technique utilizing x-rays that allows for the quantification of body tissues such as muscle, bone, and fat, and is the gold-standard for determining body composition.

Dynamical systems theory An approach to motor control and learning that emphasizes the motor system's self-organizing tendencies in response to information specifying constraints from the performer, the task, and the environment.

Dynamics A branch of mechanics that investigates bodies, masses, and forces in motion.

Dynamography Provides kinetic or force data through the conversion of one form of energy into another. A dynamograph is a device used for measuring forces produced during an activity.

Dynapenia The loss of muscle function, i.e. strength and power, with age.

Eccentric contraction A muscle contraction in which the muscle actively lengthens under tension.

Ecological approach An approach to motor control and learning that emphasizes the direct perception of information specifying affordances and the tight and reciprocal coupling between perception and action.

Efficiency The ratio of useful work performed to the total energy expended.

Electrolyte A substance that dissociates into ions in solution and conducts electricity; electrolytes such as sodium, potassium, calcium, and chloride help regulate nerve and muscle function, hydration, blood pH, and other essential physiological processes.

Electromyography A technique used to measure the electrical activity associated with the activation of motor units and subsequent muscle contraction.

Energy The capacity to perform work.

Energy availability The energy left over for normal body functions after subtracting the energy used during exercise, standardized to kilograms of fat-free mass.

Environmental physiology An area of physiology interested in studying exercise done in cold, hot, or humid climates or exercise done at altitude.

Epidemiology The study of the occurrence and prevalence of disease among the population.

Epigenomics The study of the changes or modifications that can occur to one's DNA due to environmental and behavioral factors and how these modifications can be passed on to one's children.

Ergogenic aid A substance, device, or treatment that is believed to enhance athletic performance.

Evaluation A judgment of merit based on a comparison of various measurements, impressions, and other evidence of some standard.

Evidence based practice Methodology that integrates the best available scientific evidence with clinical expertise and individual needs.

Exercise addiction Psychological dependence on regularly scheduled exercise.

Exercise adherence Degree to which an individual follows the recommended frequency, intensity, and duration in any given program or activity.

Exercise and sport nutrition A growing field that integrates principles of nutrition with exercise science to support physical performance, optimize training adaptations, and reduce the risk of injury and illness.

Exercise adherence Ability to comply with the prescribed frequency, intensity, duration, mode, and progression of a physical activity until a stated outcome goal is achieved.

Exercise epidemiology The study of factors associated with participation in physical activity and of how physical activity affects the probability of disease or injury.

Exercise physiology A specialized area of study within the broader field of physiology that examines how single and repeated bouts of exercise affect cells, tissues, and organ systems of the human body.

Exercise psychology The application of psychology to promote, maintain, and enhance exercise and physical activity.

Exercise science A dynamic and evolving discipline that applies scientific principles to understand human movement, health, performance, and rehabilitation.

Exercise snacks Frequent, brief bouts of vigorous exercise that break up sedentary behavior and may improve metabolic health.

Exhalation The process of breathing out air and expelling carbon dioxide and other gases from the body.

Eye tracking systems Cameras specifically designed to capture data on eye movement, focus of vision, head position and rotation, eyelid aperture, lip and eyebrow movement, and pupil size.

Fast-twitch glycolytic (FG) fibers Fatigable muscle fibers that favor glycolytic (anaerobic) methods of energy production; also known as type IIb fibers.

Fast-twitch oxidative glycolytic (FOG) fibers Intermediately fatigue-resistant muscle fibers that utilize both oxidative (aerobic) and glycolytic (anaerobic) methods of energy production; also known as type IIa fibers.

Fatigue A state of exhaustion or a loss of strength or endurance, as may follow strenuous physical activity.

Female athlete triad A condition affecting physically active females, characterized by a combination of disordered eating, menstrual dysfunction, and low bone mineral density.

Fluxomics The study of metabolic flux or the rate at which metabolites move through metabolic pathways.

Food science Science that applies principles of the biological and physical sciences to study the nature of foods, the causes of food deterioration, and the principles underlying the processing and preparation of food.

Forensic biomechanics Applies biomechanics to legal cases to determine how injuries or incidents likely occurred.

Force platform An electromechanical device that provides electrical signals proportional to the components of force acting on it.

Functional foods Foods that provide health benefits beyond their basic nutritional value.

Functional near-infrared spectroscopy The use of near-infrared light sent through the scalp and brain to measure changes in oxygenated and deoxygenated hemoglobin to help determine the activity levels of neurons during mentally intensive tasks.

Genomics A field of biology focused on studying the genome, which includes all the genes encoded by deoxyribonucleic acid (DNA).

Global flexibility The flexibility of multiple muscle groups along the posterior chain, including the hamstrings, lower back, and calves.

Glycemic index A system that ranks how quickly carbohydrate-containing foods raise blood sugar levels compared to a reference food, usually pure glucose.

Glycolysis A metabolic pathway that breaks down glucose into pyruvate, producing energy in the form of ATP.

Glycogen The storage form of carbohydrate found in the liver and in the muscles.

Goniometer A device used to measure joint angles by determining the static position of one limb segment relative to another around a joint axis; commonly used to assess range of motion in clinical and research settings.

Gyroscope A measurement device that assesses the rotation and direction of the sensor.

Hemoglobin A blood protein involved in the transport of oxygen and carbon dioxide.

Higher education A career opportunity that usually involves teaching and/or research at the college or university level.

Homeostasis The process by which the body maintains a stable internal environment, such as regulating temperature, blood pressure, and fluid balance, to keep everything working properly.

Homunculus Latin for "little man." Term used in neurology to describe the map in the brain of sensory neurons in each part of the body.

Hormone A chemical typically released from an endocrine gland into the blood that exerts its biological effect elsewhere in the body.

Human performance A way to characterize how well an individual is able to perform a task that reflects capabilities, limitations, and the human factors influencing their actions.

Hyperlipidemia An elevated level of lipids (fats) in the blood.

Hypertension Persistently high arterial blood pressure that may have no known cause, or it may be associated with another primary disease. It is a risk factor for the development of heart disease, peripheral vascular disease, stroke, and kidney disease.

Hypertrophy An increase in the size of a biological structure such as a muscle cell.

Hypothesis A tentative proposal made to explain certain observations or facts that require further investigation to be verified.

Independent t-tests A statistical test used to compare the means of separate (independent) groups.

Indirect calorimetry The measurement of energy expenditure via determination of oxygen consumption and carbon dioxide production.

Information processing approach An approach to motor control and learning that emphasizes the indirect nature of perception, the encoding, storage, and retrieval of information during performance and learning, and the existence of central control structures in the brain.

Inertial measurement unit A portable electronic device that combines triaxial accelerometers, gyroscopes, and magnetometers into one small piece of equipment.

Inferential statistics Techniques used to draw conclusions about a population based on a sample (e.g., t-tests, ANOVA).

Inhalation The process of breathing in air and drawing oxygen into the lungs, where it will be absorbed into the bloodstream.

Interference effect A term used to describe the activation of molecular signaling pathways due to concurrent resistance and aerobic exercise resulting in reduced training adaptations, e.g., reduced gains in strength and/or power due to too much aerobic training.

Injury and performance continuum A conceptual spectrum that ranges from an injured state to a high-performance state along which an athlete will non-linearly move through during rehabilitation of an injury.

Instrumented staircase A staircase with force plates embedded under the steps and handrail.

Instrumented treadmill A treadmill with force platforms embedded below the belt.

Insulin A hormone released from the pancreas that functions to facilitate glucose transport from the blood into cells.

Interval measurement A level of measurement resulting in values that permit the making of statements of equality of intervals in addition to nominal statements (sameness or difference) or ordinal statements (greater than or less than).

Keywords Terms from a manuscript or an article that identify the key concepts in a particular research question.

Kilocalorie The amount of heat necessary to raise the temperature of 1 liter of water 1° Celsius.

Kinematics A branch of mechanics that investigates motion without reference to masses or forces.

Kinesiology The parent discipline of biomechanics; a science that investigates movement.

Kinetics A branch of mechanics that investigates the actions of forces in producing or changing the motion of masses.

Knowledge of performance A source of feedback that indicates errors in the learner's movement pattern, not the outcome.

Knowledge of results A source of feedback that indicates whether the outcome of the practice trial was successful in reaching or achieving the goal.

Linear kinematics Motion along a straight or curved path, involving parameters such as displacement (change in position), speed (magnitude of velocity), velocity (speed with a direction), and acceleration (change in velocity over time).

Magnetic resonance imaging A non-invasive medical diagnostic technique that uses a magnetic field to produce anatomical pictures of the living body.

Magnetometer A device used to estimate direction and measure local magnetic fields.

Mean The average of a set of numbers.

Mechanical advantage The leverage obtained by using a lever system, such as bones and joints, to perform work more effectively.

Mechanism A detailed description of how and why a phenomenon occurs, i.e., a sequence of reasoning from cause to effect.

Median The middle value when data is ordered.

Medulla oblongata The lowest part of the brain stem directly connected to the spinal cord containing control centers for the heart and lungs.

Measurement The process of assigning numerical or symbolic values to members of a group for the purpose of distinguishing among the members based on the degree to which they possess the characteristic being assessed.

Mental health Psychological function on a continuum from suboptimal to optimal.

Meta-analysis A type of literature review that contains a definitive methodology and quantifies the results of various studies to a standard metric that allows the use of statistical techniques as a means of analysis.

Metabolic cart A device used to measure oxygen consumption (VO_2), carbon dioxide production (VCO_2), and other respiratory gases to assess energy expenditure and cardiorespiratory function during rest or exercise.

Metabolism The sum of all physical and chemical changes that occur in the body. Metabolism involves two processes: anabolism (the building-up or synthesizing processes) and catabolism (the tearing-down or degrading processes).

Metabolites Small molecules that are generated by cells during metabolic processes.

Metabolomics The study and analysis of metabolites in the human body.

Mitochondria A cellular organelle involved in aerobic energy production.

Mode The most frequently occurring value in a data set.

Motion recording device Captures body motion using optical lenses to provide permanent recorded images of movement.

Motivation The direction and intensity of one's effort.

Motor behavior The study of how humans learn, control, and develop motor skills.

Motor control The study of the neural, physical, and behavioral processes underlying the performance of a motor skill.

Motor cortex A region of the cerebral cortex responsible for planning, controlling, and executing voluntary movements.

Motor development The progression of physical movements and skills throughout a person's life, particularly in childhood.

Motor learning The study of the processes associated with practice or experience that lead to relatively permanent changes in the capacity to perform motor skills.

Motor neuron A type of nerve cell that carries signals from the brain and spinal cord to skeletal muscles.

Motor program A stored set of movement commands that activate the proper muscles in the correct sequence with the correct timing without the influence of sensory feedback.

Motor unit Functional unit of the nervous system responsible for muscle contraction. It consists of a single motor neuron and all the muscle fibers it innervates.

mTOR A signaling molecule involved in protein synthesis in muscle tissue.

Muscle Tissue in the body that contracts and relaxes to produce movement—there are three main types: skeletal, smooth, and cardiac.

Muscle fiber A skeletal muscle cell.

Muscle spindle A type of sensory receptor, or proprioceptor, within the muscle that is sensitive to changes in the length of the muscle and is involved in the stretch reflex.

Myokines Chemicals released by muscle tissue that act as signaling molecules.

Narrative review A subjective summary and interpretation of research results from most, if not all, of the studies in a particular area.

Neuromuscular junction The synapse between a motor neuron and a muscle where the nerve sends signals to make the muscle contract.

Neuron A type of cell that transmits electrical signals in the body for communication between different parts of the body.

Newton's first law An object will remain at rest or continue to move at a constant velocity unless acted upon by an external force.

Newton's second law The relationship between force, mass, and acceleration, expressed by the equation F=ma.

Newton's third law For every action, there is an equal and opposite reaction.

Nominal measurement A level of measurement that permits only the making of statements of sameness or difference.

Non-scientific literature Anything published in a book, magazine, newspaper, or online that is not peer-reviewed for scientific content.

Nutraceuticals Nutrients that exhibit druglike properties when taken in appropriate dosages.

Nutrigenomics The study of the interaction of nutrients with the human genome; also called nutrition genomics.

Nutrition The science of food that is generally described as the sum total of the processes involved in the intake and utilization of food substances by living organisms, including ingestion, digestion, absorption, and metabolism of food.

Nutritionists Individuals who have a strong interest in food and nutrition but have varying levels of education and training and are not typically recognized as health professionals.

Objectivity The aspect of test reliability that is concerned with the variability in scores resulting from different individuals administering and scoring a test.

Occupational biomechanics Focuses on providing a safer and more efficient environment for the worker.

Open-loop control A type of control whereby the entire movement is controlled by the higher centers without the influence of sensory feedback from the lower centers.

OPTIMAL theory Acronym that stands for **O**ptimizing **P**erformance **T**hrough **I**ntrinsic **M**otivation and **A**ttention for **L**earning. The theory stresses the need to consider the motivational and attentional influences on performance and learning.

Ordinal measurement A level of measurement that permits the ordering of the individuals measured in addition to statements of sameness or difference (nominal).

Osteoporosis A disease characterized by very low bone mass and deterioration of bone tissue that results in brittle bones and an increased risk of fractures.

Overload principle The concept that to improve fitness or performance, the body must be challenged with a stimulus greater than what it is accustomed to. This can be achieved by increasing the intensity, duration, frequency, or type of exercise.

Overtraining Exceeding a physical and psychological optimal volume and intensity over time that results in disturbed mood and staleness. Usually associated with highly competitive and highly trained endurance athletes.

Paired t-tests A statistical test used to compare the means of two related groups.

Parasympathetic nervous system The branch of the autonomic nervous system that is most active at rest and is involved in restorative functions.

Peer-review process Subjecting an author's scholarly work or ideas to the scrutiny of others who are experts in the field.

Periodization A systematic approach to strength training that involves dividing the training program into specific time blocks or cycles, each with distinct goals, to optimize performance and recovery while minimizing the risk of overtraining.

Personal training Using an individualized approach to assess, motivate, educate, and train clients regarding their health and fitness needs.

Phosphagen system Also known as the ATP-PC system, it is the body's immediate source of energy for short-term, high-intensity activities.

Physical agents A source of energy that can be used to support therapeutic restoration of tissue function including heat, cold, light, sound, electricity, and mechanical forces.

Physical education A field of study concerned with the development of the human body through movement, e.g., physical games, exercises, and sports.

Physical therapist A healthcare professional who specializes in evaluating, diagnosing, and treating movement disorders and physical impairments.

Physiology The study of the processes and functions of the human body and its parts.

Phytochemical Chemical substances found in plants that possess medicinal properties that help prevent chronic disease.

Plyometric exercise Exercise that involves quick jumping or bouncing movements which optimally invoke the stretch reflex and motor unit recruitment and maximize force production.

Pons The part of the brainstem that connects the medulla oblongata and the thalamus.

Population The entire group of individuals, objects, or events that shares a common characteristic and is of interest for a particular study or analysis.

Position The location of an object or body part relative to a reference point, providing a basis for tracking changes in movement.

Power The ability to exert force quickly.

Prebiotics Non-digestible food ingredients that stimulate the growth and/or activity of beneficial microorganisms in the gastrointestinal tract.

Pressure insole A device that consists of a matrix of small force transducers. It provides detailed information concerning load distribution.

Primary reference Original data and/or ideas that are generally the first published record of an investigation. Examples include research articles, research monographs, preprints, patents, dissertations, and conference proceedings.

Proteomics The study of the proteins coded for by the genome and produced by an organism.

Private consulting A career opportunity that involves sharing one's expertise with others (hospitals, fitness centers, and private individuals) so that they can benefit from the information.

Probiotics Live beneficial bacteria found in fermented foods like yogurt, kefir, kimchi, sauerkraut, and pickles.

Progression A principle of exercise training that involves gradually increasing the intensity, duration, frequency, or complexity of an exercise program to continue improving fitness and performance while minimizing the risk of injury.

Proprioception The sense that allows you to know where your body parts are in space, even without looking. It helps you move and balance properly.

Prospective cohort study A study where subjects are selected at random from a defined population. Baseline information on potential risk factors is then collected, and the subjects are followed over time to track the incidence of disease.

Psychology The science of mental processes and behavior.

Quality of life The overall standard of living with regard to mental and physical health, social relationships, level of independence, personal beliefs and spirituality, and relationship to the environment.

Ratio measurement A level of measurement that permits the making of statements of equality or ratios, such as one value is twice another, in addition to nominal statements (sameness or difference), ordinal statements (greater or lesser), and interval statements (equality of intervals).

Reciprocal inhibition A neuromuscular process in which the nervous system suppresses activity in the opposing muscle group during contraction to enable smooth and efficient movement.

Recommended dietary allowance (RDA) Established by the Food and Nutrition Board; represents the levels of intake of essential nutrients considered to be adequate to avoid deficiencies and meet the known nutritional needs of practically all healthy people of similar age and gender.

Recovery Restoration of mental and/or physical states to homeostasis relative to a person's position on the injury-performance continuum.

References Sources used to support various statements in a book or an article.

Regression Statistical analysis used to predict the value of one variable based on another.

Regional anatomy A system of study in which everything about a specific region of the body is studied together, e.g., all the bones, muscles, nerves, and vessels of the upper limbs are learned before moving on to another body area.

Rehabilitation The action of restoring someone to health or high performance to meet the demands of a job, sport, or daily activities of life following an injury.

Rehabilitative biomechanics Involves studying the movement patterns of injured and disabled people.

Reliability The extent to which a test consistently yields the same results when repeated under the same conditions.

Respiration The process of breathing in oxygen and releasing carbon dioxide.

Responses Short-term (acute) change in the body that occurs due to a bout of exercise.

Sample A subset of the population being studied.

Sarcomere The smallest unit of a myofibril in striated muscle made up of protein filaments that slide past each other to create muscle movement.

Sarcopenia The loss of muscle mass with age.

Satellite cells Stem cells found in skeletal muscle tissue that are normally dormant but can be activated through physical activity and are important for the process of muscle repair and growth.

Schema theory A theory of motor control and learning that proposes a performer executes an action by retrieving a generalized motor program (GMP) from memory, adapting it for a particular context using a recall schema, and making ongoing corrections using a recognition schema.

Sedentarism A term describing the situation where an individual engages in sedentary behaviors such that they sit for most of their waking hours.

Sedentary physiology The study of what happens to a human body that does not move regularly throughout the day.

Self-efficacy An individual's confidence in a specific task.

Science The systematic study of the structure and behavior of the physical and natural world through observation.

Scientific literature Reports of original empirical and theoretical work (or summaries thereof) in the natural and social sciences.

Secondary reference Information about primary sources, usually a compilation or synthesis of various ideas and data. Secondary sources may rearrange, modify, or summarize data, which include book chapters, narrative reviews, and meta-analyses.

Sensory cortex A region of the cerebral cortex responsible for processing sensory information from various parts of the body.

Simulation A technique used to provide a prediction of kinematic and kinetic data.

Slow-twitch oxidative (SO) fibers Fatigue-resistant muscle fibers that favor oxidative (aerobic) methods of energy production; also known as type I fibers.

Sport and performance biomechanics Focuses on postures and movement patterns that minimize the risk of injury during physical activity and improve performance.

Sports medicine A branch of healthcare that focuses on the prevention, diagnosis, treatment, and rehabilitation of injuries and illnesses related to physical activity and sports that often involves an integration of healthcare professionals.

Sport physiology An area of exercise physiology focused on training athletes with the goals of minimizing injury and maximizing performance.

Sport psychology A multifaceted discipline, informed by principles of exercise science and psychology, and applied within a sport or performance context.

Sport psychologist A professional who is specifically trained to address emotional problems and personality disorders experienced by athletes.

Sport science An emerging multidisciplinary field that applies scientific principles and the disciplines of exercise science to understand and enhance human athletic performance, exercise, and physical activity.

Standard deviation The spread of a set of data values around its mean (average).

Statics A branch of mechanics that investigates bodies, masses, and forces at rest or in equilibrium.

Statistics The science of collecting, analyzing, interpreting, and presenting data.

Strength and conditioning A training approach focused on enhancing an individual's physical performance by improving strength, power, speed, endurance, and overall fitness, while also reducing the risk of injury.

Stress The collection of demands that disturb the homeostasis of physiological and metabolic processes.

Stretch reflex The stretch, or myotatic, reflex is initiated by stretch on skeletal muscle tissue, activating muscle spindles embedded in the muscle, and resulting in contraction of the same muscle.

Stroke Loss or impairment of body function due to injury or death of brain cells from insufficient blood supply. Also known as a cerebrovascular accident.

Supercompensation A short-term physiological response to training in which the body adapts to a stimulus by recovering to a level above its initial baseline, resulting in improved performance capacity provided adequate rest and nutrition are included.

Sympathetic nervous system The branch of the autonomic nervous system that is most active during periods of stress and activity.

Synapse The communication junction between two neurons or between a neuron and a muscle cell.

Systole The phase of the heart cycle when the heart contracts and pumps blood out to the body.

Team A group of individuals who interact with one another to achieve a superordinate goal.

Team dynamics The process of developing roles, establishing norms, and utilizing a shared communication method to achieve the collective goal.

Temporal analysis A technique that uses time as the basis for examining motion.

Theory A comprehensive explanation of a given set of data that has been repeatedly confirmed by observation and experimentation and has gained general acceptance within the scientific community but has not yet been decisively proven.

Type 1 diabetes A form of diabetes in which the body's immune system destroys the pancreatic cells that produce insulin. As a result, type 1 diabetics cannot produce adequate amounts of insulin.

Type 2 diabetes A form of diabetes in which the cells of the body do not use insulin properly. As the need for insulin increases over time, the pancreas loses its ability to produce adequate amounts of insulin.

Ultrasound sonography A non-invasive technique that uses sound waves to assess body tissues.

Validity The degree to which a test measures what it is intended to measure.

Veins Blood vessels that carry oxygen-poor blood back to the heart from the body.

Velocity The rate at which position changes, indicating how fast something is moving and in what direction.

Videography A technique that provides a sequence of images that can be displayed as a motion picture or viewed individually.

Virtual reality systems Portable systems that create entirely new environments by displaying virtual images on a screen or overlaying digital information onto the real world.

VO_2 max The maximal rate at which an individual can take in and utilize oxygen, a measure of maximal aerobic capacity.

Wearable technology An electronic device equipped with sensors designed to be worn on the body, either directly on the skin or as an accessory. These devices can provide information related to tracking fitness or monitoring health.

Work The force applied to an object multiplied by the distance over which it is applied.

Work physiology An area of physiology that is focused on work and fatigue in industrial workers and jobs requiring manual labor.

Index